Raymond W. Waggoner Lectureship on Ethics and Values in Medicine

Edited by Philip M. Margolis MD

Copyright © 2014 Philip M. Margolis MD
All rights reserved.

ISBN: 1493680463
ISBN-13: 9781493680467

Table of Contents

Foreword
Philip M. Margolis, M.D., Professor of Psychiatry Emeritus, University of Michigan; Chair, Raymond W. Waggoner Lectureship on Ethics and Values in Medicine vii

Raymond W. Waggoner, M.D. 1901-2000 xiii

Ethics and the Changing Role of the Physician: The Coming Crisis in the Practice of Medicine, 1996
Robert Michels, M.D. Provost for Medical Affairs, Cornell University 1

Physician Assisted Suicide: Where Do We Stand? 1997
Alan Stone, M. D. Professor of Law and Psychiatry, Harvard University 23

What Is Wrong With Human Cloning? The Ethics of Technological Reproduction, 1998
Arthur L. Caplan, Ph.D., Director of Bioethics, University of Pennsylvania 43

No Place to Hide: Threats to Confidentiality and Privacy in Medicine, 1999
Paul S. Appelbaum, M.D., Professor of Psychiatry, Medicine, Law, Columbia University 67

Integrity in Scientific Publications: Implications for Research, **2000 Catherine D. DeAngelis, M.D. Editor,** Journal of the American Medical Association, and Professor of Pediatrics, Johns Hopkins University School of Medicine 87

Ethical Considerations in Research on Human Subjects:
A Time for Change... Again , 2001
Harold T. Shapiro, President Emeritus University of
Michigan and Princeton University, Professor of
Economics and International Affairs, Princeton University.........93

"Care Without Coverage: Too Little, Too Late" A Report
On The Institute Of Medicine Committee On Uninsurance, 2002
Mary Sue Coleman, PhD, President University of Michigan;
Professor of Biological Chemistry, University of Michigan
Medical School...117

Ageless Bodies, Happy Souls: Biotechnology and the
Pursuit of Perfection, 2003
Leon R. Kass, M.D., Ph.D., Hertog Fellow in Social Thought,
American Enterprise Institute, Washington, D. C.................135

Academic Science and Entrepreneurship: Are the
Conflicts Reconcilable? 2004
Sheldon Krimsky, Ph.D., Professor, Department of Urban and
Environmental Policy and Planning, Tufts University.............159

When Good Men and Women Do Nothing: Where Was the
Voice of Medicine at Afghanistan, Guantanamo,
and Abu Ghraib? 2005
Leon Eisenberg, MD., The Maude and Lillian Professor of
Social Medicine and Emeritus Professor of Psychiatry,
Harvard University Medical School 175

Contemplating Pandemics: The Role of Historical Inquiry in
Developing Migration Strategies in the 21st Century , 2006
Howard Markel, M.D., Ph.D., Professor of Pediatrics and
Communicable, Diseases; Director, Center for the
History of Medicine, University of Michigan 191

Ethics, Genetics and the Future of Sport, 2007
Thomas Murray, Ph.D., President, The Hastings Center,
Garrison, New York... .213

Beyond Band-Aids: How to Cure America's Sick, 2008 Ezekiel
Emanuel, M. D., Chair, Department of Bioethics,
The Clinical Center of the National Institutes of Health .... .229

Redressing the Unconscionable Health Gap: A Proposal
for a Global Plan of Justice, 2009
Lawrence Gostin, J.D., L.L. D., Associate Dean and Professor
of Global Health Law, Georgetown University Law Center......... .255

Old and New Ethical Problems in Innovative
Stem Cell Research, 2010
Bernard Lo, M.D., Director in Medical Ethics,
Professor of Medicine, University of California at San Francisco. . . .269

On Becoming A Physician: Stresses and Strengths of
Physicians-in-Training, 2011
Laura Roberts, MD. Professor and Chair, Department of Psychiatry
and Behavioral Sciences, Stanford University School of Medicine 289

Fixing Health Care the Ethical Way, 2012
Jeremy Lazarus, M.D. President, American
Medical Association.. 307

Myths and Misconceptions in Biomedical Ethics, 2013
Robert M. Sade, M. D., Professor of Surgery,
University of South Carolina 325

Foreword

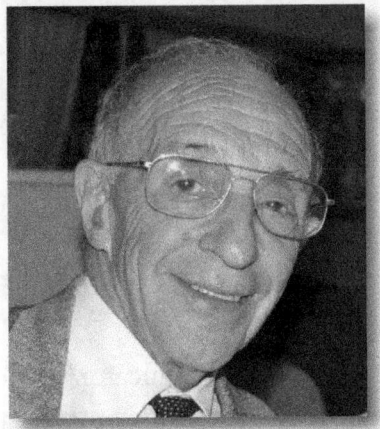

Philip M. Margolis, M.D.

This book is a labor of love and a significant document.

Raymond W. Waggoner, M.D., Sc.D., was the chair of the University of Michigan Department of Psychiatry for 33 years until 1970. He remained in the department as a most productive and stimulating member for many more years, dying in the year 2000 at the age of 98. His zealous and thoughtful work over many decades in promoting and upholding the highest ethics and values in medicine is perpetuated and preserved through the Raymond W. Waggoner Lectureship in Ethics and Values in Medicine. His legacy endures.

The Lectureship honors Dr. Waggoner and showcases the latest, most up-to-date ideas, research, debates and conflicts on a wide variety of topics within the theme of ethics and values in medicine.

Eighteen esteemed scholars were selected over a period of 18 years as The Raymond W. Waggoner Lecturer, sponsored by the Department of Psychiatry at the University of Michigan. Their defining talks are reproduced in this book. Because these chapters were originally presented as a lecture, they read as a talk. Their expression and flair remain as presented and we believe add charm, warmth and strength in the reading.

Their job titles are presented as they were at the time of their talk.

Some thoughts ---

I like the words "scholar" and "educator" to describe the Lecturers in this book. They are wise men and women, learned persons, if you will, coming from diverse backgrounds with their own unique methods, modes and styles, subject matters and most importantly, ways of thinking about life. The result is a heady burst of ideas, sometimes called philosophies, sciences, opinions and innovations, offered to us by mostly physicians, several PhD's and a lawyer. They are educators and researchers with an occasional background of history.

The intersection of the Lecturers and their thoughts/actions with one another are "accidental" but the theme of ethics and values in medicine echoes for each Lecturer, often bringing them together. I suspect that this unwitting interaction may have some influence on the reader as well as each Lecturer. At any rate, let the reader ponder and enjoy!

As I look through and re-read the lectures, I am impressed that they are all still relevant and current. Some problems may be resolved or partially so, signifying progress; others become more complex and confounding and spell regression.

In many ways, the first lecture by Dr. Michels, on *The Coming Crisis in the Practice of Medicine* set the stage for ensuing years. And the last lecture by Dr. Sade has indicated that myths and misconceptions in biomedical ethics still abound. What of the next 18 years?

Acknowledgements:

There are so many people who have made this Lectureship a reality. First and foremost are the many donors, without whom this Lectureship would not have been possible.

The Lecturers have all been selected by the Waggoner Committee - a group of diligent and dedicated medical school faculty. The Committee of 9 has remained reasonably constant over the 18 years; 15 individuals have served, composed of a diverse group of medical faculty with about half being psychiatrists. The Committee nominated candidates, discussed them and essentially made the selection via a democratic process.

The collective wisdom of the following Committee members has made this Lectureship so successful: Andrew Barnosky, Gregory Dalack, Susan Goold, John Greden, Lazar Greenfield, Laura Hirshbein, Joel Howell, Scott Kim, Philip Margolis, Howard Markel, Jonathan Metzl, Michael Mulholland, Randolph Nesse, Mark Orringer, and Kenneth Silk.

Much of the administrative work for the Lectures was skillfully handled by Adrienne Young. Murat Yashin, the Web Designer for the department, spent hours uploading videos and manuscripts and artistically designing the permanent website, He will continually maintain the internet page, enabling all of this history to be amazingly stored in a cloud somewhere. Thank you so much for your creative contribution.

Nancy Davis was invaluable in contacting and working with our generous donors.

Thus, individually and as parts of a cohesive team these people were terrific and I give each one my heartfelt thanks.

Raymond Waggoner, Jr. M.D. is Dr. Waggoner's son. He is a psychiatrist, has been a wonderful support to me and to our program.. He has traveled with his wife Nancy from their home in Columbus, Ohio, to attend most of the Lectures and has been a strong, steady friend. I am grateful to him for helping to sustain the bond between the Waggoner family and the Department of Psychiatry.

Gregory Dalack, M.D., current Chair of the Department of Psychiatry at the University of Michigan, has been helpful to me in his role as the chair of the department of psychiatry.

Special thanks to John Greden, M.D., immediate past Chair of the Department of Psychiatry here at the University of Michigan for much of the 18 years of the Lectureship. John's brilliant ideas, loyalty and support have been invaluable and are so greatly appreciated.

Extra-special thanks to my wife, Nancy, without whom this book never would have reached the press. Nancy is a journalist, social worker, and my loving wife of 55 years. She utilized all of these roles on behalf of this publication. She was essential, distinctive and completely indispensible. I am so grateful for her unique combination of skills, persistence and patience – a true helpmate!

Philip M. Margolis, M.D
Professor of Psychiatry Emeritus
Department of Psychiatry
University of Michigan, Ann Arbor, Michigan
Chair, Raymond W. Waggoner Lectureship on Ethics and Values in Medicine

The Raymond W. Waggoner Lectureship on Ethics and Values in Medicine has a Website.
You may view the video of each lecture and/or download an audio of each talk.
 Google: *Raymond W. Waggoner Lectureship on Ethics and Values in Medicine.*
 Or: http://umpsych.org/WL

Raymond W. Waggoner, M.D. 1901–2000

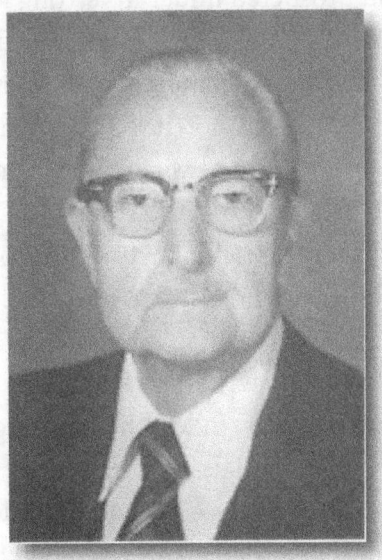

Raymond W. Waggoner, M.D.

Many of us knew Ray as a wise, dedicated leader of APA (President, 1969–1970; Distinguished Service Award, 1988) and a pivotal voice in American psychiatry for half a century. We in Michigan knew him also as a dominant force in Michigan medicine and psychiatry for many years.

Ray always wanted to be a doctor. In fact, at the age of 5 he began carrying a doctor's bag with him wherever he went. He became an M.D. at the tender age of 22 and has been a pioneer, innovator, and benefactor ever since. Ray did not really plan to be a psychiatrist; rather, he contemplated becoming a neurosurgeon. He ended up receiving training in both neurology and psychiatry and was considered a neuropsychiatrist. He was Chair of the Department of Psychiatry at the University of Michigan from 1937 to 1970. He immediately set up a three-room psychiatric unit, one of the first units in a general hospital in the country.

Dr. Waggoner built an eclectic department with breadth and class, an academic model for the nation. He was a superb administrator, and the department grew and prospered under his strong leadership.

In a tribute to Dr. Waggoner, Dr. John Greden, Executive Director of the University of Michigan Comprehensive Depression Center, and Department Chair for 22 years, noted that Dr. Waggoner's department contained "a healthy eclecticism, diversity and vibrancy, excellent clinical services, and scholarly teaching and research. Clearly, Dr. Waggoner has helped to establish the Michigan tradition of excellence that we proudly inherit and build upon." Ray was a jet setter before jets, a mover and shaker at home and abroad.

Ray has left a fabulous legacy. What I recall vividly is his caring. He has helped the careers of many, indeed he has taught an entire generation of mental health professionals—a living legacy of psychiatrists and professionals in other disciplines who trained under and with him. He has changed the field of psychiatry and has aided and supported many people in a myriad of ways. He has been a true and loyal friend!

Dr. Waggoner was ahead of his time, e.g., in his attempts to bridge the gap between the Freudian (psychological) model and biological (neuroscience) model by nurturing a healthy dynamic tension between the two. He presaged and encouraged the biopsychosocial model of today, early on seeing mental illness as both an emotional and physical problem. He always considered the patient as a total person. He was the "compleat physician," whether consulting with Masters and Johnson or integrating medical and psychiatric care by developing a first-rate consultation- liaison service.

In the 1940s, Ray helped to standardize the mental fitness criteria used in screening potential soldiers in the Selective Service. He also advised the U.S. Surgeon General on the psychological effects of World War II and the Allied Occupation in Germany and Japan. After the war, he helped devise the selection process for the Peace Corps, where I first met Dr. Waggoner and tried to keep up with this whirlwind of a man—a dynamo who is perhaps best remembered as a consummate administrator who listened to opinions and then made decisions. I remember him as an optimist, always feeling that with the right tools we could accomplish what others considered impossible. And he often did.

Ray always had a strong interest in ethics and values, which he saw as combining the human and humane. In fact, in 1995 the University of Michigan established the Raymond W. Waggoner Lectureship on Ethics and Values in Medicine in his honor. Indeed, Dr. Waggoner was a giant in his time and serves as an inspiration to us all.

PHILIP M. MARGOLIS, M.D.
Chair, Raymond W. Waggoner Lectureship on Ethics and Values in Medicine

Ethics and the Changing Role of the Physician: The Coming Crisis in the Practice of Medicine, 1996

Robert Michels, M.D., Provost for Medical Affairs, Cornell University

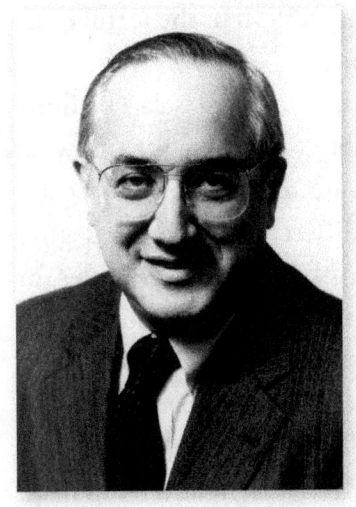

If I may start with a single slight correction to the introduction for which was very generous and I am grateful. I considered graduating from the University of Chicago the high point of my career of which I am immensely proud. I cannot imagine anything up from there. Although I am also proud of the fact that I was chairman of the department of psychiatry at Cornell University, a great one, I will argue for 17 years. That is to say I am usually proud of that. I am humbled by only two things that make me careful. One is it is very hard to be proud of having chaired a department of psychiatry for 17 years when I have the privilege of giving the first Waggoner lecture who at 17 years was halfway through his career as chairman of the department of psychiatry at the University of Michigan.

The other is, it is awesome to think about when Dr. Waggoner was chair the major task of academic psychiatry was to train physicians to do what we knew how to do. That was based on the assumption that the rule of mental health care next year would be fairly similar to what it was last year. That assumption is no longer valid and the task of chairman today, including new chairmen, is to figure out what is about to

Ethics and the Changing Role of the Physician:

happen but has not happened yet and then give his faculty, who have no familiarity with that task, an educational program for students who entered the profession expecting something else in the entirety to confront them and to do all of this while balancing his budget, maintaining faculty morale, and operating an academic institution.

Well, probably the good sign of my wisdom is that I left the chair of the department of psychiatry in 1991 to become the dean where, as you are familiar with, my job description consists of not attending a lecture such as this one because I'm negotiating with the director at my hospital about the budget. This is not a more gratifying task than the former one but it's a more pressing one most of the time.

When times are tranquil, discussions of medical ethics can be quite dull. Most of us tend to trust our gut sense about what is right and what is wrong. And in a stable world with adequate resources, this visceral morality is pretty good at allowing us to differentiate the good guys from the bad ones. Morals are different from ethics. Morals are rules for deciding who is good and who is bad. Ethics is the branch of philosophic discourse that informs us how to think about and discuss moral issues, how to consider and articulate the principles, the arguments, and the language of moral discourse. If you're sure what is right and wrong, you do not need ethics. If you cannot figure out what is right and wrong and you have to think about it, you have got to have rules for thinking and that is where ethics helps.

I believe it's the American humorist Mark Twain who captured the essence of this distinction most succinctly many years ago. Twain said, "To be good is noble. But to teach others how to be good is nobler and less trouble." It is this critical distinction between the moralist who does good and the ethicist who knows how to talk about it that will inform the beginning of my discussion today.

A few decades ago we thought the big problem facing medicine was that we didn't know enough. We thought when scientific advances finally taught us how to cure cancer or heart disease or schizophrenia we would not have much need to worry about subtle questions of medical ethics. We might still have moral concerns. We still have to identify the bad guys and kick them out of the profession. But you don't have to have a PhD in philosophy to do that. Our problem, we thought, was to develop the resources essential to scientific progress and to use them. At most, perhaps ethics would be a distraction to concern while the science was doing its job. Until we knew how to cure those diseases, we would have to worry about what to do when we were only halfway. We recognized that we might be too poor to move as rapidly as we wanted to.

But it never even occurred to us that we might not be good enough to make the right choices or the right decisions when we got there.

Today things look quite different.

It is beginning to look like the more we know, the bigger our dilemmas and the greater our ethical problems. Who is going to get a heart or bone marrow transplant and who is not? What do we do with the information we get from prenatal genetic diagnosis? Who deserves to know and who should not? Or for that matter, with an HIV test. A case that has occupied my home, New York City, for the last ten days, how long do you support the beloved body of a brain dead child who's religious parents don't want to pull the plug. A question that is complicated in this case by the fact that their district attorney believes the child died of child abuse and the corpse, now on life support, is vital evidence in the case and the corpse cannot be investigated until the plug is pulled. This is a complicated and interesting problem that involves hundreds of thousands of dollars of social resources, ethical, religious, medical problems. What do you do? Somehow our visceral signals aren't always clear anymore. Furthermore, although we always knew and still believe that we're the good guys, even that is now being questioned.

Some members of the public believe that we, by practicing the very highest quality of clinical medicine, are wasting valuable social resources, misallocating what should be applied to support public health preventive medicine and adequate minimal care for the underserved. They

Ethics and the Changing Role of the Physician:

even suggest that we are motivated in our doing this by personal gain rather than by professional standards. Our moral intuition may be less clear than it was before, but the public's moral intuition is getting down right scary to some of us. Perhaps it would be a good idea to get some of those ethicists in to help in the dialogue.

Now most of our ethical principles have been around for millennia. However, each new historical period, each new practical situation, each new advance in medical knowledge or in medical care raises new ethical problems. Some of these test, strain, and occasionally though infrequently destroy the ancient principles that we have honored and help to generate new ones. Most often those principles survive and help us to understand and cope with our new problems, drawing on the wisdom we've accumulated by coping with the old problems.

I am going to talk about a new challenge, the coming revolution in the healthcare system. I am not sure. I think the title for this paper in New York is, "The Coming Revolution in the Healthcare System." In Ann Arbor, it may be that the title should be, "The Current Revolution in the Healthcare System

There are two major themes in medical ethics in general. The first of these focuses on what is most familiar, the doctor patient relationship, clinical ethics. This discusses issues such as confidentiality, informed consent, the physician's obligation to maintain clinical competence, to serve the patient's interest and it's fiduciary relationship with the patient to advocates for the patient's need and not to exploit the patient for any of the physician's interests or lusts or desires. These are the issues that most people think of when they think of medical ethics. These are the ones that the public associates and the profession with the oath of Hippocrates.

The second theme of issues in medical ethics relates to medicine as a profession. An organized group of individuals who are in possession of socially valuable knowledge and skills, and therefore, who are granted considerable autonomy and privilege and authority by society ranging

The Coming Crisis in the Practice of Medicine, 1996

from being able to park your car where no one else can to performing assault and battery in an emergency without permission on an unconscious person because you believe it to be in that person's good and to be praised rather than damned for doing both of those things. The reason we get those privileges is because society believes it is in society's interest to give us those privileges. If the first theme of medical ethics, clinical ethics has to do with the doctor/patient relationship, the second theme has to do with the profession/society relationship. It includes the profession's obligation to educate new members. That doesn't grow out of the doctor/patient relationship but of our obligation to future potential patients who must also have care. The profession's obligation to develop new knowledge, to assure access to its service by those who need those services, to advise society about the allocation of scarce resources, to ensure the integrity and the competence of its members and to educate the public at large.

I'm going to today discuss the coming changes in the healthcare system, the challenges they present to our traditional principles of both clinical and professional ethics, some early thoughts about how we might cope with these challenges, what we might learn from them, and in passing, what I'm scared of. What justifies the word crisis in the title of my talk.

But first, let me talk a little bit about what changes we are anticipating in the healthcare system. What is going to happen, what has happened already, and what's likely to follow. I'm certain, particularly since arriving here last night, that you and Ann Arbor are at least as familiar with these issues as I am or the citizens of any other large academic medical center. Indeed, based on some of your recent publications in the New England Journal, you are more familiar with some of these issues than most and you have actually done some of the arithmetic, which is better left undone as far as I'm concerned. I'm thoroughly in agreement with those consultation liaison psychiatrists who have pointed out that denial is not always a pathological mechanism and some things are better not known.

Ethics and the Changing Role of the Physician:

I'm going to describe these changes as I see them from a very particular perspective. Not from the perspective of healthcare or the efficiency of the system or economics, but rather in terms of their implications for the clinical and professional ethical issues I have talked about. I suspect none of them will be new to you so I'm simply going to recast them in new language to help us think about them from this perspective.

First, healthcare has always been a cottage industry in this country where a single health professional or maybe a very small group of them took care of a small group of patients without much regard for the system. We didn't think about the healthcare system. We thought about doctors and patients. Furthermore, woefully, except for a couple of visionary academics or political leaders, nobody cared much about citizens who were not patients. They were not part of the issue as we framed it. We are shifting to where there will be large organized groups composed of many different types of health professionals, para professionals, administrators and staff who care for huge groups of patients. And increasingly, not only care for those patients but accept responsibility for entire segments of the community, including both patients and potential patients. The current jargon is covered lives.

I'm the head of a faculty practice plan of about 500 full time positions in my medical school. I think it is about the same size as yours, roughly. A decade ago, I was one of the largest organized groups of physicians in my community. We're rapidly terrified that we are so small that we may be edged out of the marketplace unless we affiliate with, combine, merge, or something else with even larger groups of physicians of somewhat dubious quality that cover sheers of our market. I would not tell you this secret of mine except that I know you already know it because it is your secret too.

A second change, we are shifting from viewing our clients as being equivalent to our patients, to viewing them as all members of the community. Current patients, past patients, and potential future patients. We have had a clinical ethics of the doctor/patient relationship but I've never seen anyone even discuss the clinical ethics of the doctor covered life relationship. How do we think about that one?

It is only in the last few years in our country that the average physician became either an employee or a member of a group rather than a solo practitioner. But that rate of change is accelerating so rapidly that my medical students and residents do not anticipate ever being solo practitioners in their careers.

The daily social world of the physician has always been a world that included contact with peers and staff, as well as patients. But the social organization of the new emerging system, as viewed by an anthropologist, is a little scary. There is a corporate structure in which the patients are customers and in which the casual social relationships of the caretakers are with administrators and with each other with the patients passing through as customers do in a large enterprise. This changes the feeling of what is going on with some good but a lot of concern.

If one shift is the shift from cottage industry to organized system and another from the patient as client to every citizen in the community as client, a third shift involves not organizational structure or the definition of the client, but rather power. Doctors used to have all the power. Some of us think of that as the good old days. We decided what to do, who to do it to, how much to tell them about it before we did it to them, and then we did it. We did it because we knew it was in their best interest. Now for some years we've been forced to share this power with patients. We have been taught, and more or less believe but anyway accept the inevitability, that patients have a right to decide what should be done to them and their bodies and their lives. The doctrines of informed consent and the right to refuse treatment reflect this change. You know, I'm immensely proud of the fact that the doctrine of informed consent was first formulated in a law case involving the New York Hospital in 1912 or 13. What I don't always add when I mention that is we were losers in that case and the doctrine was established in order to not let us do what we had customarily done before that, which was not bothering with informed consent. So we play a critical role in the history of this particular ethical principle. We were the devil.

The patient's autonomy has come to be recognized as more important, more ethically valued than the doctor's. But now both of us are losing our autonomy to external organizations, manage care companies, third parties, fourth parties, regulators, committees, and those who write and formulate clinical pathway guidelines. Decisions that used to be made badly--I don't mean poor decisions. I mean ethically offensively by the doctor alone then were made in consultation with the patient, then were made by the patient with the advice of the physician, are now being made by some anonymous person who will graduated high school who is at the end of an 800 phone line number in another state in front of a computer screen and who tells the physician what the decision is. And the autonomous, free discussion between physician and patient and the consensus they reach has less determining force in what happens than the decision made by this other person at the end of the 800 number. This is a serious change in where power has been placed in the system.

So one change is the shift from cottage to industrial organization. A second from patient client, the community citizen is client. A third from physician and patient autonomy to corporate control of medical practice. A fourth shift involves the economic context of the doctor/patient relationship. For centuries we've been accustomed to a system in which the physician might be tempted to advise and deliver excessive treatment for personal gain. This was a risk that was formulated as clearly as ever by George Bernard Shaw in The Doctor's Dilemma that pointed out the absurdity of paying a doctor to treat you when you were sick and not when you were well, thereby motivating him to keep you sick. Shaw saw the problem and favored capitation as a solution.

We are moving toward a system in which the physician may be encouraged to under treat by the so called delivery system, which is either the physician's employer or the patient's insurer or both. On the surface to an ethicist, these seem to be symmetrical risks. In either case, there is

The Coming Crisis in the Practice of Medicine, 1996

a conflict of interest in which monetary gain may lead to an erroneous decision, either too much or too little. But they don't feel symmetrical to practicing doctors. Why is that? The least charitable explanation would be that this only reflects the greater economic concerns of contemporary physicians today, their dismay at the reduction in their perceived future incomes, and their displacement of this unhappiness to a negative view of the structure of the system that's failing to reward them appropriately. They are really mad, not about the structure, but about the fact that they are making less money and they find the structure an easy thing to blame it upon.

But perhaps there are other factors as well. The old system allowed the doctor and the patient to feel like allies. The new one can lead them to cross purposes and direct conflict. With the patient seeking the treatment that although the doctor may believe to be desirable is one that, "Isn't covered by the plan," or, "Isn't part of the contract," and one where the doctor either chooses not to or is contractually prevented from describing to the patient as an alternative.

One of the early ethical issues being confronted in the new system is where the doctor's primary loyalty should fall in such a situation. Does he tell the patient what he really thinks or does he defend the company line? Or let me rephrase that very biased phrasing. Does he accept the wisdom of his peers in their collective judgment about the optimal clinical pathway or does he advocate his personal and perhaps idiosyncratic treatment plan in spite of its rejection by the collective? I think most physicians' attitudes between those two ways of describing that situation would be heavily colored by who the peers happen to be. Were they respected colleagues or expert in the field? Or were they accountants trying to optimize or maximize the bottom line of a for-profit corporation. Somehow that seems to be different.

This may be where the old system and the new one are no longer symmetrical. We are certainly accustomed in medicine to individuals who are motivated by profit. But we are accustomed to they're being ashamed of that. We've never before had large powerful organizations that were proudly announcing their success in maximizing their profit while delivering healthcare, that had profit as their dominant or primary motive as their responsibility to their stockholders. This is new and this may make a difference.

There are other changes underway in our healthcare system. But for the moment, let me stop with these four basic ones that I have described already. From cottage industry to large, organized system, from patient to covered life, from autonomous to physician, to a physician who is a subordinate, perhaps an employee and from a subtle financial incentive, for the selfless physician to over treat to an explicit financial incentive for the dutiful physician to under treat. Again, there are more, but if those don't remind you of what is happening in recent years, you are in the wrong room, I suspect.

What will be the impact of these new developments in the healthcare system on our medical ethics? I'm going to talk about five different types of impact. And it's a very simple-minded set of five.

First, there are some really good impacts and I believe as a profession, we should be the first to recognize them, applaud them, and point out to the public how valuable they are. For example, one of our professional responsibilities is to maintain the competence of ourselves and assure the competence of other members of our profession. On the whole, we have done a lousy job at that. Our guild concern with protecting other members of our profession has led us often to conceal their incompetence from the public and our willingness to impose on their voluntary participation has generally led us to make competence enhancing activities totally voluntary rather than required. It was only in the last few years, in the year that I was president of the American Board of Psychiatry that we reluctantly were forced by public pressure to require time limited certification of psychiatrists. You now can only be certified for ten years and then you have to get recertified. When I was certified, I was certified for life and it seemed to be perfectly reasonable

The Coming Crisis in the Practice of Medicine, 1996

from the point of view of profession that at the age of 26 I could pass an exam meant that at age 76 I could practice psychiatry with any willing subject because I was certified as an expert in the field that had probably moved beyond anything I knew by that time. That is not right. We allowed it and the new system won't allow it. We should probably applaud the new system for getting us to do what we failed to do well.

We have not been super at monitoring the most egregious, unacceptable, immoral, or financially wasteful behavior by members of our profession and the new system is extremely good at smoking that out and doing something about it. And we should recognize that. There are some good things.

Second, there are some bad things, some clearly unacceptable intrusions on the ethical core of the doctor/patient relationship by some of the changes that are going on in managed care. For example, confidentiality has been a core value of our profession, certainly going back to the oath of Hippocrates. There are legitimate things that it is reasonable for a payer, a third party or a fourth party to know. But they are far fewer than the information they request. Furthermore, the consent to procedures that are used are so patently coerced as to be ethically offensive. No human rights review committee for a research protocol would accept a consent form signed with the same contingencies that we casually accept consent forms for disclosing clinical information to payer. If it is not acceptable for consent for one activity, it is probably not acceptable for consent for the other activity. The profession has a responsibility to define the appropriate limits by which others can intrude in the doctor/patient relationship and then to defend that boundary ferociously. We have not done that well.

Secondly, the new system has challenged the physician's primary fiduciary responsibility to concern for what is in the patient's best interest. In an at least one dramatic set of cases has explicitly stated that the physician's employee relationship takes precedent over that fiduciary interest. I'm talking about the so called gag rules that have been included in a number of managed care contracts in which the physician provider is not allowed to tell the patient anything that is inconsistent with the position of the managed care corporation on the delivery of that specific area of healthcare. I believe that any physician who signs such a contract is doing something unethical. Even if he doesn't go on to do it, to agree to it is unethical. And I think our profession should make that so explicit that you get brought up on charges if you do that just as much as if you spoke out about a secret you learned in the clinical relationship or if you violated a patient's body for your personal amusement rather than for the patient's welfare. Those are all violations of our core contract with what we're doing here, and I think we have immense power. I think if we announce that this contract is unethical if a doctor signs it, those companies would back off awful fast. A recent brief article in the New England Journal of Medicine about such a contract forced one of the biggest HMO's in the United States to reverse itself, announcing that it was clarifying its contract and totally reversing it in the process. I don't know if you have a lot of U.S. Healthcare business around here, but it was U.S. Healthcare. I think we haven't taken a stand where we have to on that.

Thirdly, everyone agrees that one of the potential powers of the new system is to monitor, assure, and enhance the quality of healthcare. But not everyone agrees on what the definition of quality is. To a large organization selling healthcare, the definition of quality is what customers want. To a profession, the definition of quality is what patients need. And we're not so good at educating the public that they want what they need. Therefore there is a gap between the organizations that sell healthcare who define quality in terms of the attractiveness of the waiting room, the length of time before your phone call is answered, and the pleasantness of the relationship with the provider but aren't as concerned as we are about markers of the quality of the care that's delivered in terms of the biomedical sophistication, particularly if it is care that is involved in ruling out, diagnosing, or assessing rather than delivering treatment. I do not know how to initiate a psychiatric treatment plan within 24 hours of meeting most people I have never met before. I have had many years in the field. I am a clinician more than a researcher, and I do not know how to do it. But there are a lot of contracts that force one to do it. I think we have to talk about that.

In the old days, physicians defined quality. Recently in the political process, we have moved to public definitions of what is priority, what is most important, which is one part of quality. You have seen that in the fascinating Oregon experiment with having a priority list of what is most and what is least important in healthcare defined by a public organization in a democratic dialogue. One of the first decisions they reached, one dear to my heart, is to exclude mental healthcare from healthcare in that process, and the courts forced them to back down and reverse themselves on that one. But the new system is not primarily interested in either the democratic dialogue or the profession's views. They are interested in the market's views of quality. The market does not value public health as much as personal healthcare so it is far more concerned about the ready availability of a useless visit with a doctor than with the use of the same resources for public health interventions in which the client will benefit but will not be aware that anything happened. It is much easier to get public support for readily available house calls than for inoculations for measles. But ask anyone what the relative cost-effectiveness of those two procedures is who knows the data.

So as we move from physician based quality to public based quality to market based quality, we move toward anti-public health, pro-user friendly, anti-access for the underserved, a very special package that professionals ought to be uncomfortable with. I've talked about some ways in which I think the system is potentially good and others, perhaps more in which it is potentially bad. But frankly I think both of these are fairly self-evident. And I want to close by going into some areas where I think it's neither good nor bad and where it is not quite so obvious.

First, of special interest to people in this medical center or mine is there are a number of areas in which the new healthcare has decided it is irrelevant, but we as a profession are not irrelevant and we have to think about those and not let them fall off our plate. The most obvious ones are

Ethics and the Changing Role of the Physician:

the profession's responsibility for educating new members of the profession and for creating and generating new knowledge. That is not a concern of organizations delivery healthcare, but it is a concern of a group of physician or experts on health and who are supposed to advise and counsel the public on what to do in this area. The resources that support our educational and research enterprises have long been stolen or borrowed from a hugely inefficient, highly lucrative healthcare system. As we make that system efficient and streamlined and cost accounted, that source of stolen resources will no longer be available. That is already happening in places such as this. Either we have to educate the public and help them generate new resources for us or we have to downsize our system, or both. Or we have to recognize that we are going to have a very, very good healthcare system for ten or fifteen years and then no system at all.

Some of the planning has about a ten year window. The original Clinton set of task forces on the future of healthcare included 42 committees, none of which were interested in academics. We added one three months later on academic medical centers. So the public needs help in research and education. The profession is concerned with help in research and education, and we are not assured that the major providers of healthcare in the new system share that concern as did the less efficient but more socially minded providers of healthcare in the old system, the great non-for-profit community based hospitals with boards of directors who were concerned with what is good for the community rather than with their bottom lines.

If our major academic centers become links of highly efficient provider organizations which compete in the market and medical schools that survive off of their tuition, we will see a dramatic demise in the quality and value of those academic institutions for our nation. This is a scary and not totally impossible prospect confronting us at this time.

In addition to education and research, although our public governmental leaders have had some interest in assuring access for the underserved, it does not seem to be an important priority for corporate healthcare in general. Another type of access, access that involves the continuity of care, access to the same doctor one had last year this year, particularly important for chronic patients and for a special group of chronic patients that I have an interest in, the mentally ill, that type of access is also not defended by the new system. In a commercial model with customers, you can change providers at will. There is no value added in the mind of the organization providing the care to having a continuity of the provider/customer relationship.

Fourthly, the new healthcare system, as I've said before, is probably a very good ally in ensuring the competence and continued growth of competence of those who are working within it. It has little interest, and perhaps negative interest, of competence of those who are not working within it. Therefore, we have seen the growth of proprietary attitudes toward advances in scientific knowledge relevant to healthcare, companies keeping secrets about new drugs or new treatments so it will have commercial advantages over their competitors. This is not exactly what most of us thought was core to the Hippocratic medical ethical tradition. The profession has a responsibility to ensure not only the competence of all the providers in the specific healthcare system in which the individual himself belongs but all the providers in the profession whatsoever. It is part of our core definition, and we do not have good ways of doing that.

And I have talked about what is good, what is bad, what is left out, and we have to attend to because it is irrelevant to the new system, but we are in danger of being so distracted by the new system that we do not spend time attending to issues that it leaves outside of its purview. I believe that one of our major responsibilities as a profession, part of the professional ethics rather than clinical ethics, though we've only begun to recognize is if healthcare is going to be delivered by large, often for-profit organizations led by administrators and business people and financial people, then we have a major responsibility for advising the public on how to cope with such organizations, for helping governments write the regulatory rules, for insisting that just as it was prudent for

Ethics and the Changing Role of the Physician:

a community hospital to have businessmen rather than doctors on its board 30 years ago or it would go bankrupt, it is prudent for the government to require that they are real doctors as well as businessmen on the board of any organization that delivers healthcare to assure that it will not only not go bankrupt but will also take care of its patients. I cannot imagine any valid reason for not requiring professional caretakers in governance roles in any organization that is going to be chartered to give professional care. But we do not now have those requirements.

Advising the government re-regulations is one of our obligations as the advocates for health concerns in our community regardless of who is providing the healthcare and who is making or not making money in the process of doing it. So I have talked about good things, bad things, things left off the plate, new charges for the profession's ethics, and I will have one other new charge.

Medical ethics has been the ethics of doctors and other health professionals. But we need a new kind of ethics that we have never needed before, an ethics of organizations. If organizations are going to have the power to make decisions that affect people's lives, then we have to have codes of conduct for organizations and teeth attached to those codes. An organization that comes into a community and develops a healthcare system that wins out over all of its competition cannot then close and leave the community with no care at all. That is offensive, but that has happened. And our regulations and rules have allowed it to happen. It is different if you are selling healthcare or automobiles in a community. It is okay if the only automobile agency closes but not okay if the only doctor closes. An organization that owns the only gamma knife in town cannot use it to care for its patients and not others in order to have a market advantage in that town without offending something that is core to our culture. So we need a way of thinking through that so there will be organizational ethics as well as individual professional ethics if organizations are going to be allowed to play in this field. And they are being allowed to play in the field.

I believe that we have great power that we have not used because of our professional credibility with the public. We are in danger of losing it if we appear to be too clearly a guild interested in advancing our own welfare. But if we maintain reasonably concerned with the values of the public in receiving healthcare and in maintaining the quality of our relationship with them, they will be immensely interested in the profession's score cards on which providers follow the rules and which ones don't, which ones adhere to ethical standards for healthcare organizations and which ones don't, and if we do a kind of good housekeeping or consumer's report evaluation of the various organizations in the market, we will give immense market advantage to those who play by our rules. I think it is vital that we figure out a way to do that.

What are the rules we must, at all costs, preserve? I would say that I cannot imagine a profession that deserves the name of medicine that allows doctors to keep secrets from patients for other than the patient's benefit. I would say one rule is nothing can interfere with the--I wouldn't trust a doctor who I thought had a motive to keep a secret from me because of a contract with his employer. And I would not entrust anyone to trust me in that situation. We cannot allow that.

Secondly, we need something equivalent to academic freedom that protects physicians who advocate for their patients needs from retaliation from the organization in which they are working. The doctor should have no constraint and should be protected legally from any constraint on his ability to fight for getting the patient what he thinks the patient should deserve. I am not saying he should always get it. Doctors, as any advocate, may be misguided and may be making poor scarce resource allocation decisions. But they should never be told to shut up and not pursue what they believe to be their patient's interest.

Thirdly, I think the profession has to be very clear on delineating what are the limits of the kinds of situations in which we are willing to work. What is too evil for a physician to participate in? Let me give you some examples from our history. The psychiatry profession decided

Ethics and the Changing Role of the Physician:

that, a decade or two back, that there were totalitarian governments that were asking psychiatrists to play roles that were not professionally acceptable. You could not be a good doctor working in a totalitarian country where your job was to suppress descent rather than treat illness. And we ran out of the profession leading practitioners in those countries who didn't accept that.

Let me tell you an anecdote. We at Cornell, as I suspect you do at Michigan, have a course in medical ethics for second year medical students and we presented a case seminar two years ago in which we had a panel discussing a case with a class of 100 second year students and it was a simple and interesting case. It was a man who came to see a generalist physician in our clinic, a real case, who had been transferred there because he had just--his employer had switched contracts with HMO's and the new HMO had a contract with our clinic. And he had a cough and a little hemoptysis which he'd had for several months and he was a little worried about it. He was a chronic smoker. He knew what it might be. He hoped it was not that and he told the doctor that he wanted to have a checkup and he also told the doctor that if it was cancer, he had thought about it and he was going to kill himself. He came with his wife to the appointment. The clinician arranged in our system to get a quick x-ray and went to look at a wet reading and saw at least what was on wet reading an unequivocal neo-plastic diagnosis. That was the case. And we talked about a number of fascinating ethical issues. We asked the student, "What are the issues?"

We talked about the patient's right to know. We talked about the ethics of suicide and the doctor's potential role in suicide. We talked about the confidentiality and whether the wife who was in the waiting room should be called in and involved in this before or after or during exposing it to the husband. We talked about questions of competence and the fact that we had a wet reading by a primary care doctor. Did he have an obligation to talk to a radiologist first before basing his judgment on his less than state of the art knowledge of how to read that

The Coming Crisis in the Practice of Medicine, 1996

film. And I was the last one to speak and I chose not to do what I was supposed to do. I was playing psychiatrist that day rather than dean, but I chose to play dean rather than psychiatrist and I said, "Did anyone worry about whether the guy who makes our contracts with managed care companies should have agreed to sign a contract in which he was forced to switch doctors last month? This was a man who had seen his physician recently for the same symptom, had a good relationship from that physician and was told, 'You are no longer being cared for by this person in this clinic but by that person in that clinic.' And we signed that contract. Was I ethical in putting my signature on that document and accepting a bad pattern of healthcare so that I can increase my market share a little bit and my bottom line that year?"

The students were nervous with that dialogue, but not nearly as nervous as my faculty. Nor as I that night at home when I thought over the case. So I think we have to outline what the rules are that we are willing to play by and be a little less passive in accepting rules that have been imposed by the market upon us.

Fourthly, I have talked about full disclosure. I have talked about freedom for advocacy. I have talked about the separation of our clinical--I'm sorry, I have talked about the limit of our participation in evil. A fourth one is the clear separation of clinical and administrative roles. I think it is perfectly reasonable for physicians to function as reviewers and refusers of treatment but not for their own patients. I think the patient has a right to know my doctor is my doctor and if my treatment plan is rejected, it was rejected by some other guy, not by the guy who is taking care of me. That no one is ever in the position of deciding not to do what he thinks is best because he is worrying about covered lives rather than about his patient. There are many who would take a sharp public health difference of view with me on this, but my argument in response to them is, "If you had two doctors who were honest with you, one of whom was simultaneously monitoring the use of resources while caring for you and the other one was totally working for you and only someone outside was monitoring resources, which one would you continue to see after your first visit?" I have yet to find someone whose attitude toward the value of public health was such that he would rather see the doctor who was a resource monitor rather than the doctor who was a personal advocate for the patient.

Fifthly, I think we have to systematize the profession's ability to cope with these new strategies. We have to strengthen our professional organization, improve our communication to the public to protect the value of our core principles of clinical ethics. We have to greatly strengthen our professional ethical activities. Medicine has come out of a period of half a century in which there was a love affair between medicine and the public and we could comfortably sleep without much concern for the public's regard for us and protection of us. That is over. And we now have to struggle to protect our values and that requires the effort of members of the profession.

I think that medicine will survive and will outlive the current revolution in the healthcare system and the next one and the one after that. I believe healthcare executives will, when they get sick, come to our ICUs and we will take care of them there, both in this system and probably after it is over. But I think it is important that in doing that, we preserve and enhance our core ethical values that go back to a second theme in the Hippocratic Oath. I talked about the most famous theme, the obligation of the physician to the patient, not to do harm, to call in consultation, to maintain confidentiality, the obligations we all know so well. But a second theme in that oath is the professional ethical theme.

The Hippocratic physicians succeeded in a market competition. They were one of a number of groups of physicians in the ancient world more than 2000 years ago. They were composed of a group of itinerant practitioners who went around from town to town, set up a booth in the marketplace and cared for patients. Not too different from a modern managed care system. If you read the oath, they have to be good doctors not so much because it's patient ethics stuff but because it is a good marketing strategy. What they learned is that the other doctors, the non-Hippocratic ones, would seduce the slaves, would sell poisons, they would do all kinds of other things that meant when the next one came to town instead of trusting them, all the citizens ran the other way. The Hippocratic docs figured out that if we are honest, ethical doctors, then even if we have never met them before, if we wear that logo on our jacket, when we show up in town and we tell them we are Hippocratic, they will know we are sworn not to do those things. And the oath tells you that if you break the oath, the punishment is that you are kicked out of the club. You also swear to train others to do it your way. We have to make medicine a profession where once again, the public knows that we do not do bad things no matter what the reward is, that we do good things because that is the way we have been socialized to practice, and that those core values are more important than our employee/employer relationship.

Ironically in 1996, as in 400 B.C., nothing will enhance our value in the market more than our being perceived as placing our ethical values above all else. So I appeal not on ethical grounds, but on shrewd entrepreneurial grounds that we reaffirm our core values in medical ethics. Thank you.

Physician Assisted Suicide: Where Do We Stand? 1997
Alan Stone, M. D. Professor of Law and Psychiatry, Harvard University

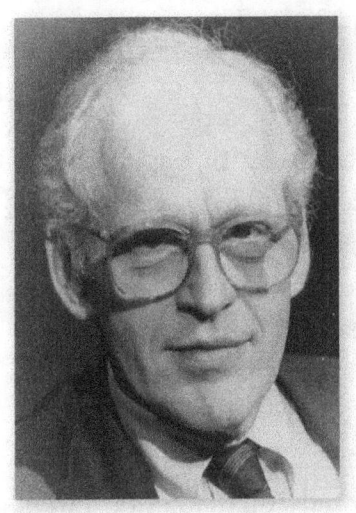

This introduction reminds me of my favorite Jewish story. It's about this old Jew who was trying to get from Minsk to Finsk. And he couldn't get on the train so he had to stay overnight and he went to the inn and there was no place at the inn. But this all has to do with the introduction. So he begged and implored the innkeeper if he would let him sleep somewhere in the inn. And the guy says, "There's no room." So finally he says, "Well, I'll tell ya, there's a Russian general. He's drunk so much that he's probably out on his feet. You can sleep in his room. I'll wake you up early in the morning and you have to get out of there before he wakes up." So the old Jew sneaks in. He falls asleep. Early in the morning somebody grabs ahold of him and he jumps into his clothes, rushes down to be first in line at, at the train station, goes in for his morning abalutions, looks in the mirror, and he's wearing the uniform of a Russian major general. And he says, "My God, they woke the wrong man."

Now for me to come here and talk to you people in Michigan about this subject is like bringing coals to Newcastle. And it's very, very presumptuous on my part so I approach it with a certain amount of caution. I come partly, I must say, because of my great affection for Dr. Waggoner, with whom I actually overlapped some time on the American

Physician Assisted Suicide:

Psychiatric Association board and I will say something further about Dr. Wagner when I discuss the question of medical ethics. Then I now say something about how I got into this. This article that is referenced is actually the second article a group of us wrote on taking care of hopelessly ill patients, which was published in the New England Journal. The first made the proposal, which some of you may remember that with patients who are second or third stage Alzheimer's that if they refused food and water, you did not have to automatically tube feed them and begin tube feeding. That article by itself was incredibly provocative. And I must tell you I got a number of letters accusing me of being a Nazi doctor.

The group reassembled two years later and went through much of what the AMA has been going through recently in describing the importance of terminal care. And the basic idea that the doctor's responsibility, which is to cure those who can be cured and to ease the suffering of those who cannot and we went in at great length to emphasize the rule of double effect of which I will speak. Now we had prepared something. We all gave papers. We were going to write this paper for the New England Journal. And then the chairman of our group, a dean at Harvard Medical School and a wonderful, wonderful man said, "I want you all to know that although I've proposed a regime with you of titrated care to ease people's suffering that I myself have a bottle of pills, and my wife who is a nurse has an understanding with me that if I get to this stage, she's going to bring in the pills so I can avoid all of this terminal care that we are proposing for patients."

Now that was a very strange moment in these deliberations because then the doctor sitting next to him said, "You know, I have the same agreement with my wife that if she's in this situation I'll bring in the pills for her." And then it turned out that those who didn't have the plan already were very enthusiastic about it. Now it's very strange because the standard ethical question the doctors ask, "What would you want if it was your mother?" Turns out that's the wrong question. You should ask, "What would you want if it's you?" Now it turned out that ten of the

Where Do We Stand? 1997

twelve people in this room, we were sort of the disciples without Christ. But ten of the twelve decided that that's what they would want. And we published an article in which for the first time we said, "It might be ethical for a physician to assist in suicide."

Now, the whole--everything we were proposing is just what the American Medical Association is now proposing of comfort care end of life. But these doctors thought, and I want to tell you, the doctors were-- who is the leading person taking care of cancer patients at Mayo's? Who is the leading person at Smith? Anderson Smith taking care of children with cancer? These were not just a group of people that were rounded up. These were very distinguished doctors taking care of terminal patients all the time. And ten of them were prepared to say, "This is what they wanted." As it turns out, I was not prepared to say at that point that I thought that physician-assisted suicide was ethical. Although, I am not sure that if the first question is, "What do we as doctors want for ourselves?" that everyone in this room who is a physician is prepared to go through a terminal illness and accept the comfort care that organized medicine promises us, which I believe is a very important question with which to begin the discussion.

At any rate, whatever we as doctors were pontificating about in the New England Journal of Medicine, events moved on as they do and as has happened to most of medical ethics, namely they've been replaced by the law so that although we still talk about medical ethics as I shall discuss, what we're doing is mostly what the law has told us to do. Twenty years ago, most doctors did not believe in informed consent and most doctors did not tell patients they had cancers. There were polls which said, "What is your practice?" I don't tell patients they have cancer. Now everybody tells patients they have cancer and they think this is the medically ethical correct thing to do but it did not come from medicine.

The important thing about these two decisions--let me speak about the second circuit opinion first because it's very much what I had written about in my editorial--actually for the American Journal of Psychiatry.

Physician Assisted Suicide:

You just imagine two patients who both have had a fracture and are paralyzed. And it may be there's a centimeter difference in where their fracture occurs and where the spinal cord is injured. One is on a respirator and the other is not. Under the law of the United States now, the person who is on the respirator can refuse the respirator and die. The person whose injury is one centimeter lower has no treatment to refuse and therefore is that kind of problem. So, so you can argue, and I think the argument can be made, how do you distinguish those two human beings and their right to end it all?

At any rate, the second circuit made an argument saying there was no rational way to distinguish between people in those situations who needed the doctor's help to die by some pills and somebody who could just have the treatment stopped, right? The Ninth Circuit opinion was more ambitious, more politically provocative and complicated. It went in the direction of the thinking on the right to abortion and found a new right to hasten one's death. Now when the cases were argued before the Supreme Court, one of the first questions asked by Justice Kennedy was, "Are you asking us to outlaw - to overturn on constitutional grounds all these state laws which presently prohibit assisted suicide?"

Now, I want to emphasize to you that's just what happened with abortion. Every state had a law against abortion and the states that had regulated and permitted it to some extent still had laws. All of those were overturned by the decision, right? Now I would say although it may be unpopular in this group, I would say the most important decision in medical ethics in this century was Roe vs. Wade. You may not know it, but in this century, most doctors went to prison for performing illegal abortions in this century. Okay? That's the chief reason for doctors going to prison, okay? Now Michigan, the statutes that were overturned, the first is the Washington statute, that the person is guilty of promoting a suicide when he knowingly aides another person was the part of the statute that they overturned. And in New York where the law is if he intentionally aides another person to commit suicide. Now, as you know,

Where Do We Stand? 1997

Michigan does not have a law against it. Like many states, you did away, apparently, with the law against--that, that made committing suicide a crime. It used to be a crime. And in this--I doubt, perhaps if anyone will know whether anybody seriously thought about the problem or it's like I actually served on the Massachusetts commission for the reform of the criminal law and they were just package deals they were made. And I'm sure no one focused on it but perhaps they did. But you have, you have both Dr. Kevorkian and Professor Kamisar so you know everything there is to know about this subject since you have the advocates on both sides. In common law, it was a crime to commit suicide and to assist in suicide. And so that's the basis which people have tried to proceed here against Dr. Kevorkian.

A lot of the impetus for physician-assisted suicide has come from people with AIDS who are dying of AIDS and when their T-cells get to a certain level, they would like to be able to check out. And this has become a much publicized situation where they invite people to actually be with them when they take medication and end their lives. The plaintiffs in the constitutional cases were HIV patients, a physician with cancer herself who had metastasized to bone and she was in incredible pain. Every time she tried to move she would get fractures and so the cases are very compelling. The cases are very compelling. Who could be more understanding of their situation than a physician who's got advanced metastasized to their bone? They know just what the medication is and they're still asking for it. So what they are asking and the doctors in California said that the prescription of drugs to competent terminally ill patients is consistent with their best professional judgment and the standards of medical practice. So here are doctors saying, "Look, this is okay."

Now, what basis do we have to say it is not okay? "I will give no deadly medicine to anyone if asked nor suggest any such counsel and in like manner, I will not give to a woman a pessary to produce abortion." So the Hippocratic Oath, in my view, is built around sort of not giving physician-assisted suicide and not performing abortions I know some of you feel these subjects should be kept totally apart, but I do not think that they can be. And I don't think it's any mistake that, for example, of Ronald Dworkin's book deals with those two subjects together. Now I want to point out to you that the Hippocratic Oath is not part of--it's not enforced anywhere. Whether we took it or not, it's not enforced by anyone. And I want to now show you the next which is the AMA's principles of ethics. And I would say--that's right. Now I don't know if you can read the AMA's principles of ethics, but unfortunately, there's almost nothing there to read. They have almost no content. I want to emphasize that to you. It doesn't say anything in the principles of ethics about do no harm, for example. And although the AMA has in its newspaper and in its editorials emphasized how they told the Supreme Court that the basic tradition of medicine is do no harm, it is not in our principles of ethics. Okay?

Well, I put that on because that's a small university on the West coast that some of you may have heard of. And, you will see that they have, in fact, over their hospital put these ethical principles. Now I would say about that, this is part of the problem of ethics in medicine. Whose ethics? Who's got it? Where do we stand as a group on medical ethics?

Now the line being crossed, as far as the law is concerned and as far as the AMA in their brief is concerned is this comes from the AMA's council on judicial and ethical matters and it was first dated 1982. And those of you who were lawyers will recognize that it is very legalistic indeed. It says that we should not intentionally cause death. It's almost like a statute. You should not intentionally cause death. Now that's because we were then, as our group who wrote in the New England Journal of Medicine, we were welcoming the double effect. And basically the idea is that if you're trying to ease pain and you give a huge amount of medication and the patient ends up dying, that's alright because you did not intentionally cause death. Your intention was to ease the pain. So the AMA has accepted that. The line being crossed in these briefs is whether you can write a prescription for a lethal dose

Where Do We Stand? 1997

of medication therefore. Not what Dr. Kevorkian has done, but what Dr. Quill has done. Can you use your power to prescribe a lethal dose, explain it to the patient, and give them the prescription? Now as I said, you cannot escape the connection, legally certainly. The Ninth Circuit wrapped itself in the abortion law arguments in ruling that there was a right to assisted suicide. And I want to point out that when the court dealt with abortion, it also had to deal with the Hippocratic Oath. And the way the Supreme Court did it was to say that that part about--and this is very interesting, that part about abortion was from the Pythagoreans who were a strange subset of the group of doctors at the time. And so, therefore, this should be distinguished from the rest of the Hippocratic Oath. Okay?

Now I think that Hippocrates, the Pythagoreans, and other Greeks are all going to--have all fell in the court of appeals. So the important thing for us to realize is that the law looks increasingly, in my view, and I will try to demonstrate this, increasingly disdainfully at medical ethics as a reason not to do anything for the law. In fact, in one of the most compelling arguments, the court said, "Well, what the doctors are supposed to do with informed consent is what the patient wants. So what are the doctors complaining about? They're supposed to do what the patient wants." Now public opinion on assisted suicide is rapidly, it seems to me and perhaps wrongly, but rapidly moving in the direction of greater and greater public acceptance and approval of it. The Roper poll in 1990 had 64 percent, the Harris poll had 73 percent in 1994, the Oregon Referendum actually passed in a plebiscite. The Oregon MD's were said to be 60 percent for it. The Washington and California referenda lost but many people say that in the future they will pass again. I have 125 students who take law and medicine at Harvard Law School. Ninety percent of them favored physician-assisted suicide and they will be part of the elite class of lawyers running the country. Ninety percent of them favor physician-assisted suicide. I am told that the Michigan Medical Society recently came out opposed to it, some 56 percent but

Physician Assisted Suicide:

earlier polls showed that doctors in Michigan, 56 percent would prefer physician-assisted suicide to a law that was an outright ban.

Now why does the public want PAS? In my view, I'm giving you this from my reading of legal opinions and from medical writings. First, there's a strong argument made by many doctors that many of our treatments actually prolong suffering and cause people to have a more painful death than they would otherwise have. Some of you may have read Ben Ruby's column to that effect in the New England Journal of Medicine, that patients who would have died a relatively quick, uncomplicated death say from leukemia now go through a prolonged treatment, very painful and perhaps in the end, die a more painful death. Second of all, there is the growing recognition that we can prolong life but we cannot prolong the quality of life. And so there is a huge sense among the public of, "I'm gonna end up with some chronic disabling disease and the doctors are gonna be able to keep me alive but they're not gonna be able to give me what is necessary for me to enjoy life." Then there is this horrible situation that if you work in a nursing home or visit a nursing home you discover that most of the patients are quite isolated. Many of them have--half of them in a standard nursing home have no known relative and nobody has visited them in years. This is standard sort of public nursing home. So there's this incredible isolation. There's the dementia, of course, and the concern has been a very important part of the literature. If I don't decide now and do it now, I'll be incompetent to decide it then. So there's this fear of dementia. I, I think judges are very much, when they write about this, their sense that they're gonna be lying there naked, incontinent, dependent on people for their basic needs is a horrifying picture to them.

Now adding to this list of woes is the recent study by the Johnson Foundation which found that in many hospitals, the quality of comfort care for terminal patients was not getting better and that many people were in hospitals getting poor comfort care. Now Emanuel claims--now there's a certain Harvard spin to this presentation which is not entirely a, a result of my egomania. There's, there are the Emanuels, Ezekiel and Linda Emanuel. Ezekiel is gone to be the head of ethics for NIMH from Harvard and Linda has gone to be the vice president for ethics of the AMA. And they are organizing sort of the organized medicine's response against physician-assisted suicide. Ezekiel Emanuel has lots of data and he claims that the patients who want--and this is what puts it into our category, who want physician-assisted suicide are depressed, not in pain and that medicine can handle pain. But what is going on is that people become depressed.

Now if you will forgive me, I want to just describe to you the reasoning of the court and how it gets from the Cruzan decision in the Supreme Court to physician-assisted suicide. Now what happened several years ago as many of you know, the Supreme Court was--dealt with the Cruzan case and it said that a patient who was permanently unconscious, is the current language, had a right to refuse treatment. The question was whether they had also a right to refuse food and water, whether that was to count as treatment. The AMA presented a brief saying it should count as treatment. And in the concurring opinion of Justice O'Connor, she made clear that it was meant to include food and water. So then the argument goes, if you can do those things, you are in fact being given a right to hasten your own death. Now this is related to the question: How do we speak about it? Do we speak about it as physician-assisted suicide or hastening your own death? The logic chopping view of the Ninth Circuit is everybody has a right now to hasten their own death. Right? That's what Cruzan is about, the right to hasten one's own death. So the holding in Cruzan can be read as doctor assisted suicide because you pull out the tubes and then Nancy Cruzan starves to death or dies of thirst. That's how she dies, right? And so you're assisting her in that way of committing suicide. That is hastening her death by withdrawing treatment. Now the irony is that the most conservative member of the court, Justice Scalia, said, "You know, this letting Cruzan refuse treatment is nothing but suicide." And now the liberal judges have

Physician Assisted Suicide:

jumped on his language and say, "Yes, that's right. You said it yourself." And if you remember the grave digger scene in Hamlet, there's the question of whether the water comes to you or you go to the water depends on whether you're gonna get buried on holy ground or not, whether you've committed suicide or something else. The grave digger is debating whether Ophelia is going to get buried in holy ground or not. Actually, Justice Scalia rehearsed that argument in his opinion. Now the point then for this court was that Cruzan is really about hastening death and with the assistance of the doctor who removes the tubes. So then this court had to look at the standards of medical practice. And this is my reason, along with others, for talking about the disdain. They said, "First we did do not resuscitate. And that actually means letting the person die. Then we let them refuse extraordinary care." That's what Quinlan was about. Then we said, "There's no difference between ordinary care and extraordinary care." That's what Cruzan was about. Then we said, "Ease the pain and suffering even when it hastens death." The AMA said that. So why is the AMA objecting now? This court found no ethical or legal distinction between double effect and single effect. You're giving these drugs so that the person will ease their pain but you know the patient is going to die. That's what you want to happen. Indeed, I don't know how many of you work in hospices, but if you are around hospices, basically the nurses start giving more scopolamine and whatever and they really are expecting the patient to die. There isn't any question. They're waiting for is it tomorrow or the next day and they're upping the dose. And that's what's happening. Now you can continue to call that not intending, but that is just, I would say, pretending. Then the court said, "Pulling a plug and prescribing to allow death are legally equivalent.". I was consulted about a woman who was on a respirator that had neurosurgery. It'd gone badly. She'd been on a respirator for several years and she wanted out. And so the question was, would somebody go--some doctor go to her house and shut off the machine? She had adult children. She talked to her adult children. They all thought it was the right thing to do but they didn't want to be the ones to shut off the machine. So they wanted a doctor to go and shut off the machine. So the doctor who had operated on her said he would shut off the machine but he wanted her to come in the hospital to shut off the machine. He didn't want to go into her house and shut off the machine. She was living at home. Then the hospital said they didn't want her in the hospital to have her machine shut off. Okay? So finally they went to court and under the Massachusetts law, they were told they could shut off the machine. Then with a court order the doctor who had operated her went to her home and first gave her medication. Of course he was not going to shut off the machine and just watch her suffocate. So first he gave her medication so she wouldn't go through the experience of feeling that she was suffocating to death. Now the critics of the AMA's position said, "You know, doctors are already doing much worse than physician-assisted suicide in these cases. This is a woman who had a life expectancy of twenty years on her respirator. So she was not imminently dying. The court said she has a right to refuse the treatment and the doctor goes and gives her medication first so she won't feel it and then shuts off the machine. And as you know, there is an article now in the literature about treating terminal pain patients by giving them huge doses of barbiturates to put them in barbiturate coma and then turning off the fluid and food so that they will die peacefully in their sleep which is sort of an incredibly roundabout way, again, to get to involuntary euthanasia.

At any rate, the court looked at all this and said, "We can't see the difference between acts of omission and acts of commission. We're not talking about assisting suicide, rather terminally ill hastening death by refusing a treatment." Now the Ninth Circuit also looked at our medical literature and the pleadings of the plaintiffs and said, "First we're making criminals out of compassionate physicians." Right? Dr. Quill being an example. You all know about Dr. Quill. I'll say a few words later on if--now the truth of the matter is that physician-assisted suicide and voluntary euthanasia have been done for centuries and there are many descriptions in the literature. There happens to be a very moving description of Sigmund Freud's doctor performing voluntary euthanasia on Freud after Freud asked for it after he'd suffered for years from cancer of the jaw. And he says, "You know, doctor, you promised me that when I got there you would do this. I've gotten there. Do it." And the doctor did it. So Emanuel had written an article earlier on before he got on this particular kick, which I think was true that doctors all over America were doing all sorts of things like physician-assisted death, voluntary euthanasia and so forth. And there was really an information problem. If you could get to the right doctor, you could find a doctor who would do what you wanted. And so there's the question of what is this slippery slope that people are talking about? We're already doing everything. There is no risk to the integrity of the profession.

If you look at doctors who oppose assisted suicide, you find they do not give ethical reasons. They give their own personal religious reasons. And so doctors who are opposed to suicide are usually Catholic or they live in small towns and are fundamentalist Protestants. They are not objecting to these things on the basis of their ethics. Now Yale Kamazar has written that one can object to it on non-religious grounds and I agree with him. But that is not the reason that doctors give. And then I quote from the Ninth Circuit, "Twenty years ago the AMA contended that performing abortions violated the Hippocratic Oath. Today it claims that assisting the terminally ill patients to hasten their death does likewise. The AMA's contention had no constitutional weight then and it has none now." Most doctors can readily adapt to a changing legal climate and if you look at abortion, we certainly did.

Then the court goes on to say, "And furthermore, if you don't want to do it, you don't have to do it. We're not forcing anyone to do it." Now at this point, I want to deal with the question of, could this be regulated?. I told you about the kind of cases that were presented to the Supreme Court but I want to remind you of the cases. First, you all know Dr. Kevorkian's first and most famous patient that we know of which was

Janet Atkins. And Janet Atkins was in early stage senility. She could still beat her thirty year old son at tennis but she couldn't remember the score, right? Now I want to tell you I play tennis with people all the time who can't remember the score. It's a question of whether it's their age or--it's a great temptation to cheat but I don't--they don't usually think it's a reason that they want off if they can play tennis, right? Now she was actually in a clinic in Washington which treated people. She was unhappy with it but she is a long way from the test case of somebody who's got advanced metastasized to bone marrow and can't move in their bed without breaking a bone, right? That is a long way. Now Dr. Quill's famous case was a woman who developed leukemia. She had a one chance in four of a five year cure and she refused it with consultation with Dr. Quill. Okay? So she had decided not to take it and then she was dying the less painful death that people die from leukemia. And at that point Dr. Quill went over and he actually wrote a prescription, as you know, for a lethal dose, explained to her that this would be a lethal dose in a sort of double talk and then signed the death certificate saying that she had died from leukemia. Now I don't object to Dr. Quill doing this morally as a human being. But I do think it's rather asinine to then write it up in the New England Journal of Medicine and wave it in people's face and not expect the prosecutors to attempt to prosecute him, particularly since he lied on the death certificate. I don't think doctors are supposed to lie on the death certificate, right? So I can understand he was trying to avoid a conflict, but I don't think this is quite the way to go about it. At any rate, I want to emphasize that this was not a patient then who we, from our treatment, had cause to suffer. She was dying the way people have died for centuries from leukemia or other diseases. So now I give that as an initial statement about the problem of regulation. Could we really regulate? These are the cases--if you look at the cases Dr. Kevorkian has done, could we regulate?

Now what is the role of psychiatry in this? I wanted to say a few words about that. In the Ninth Circuit and as I will show you, the expectation

Physician Assisted Suicide:

was that physicians, psychiatrists would determine whether a patient's request to hasten death is rational and competent or motivated by depression or other mental illness or instability. So what is the concern that everyone has is the concern about irrational suicide and the psychiatrists that are supposed to check the people out that they're not irrationally suicidal. There's been much debate about what model statutes should provide in this respect. Dr. Kevorkian thought that every patient should be screened by a psychiatrist. He has written up some material, actually, and calls for everyone to be evaluated by a psychiatrist. And it's my understanding that he has a psychiatrist who is now assisting him. Dr. Quill thought it would be up to the primary practitioner to decide and the language of the various statutes goes all over the place. There are now many of these statutes. I just give you a sample of them to give you a sense of what role the psychiatrist might play. Could I have the next transparency?

Now let me just emphasize to you as a clinical matter that there are these huge problems of overlap in our DSM-IV criteria for depression, for major depression and the symptoms of terminal illness. Three--as psychiatry has become more biological, three of our categories involve weight loss, sleep disturbances, and fatigue. These were all things that patients who have terminal illness will have. Now complicating the picture and I think quite interestingly complicated, oncologists are routinely now prescribing tricyclics for all their patients. And a very interesting development in oncology. They think that tricyclics one, help patients to sleep. Second, they keep them from losing weight and maybe as a side effect, they lift their depression. That's how they tell patients. I'm gonna give you this mediation. It'll help you to sleep. It'll keep you from losing weight and it might even cheer you up. Some also prescribe Ritalin. So you would be evaluating a patient who is already on medication. Now even as a further clinical problem, I want you to know that the MacArthur study has shown that most depressed patients are competent on all tests of competency to make medical decisions. So even if

Where Do We Stand? 1997

you decide someone is depressed that does not mean they are not incompetent. The only test which has been proposed is the question of whether they appreciate what they're doing. And I would say we have no reliable basis for determining whether somebody's feelings of hopelessness when they have cancer and they have a few months to live is irrational or rational. And we certainly, I don't think, can claim to have that wisdom. So now there are--for our profession, for psychiatrists as part of medicine, we--in the atmosphere of managed care, do we now become like the competency gatekeeper? They call us in and if we say the person is competent, we give them the stamp of approval and then they get to commit suicide. Is that ethical? Is that how we--should we play that role? Or shouldn't we prefer to do--well, if I'm a doctor and I'm called as a consultant, I want to give a trial of treatment. I want to try some other anti-depressants. I don't want to just say, "Yes," or, "No." And I'm the gatekeeper for suicide. This is a serious ethical problem within the profession about how they would go about that. And if you compare what we have said about participation in capital punishment with participation in this, you will see the incredible discrepancy.

Now, I want to now tell you about the Oregon Death with Dignity statute which was passed in 1994 by the voters. That provides that no professional organization, association or health care provider shall censure any doctor who does it. So the basic thing I would like to convey to you is if these laws pass, we are out of the loop. Nobody cares what we think. Now we might hire Yale Kamazar and say, "We have a right, some Constitutional right to condemn these people." But the statute forbids us from admonishing our colleagues if they do it even. So I want you to see how far out of the field of play we have gotten. We would be unable to sanction our own members. The AMA would not be able to throw somebody out of the AMA. They might be able to throw them out of the American, but they couldn't throw them out of the Oregon. Or they certainly couldn't do anything that would affect their economic livelihood in any way.

Physician Assisted Suicide:

Now here's the idea that is the key idea, my contribution to all this. And I want to emphasize to you that I am not trying to change anyone's view one way or the other. There is this great book I recommend to all of you written by Nisbet and Roth called *The Structure of Human Inference*. I think that's the title of it and the book, which it should be required reading for all doctors and lawyers, describes one of the remarkable things is when we have some deeply held belief and we hear evidence that is equivocal, we go away even more deeply convinced of our original position where if we were rational, we would be less convinced because we would know that there is no good evidence, right? So one of the problems of listening to all this kind of talk is everybody just hardens their pre-existing attitude. So I hope only to enlighten you. I'm not trying to push you one side or the other.

Now what has happened is that American medicine has lost its ethics. We did it partly to accommodate to legal restrictions, partly specific laws which took the lead away from us. But despite that, we had a very strong tradition of ethics which was what--those of you who know fancy words I would call a praxis. We didn't have a theory of principles that we could look to and say, "Here, we've thought it all out. We've got all these qualifications like the lawyer's code, but we knew what a good doctor was." We had good doctors who were our role models who embodied excellence and compassion and caring. And they are the people from whom we learned our ethics. There were real, practical examples when you went on rounds with this person. This was an exemplar of what it was to be a physician. Those doctors are now all outliers under managed care. I mean that. That is a serious problem. They're outliers. They gave more time and care than was economically efficient to their patients. I remember going on rounds. A lot of you probably went on rounds. Who was the guy who taught us about diabetes? John Peters, he would take us on rounds and he would start putting cotton batting on the feet of the diabetic patient who had sores and would make us all stand there and watch as he did this. So by an example, he was showing you, you know, we were all very busy but I'm showing you--he was not a nice man. But he was showing us what being a doctor was about. That is not permitted under managed care.

The real organized medicine has written briefs in opposition to physician-assisted suicide and the Supreme Court. I've gone through the whole debate when the AMA came to the APA and argued that we should get on board with them and join them. I would say--Linda Emanuel came representing and she went through the entire literature and gave her reasons. I would say--now, this may be unfair. I would say that oncologists have a special view about taking care of dying patients that the rest of us don't have. And I said to her, "Well, you know what? This sounds right but what are you gonna do with a patient who's demented?" And, you know, basically she said, "Well, if the patient gets pneumonia I would just withhold treatment." And, well, I understand that. That's something one could do. It's hardly an organized approach. I believe that oncologists increasingly are concerned about giving care but I now refer you to all the oncologists who didn't want that care themselves and wanted to be free to take a lethal dose of medication when they got to that point.

At any rate, I would say to you, and this is part of my agony about how I stand on this is that in a strange way, the stand against physician-assisted suicide is the last stand of medicine as a profession. For agonizing, you want to know what is at the cutting edge. If we don't control this in some way, if we don't rally around and say, "No, we're not going to sit." Patients who say they want the pills and it may be the right thing but I would say it will be the end of medical ethics. And so I see what is going on as having a political dimension to it that organized medicine is saying, "No, we've got to--we've found something we can agree to. Now, it's not that hard. It's not that easy to get people to agree. They have agreed on this."

Now I already described to you why I thought regulation was unworkable and the AMA thinks so and I think this is one of Professor

Physician Assisted Suicide:

Kamazar's argument. And I think it is a valid argument. When the abortion decision was going through the Supreme Court, Justice White said, "This is nothing but abortion on demand." Chief Justice Burger said, "No, you've got that wrong. Justice Bachman has assured me that doctors know what they're doing and doctors will regulate abortion." Well, it turns out Justice Bachman and Justice Burger were wrong. And Justice White was right. And if you read Roe versus Wade, you'll be amazed. You think they're talking about doctors but what we really know is it is about choice. Now I'm all for choice. I'm not against choice, but I don't think choice is regulated. Okay? I've already discussed the famous cases of Dr. Quill and Dr. Kevorkian and I don't think on any scale of regulation, they are cases that should be given physician-assisted suicide. And yet patients like that will want it. Herbet Hendon who studied the Dutch experience is--and is a very eminent suicidologist is totally opposed to it and claims that although the Dutch report in the New England Journal of Medicine it was working fine, he claims it's working very badly. They do about one a year, a psychiatric patient who they give physician-assisted suicide to in Holland who we would not think had a terminal illness by any definition we use. They might have an illness that they'll have for the rest of their lives, but we would not consider it a terminal illness. So Professor Kamazar has made the point which I think is absolutely right that there is a difference between act and omission. If you withhold a treatment, there are only so many people who die. But if you give a treatment then everybody becomes somebody who can die. There is a real distinction between physician-assisting suicide by giving a pill and taking things away. We take away things from patients and they go on living, much to our dismay day in and day out. So I think there is a distinction. This is a line that if it happened that next year 20,000 people did physician-assisted suicide, how would we feel? How would we feel as physicians if 20,000 people next year did it? Or 40,000 or more? So there is the external consequences of these decisions which Professor Kamazar can describe even more eloquently.

Now in this case that is before the Supreme Court, a group of moral philosophers submitted a brief. Among them, Professor Dworkin who is without doubt a brilliant man, and I know most of these gentlemen and I consider them all would get an introduction like Phil gave me. They argue powerfully that there has to be a right to physician-assisted suicide. I would say the first argument is the argument of autonomy. That's what informed consent is about. I would say autonomy is symptomatic of our society. We don't trust anyone, therefore we want autonomy. If a guy tries anybody else, the one thing you can all agree on is autonomy. Autonomy is the chief moral value at Harvard Law School. You don't trust anyone but you trust yourself. Autonomy rules. This is the most important value in contemporary society is autonomy. Individual choice, that's the value [inaudible] and trumps anything else. You gonna tell me what to do? Now Dworkin also has this very brilliant but I think wrong-headed argument in which he says that the way we die should somehow be the last line in the poem of our life. It should be like--it should be a fitting end. And we don't want to die in this demented, degraded way. And then he divides it up in terms of what he calls critical interest and experiential interest. And he says, you know, sitting in front of television is just an experiential thing. It doesn't count. It's not part of our critical life plan and it is possible to distinguish what is in person's best interest and saying keeping someone alive when they're demented to say that is in their best interest is an insult to their humanity. And then he makes another brilliant argument about the sanctity of life, to capture it away from those who believe that sanctity of life comes from religion or from God. His argument is, "I'm an atheist but I believe in the sanctity of life and the sanctity of life is from my human investment in my life. That's what makes it sacred." And then there is, I think, the most powerful argument in the arsenal of arguments which can only be overturned by an argument like Yale Kamazar's which says, "But the consequences are so terrible. And that is the idea that the state is going to make you suffer three, four, five years because they believe that life is sacred. That it is incredible tyranny for those of you who think you have to live out until you die to impose this on anyone else, that this is an odious form of tyranny. That is the last line of the Ninth Circuit argument is, well, however you say about this, the idea that you would compel somebody to go through what they're going through for those months, that is tyranny. That is not justice. Now what is going to happen in the Supreme Court? I will say to you, I am willing to bet money that the Court overwhelmingly rejects physician-assisted suicide.

So what does that mean for the medical profession? It means that in every state, we're gonna have proposals to change the law to allow physician-assisted suicide. And so the medical profession for the next ten years is gonna be consumed with this issue, which is going to be a matter in every state over and over again. Well, with that bad news, I'm gonna end and thank you for listening.

What Is Wrong With Human Cloning?
The Ethics of Technological Reproduction, 1998

Arthur L. Caplan, Ph.D., Director of Bioethics, University of Pennsylvania

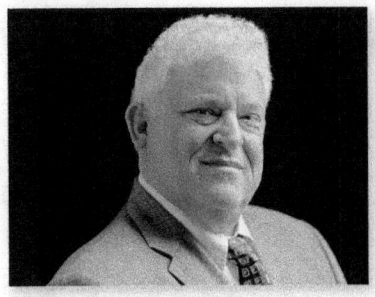

Well, thanks. Actually, Dr. Margolis did not say it, but the reason he and Dr. Greden had me here is I am the third Viking fan that they've ever met in their life so there's three of us left. Actually, this is a good year though. They are going to do very well this year.

It is an honor to be here to give this particular lecture. The importance of having an ethics and value talk, I think, is self-evident at times at which things are moving fast in bio-medicine and I know that Dr. Waggoner played a pivotal role. I have been listening to some of the things he did in the department of psychiatry here and in for the medical school for many, many, many years and it is really a thrill to be able to be part of this series and watch it grow and evolve.

I am going to not leave you in suspense about what's wrong with human cloning. My own view is not much. Things are wrong. Things need to be thought about, but I am not of the opinion that human cloning is so fundamentally wrong that it is something we ought not do. That is interesting though because we're in a state that has banned it. California has and so has Michigan. There are certainly other states moving in that direction. As you know, there's a federal moratorium on research on human cloning. Federal funds are not to be used for that purpose. Some

What Is Wrong With Human Cloning?

other nations have banned human cloning. France, Germany, Japan, Portugal, Denmark, just to name a few, have all banned human cloning. So it is certainly something that a lot of people think apparently there's a lot wrong with. What I'd like to do for this lecture is tack in the following direction. I am going to tell you a little bit, just a quick reminder about what some of the interest in cloning is all about as best a philosopher can describe. Science and the question/answer period people can jump up and correct the things I get wrong, but I will feebly try to say something about why people were so excited about adult cell cloning. And then say a few words about something very different from human cloning. And this is partly just the philosopher's trick of getting you to think about something with some of the emotion detached.

I am going to spend a little bit of time asking you why you shouldn't clone your pet. Some of you know that there's a project underway at Texas A&M that just got funded to clone a dog named Missy. Has anybody been to the Missy site on the Internet? It is an interesting website. It leads off with a code ethics about cloning your dog and what you should do, what you shouldn't do, and why it should be done. A wealthy family has said they would put forward 2.3 million dollars to have their dog, Missy, cloned. A friend of mine that I know at Texas A&M and the vet school has agreed to set out to do this project. So is this a good thing? Would we be well-served by cloning our pets? It might give us an angle on the issues of ethics of human cloning that maybe gives us a little distance so we can talk a little bit more about the rights and wrongs of it. Then I will come back and offer you a few thoughts about the ethics of human cloning having set the stage in that fashion.

Well, some of you may recall that what has set off the current frenzy about cloning was the appearance of Dolly, who actually was born in July of 1996 but whose birth announcement became public in February of 1997. I was always a little befuddled about why people were so excited about Dolly just as a clone because as some of the scientists in the room will know, it has been possible to make clones, and indeed, a number

The Ethics of Technological Reproduction, 1998

have been made of animals, even mammals, doing embryo splitting. You can divide an embryo and produce copies. It has been done, certainly not considered remarkable around veterinary schools to divide embryos at four and eight cell stages and make duplicate copies of animals. So it is not just that we copied an animal that is the source of interest. It certainly was true that for adult cell cloning, the kind of cloning that Dolly represented, people had done it with frogs.

I remember myself being forced to read J.B. Gurdon's articles in Scientific American reprints in college biology class and understanding a little bit about what some of the techniques were for nuclear transplant cloning from adult cell DNA sources. And Dolly represented a mammal and that was certainly the first mammal to follow that technique. But again, it was a little puzzling about why the reaction. And just in case you forgot, the reaction was incredible.

The front page of the New York Times on the day they announced Dolly's birth had three ethical speculations about why this might not be a good idea. One was it might be bad to generate a means to immortality. Another was it would be bad if you could use this technique to make armies of fiendish soldiers who would attack Washington, D.C. By the way, subsequently I noticed that when that objection was brought up, the location of the attack was changed because people did not seem to mind attacking Washington, D.C. So they found other places to talk about. And there was a third objection that showed up on that same initial spade of reactions in the New York Times and the Washington Post, in addition to immortality, in addition to having clone armies, this was actually my favorite, it might be bad because we'd use this to make clones to use as sources of organs and tissues. That later evolved into an even weirder objection which became what I sometimes call the headless clone phenomena that we would make mutant creatures.. We would make these headless things and form them, but that day, the first day, people worried that if you had cloning techniques, you might create basically portable organ farms of clones who would be around to keep you alive if one of your organs failed.

What Is Wrong With Human Cloning?

And things got worse from there. Something about cloning has to go beyond the technology. I mean, if you look at it from a scientific point of view, people were thrilled to find out that you could pull genes out of an adult cell from a mammal, somehow insert them into an enucleated egg, fire it up with a little electricity and get the darn genes to turn back on again and govern the development of another creature. And that was very interesting. I think that people thought that mammalian DNA would not do that and Dolly did that. But that is not what got the media excited about human cloning.

Human cloning has continued to represent a much broader set of issues. It is not about human cloning that the ethical debate has swirled. It is about genetic engineering. And I think cloning is a stand-in or a kind of place holder for a lot of concerns about where is genetics going and what are we going to do with genetics? The reason I say that is in some ways, you're not going to ever be immortal by cloning yourself. Having a DNA copy--well, let's put it this way. If you have a twin and your twin dies, I am sure they take very little solace in the fact that you're still alive in terms of their views about being on this earth. They consider themselves--we consider them very dead even though their twin may continue to go on. We have no problems with personhood or personal identity in saying that even though people are absolutely genetically identical, when one of them dies, a person has died. And they do not continue to exist because their genetic copy in bodily form, imitation still goes on. There's never a doubt that the road to immortality is not through cloning. You might have the road to vanity which is a separate problem, but you do not have the road to immortality.

It is also the case that I know we cannot get far in our society about consensus on matters of morals, but it is probably the case that even this society in love with self-determination and autonomy could bring itself to think that it wasn't a great idea to make a person to kill them for their parts. This probably is not a cutting edge type of policy solution to the shortage of organs and tissues. To breed people to kill them is probably

The Ethics of Technological Reproduction, 1998

not going to fly very far so I would not worry about seeing clones made, even the headless ones who, somebody pointed out to me, maybe they do not have rights. Maybe we could kill them. They couldn't consent.

And certainly the clone army business presumed a kind of genetic reductionism about what you would have to do to get people to turn into battling mimics. I do not know that we have any idea how to create the developmental circumstances, the environment, the surrogate mothers, the apparatus it would take to breed tens of thousand of soldiers or killers or something that would come after us. I do not think that that kind of picture is accurate to what the role of genes versus what the role of environment is for forming behavior and character. I am not saying it could never be done, but it would be one massive undertaking to get it done and it certainly would be beyond the capability of anybody to do it now.

Probably more indicative of how bereft we are for dealing with the impact of the announcement of Dolly and cloning and what genetics is doing was the fact, and I was going to sneer about this for a few minutes and then get past it, but I cannot because he's back. Richard Seed, the most felicitously named exponent of genetic views in the history of biology announced--I will tell you this story. It started the complete frenzy about human cloning. I gave a talk in Chicago, something similar to what we're doing here about the ethics of cloning. I was trying to say, "Look. Let's be reasonable about what cloning can do and what it cannot do and there are things to think about. But let's not sort of go out of our minds about what the real dangers are in terms of making robot clones and organ farms and this sort of stuff."

Richard Seed got up from the audience at the end of that talk and he announced after my talk that while I had raised some issues about why it might not be good to make a human clone that he was going to make a human clone and no one would stop him. I thought that was a very interesting comment. I did not spend a whole lot of time answering it. I thought, "Well, good luck to you. I wish you well on your mission." My talk was taped. Some of you may have heard it. It was broadcast

What Is Wrong With Human Cloning?

on public radio. So was Richard Seed's question or declaration. At that point, Richard Seed became legitimate because public radio had broadcast his plan. And so the rest of the media rushed in to ask Richard Seed about his plans. Now Richard Seed is an indication of what we're worried about with genetics, represents what I am going to refer to throughout these remarks as the nut factor. That a nut will get this technology and do harm to us and you couldn't get a better nut than Richard Seed. He was the paradigm of sort of the nut factor in genetics.

Richard Seed had no background in biology. Richard Seed had no training or skills. I am more likely to be able to clone something than Richard Seed is and I have no chance. I mean, I have watched people do sort of cell cloning and I once went to Robert McConnell's lab in Minnesota and watched some frog cloning, but I cannot do it. And I have no doubt that Richard Seed cannot do it. Moreover, even if you wanted to start a project or a company to do cloning of humans or anything else, you probably would not find a man who has no money and is bankrupt to affiliate with to launch your organization, and that is Richard Seed. He has no money. His house was seized for taxes. He has absolutely no ability to raise money. I do not think venture capitalists are hanging around his small, under court order house in Chicago waiting to partner with him. So he is probably not the guy that is going to be the first to clone a human being. I thought he'd gone away. In fact, it was the one reason I was grateful to Monica Lewinsky. She took his microphone away and it was the end of Richard Seed. End of the chase Richard Seed around and tell people, "No, he is not going to clone anyone. No, he does not know how. He does not have any contacts. He does not have any money. He does not have any science. Nobody takes him seriously. He is not." And then he announced two days ago that he was going to clone himself and that he had asked his wife to serve as his surrogate mother. And there are wire stories running again. And people are calling me up saying, "So what do you think now about--can he really get this done?" His wife is post-menopausal. She is seventy years old. It is patently immoral to even

The Ethics of Technological Reproduction, 1998

ask her to even contiplate pregnancy carrying anybody's child. So in some ways, Richard Seed, the only way I can explain him as a phenomena aside from wanting to know why public radio kept telling us that he was a legitimate person, thereby putting him into the national dialogue is that he represents a fear. He represents a fear about what happens when technology falls into the wrong hands. What happens when you cannot stop technology? What happens when genetics is put in the power or the service of someone with no ethics, no morals, no values and basically someone who is going to go ahead for business reasons or personal reasons or whatever. That is something we are worried about with genetics, although it is not really something we really worry about with cloning. It is what we worry about with genetic engineering. Who will be in charge? How can we control them? Can we ever stop anything?

There is a cousin to this fear, which I do think is interesting the reactions, and that reaction was what I am going to call, for those of you who spend any time in the state of Iowa being punished or for cultural exchange reasons. Minnesotans understand Iowa is a barren wasteland far, far below us. The problem with the state of Iowa, if you look down that way, is that it has a senator by the name of Tom Harkin who normally I like and admire and think is a fine fellow. But Tom Harkin jumped up right after Dolly's birth was announced and some of this controversy begun and he said, "Well, there is really nothing we can do. Science is basically going where it is going and all we can do is get out of the way." I mean, I am not paraphrasing, or we will be crushed under the juggernaut. But there is no stopping it. He said--I mean, the metaphors were, once the genie's out of the bottle you cannot get it back in. And once science and technology take off, no one, no mortal being can ever do anything to bring it to a halt.

Now Tom Harkin clearly has never sat on the appropriations committee for the NIH because I can tell you, I have seen things brought to a screeching halt, things that I thought shouldn't be halted in this country. Embryo research, fetal tissue transplant research, we were talking this morning about research that is been stopped in New York State on

What Is Wrong With Human Cloning?

institutionalized children with severe mental retardation stopped cold. It is not true that you cannot bring things to a halt in science. And in fact, if you take a broader historical perspective, you can see that there are many areas of research where because of human subjects protection, informed consent requirements, and peer review, a lot of experiments have been slowed if not stopped. It is just not true. It is a false sense in the history of science to say that science goes where it wants to go. Science needs money to get there. These days it often needs teams of people to take it there. That is why also I am not too worried about Richard Seed and his home cloning company. And it is simply false to suggest as Harkin did take the position--I will name it Harkinism that we cannot do anything, that we're just--the only thing we can do is get out of the way once genetics gets rolling.

But the Harkinism view and the nut factor view are very important in trying to understand what was going on with cloning because I think they are the legacy of something else. And they are the legacy of the age of physics, and specifically, nuclear physics. What happened to cloning is it got caught up in the cultural phenomena, I think. The cultural phenomena was we were told in the forties and fifties that atomic power would be a wonderful boon to humanity, that it would produce electricity so cheaply that it would not be metered. Remember that phrase? And then a large number of Americans spent the rest of the century hiding under their desks and digging big holes in the basement because of the Cold War. It was not a technology that delivered. And then the fear was, if you want to take it in two directions, one, once the nuclear genie is out of the bottle, anybody can get it and terrorize you with it. And two, if a nut gets it, they'll do terrible harm. Those are the fears of nuclear power, of the misuse or misapplication of nuclear knowledge. I do not believe they have any relevance to what cloning is all about.

Let's say, just for the sake of argument that I am a clone. Could be. Do not know. If I am, I actually pose no threat to anybody here. I am just a person who was made in a different way, but I am not a threat, a public

The Ethics of Technological Reproduction, 1998

health threat. No one could take me and use me to their evil purposes particularly just because I am here. The metaphor that genetic engineering or cloning, if it fell into the wrong hands could be used to imperil the rest of us, I think is a false metaphor. It is from a different technology and a different situation. Even if a nut were to make 100 clones, one might say, "Well, is it good? Is it bad? Is it safe?" Some other things we will talk about in a little bit, but the one thing I would not worry about a whole lot is that they would endanger the world or pose a public health threat to the rest of us. That is not what cloning is about. That is now how it works. That is not where its ethical punch is. But because our society has a legacy of dealing with atomic power, nuclear weapons, if you will, nuclear power, the dangers of that plus the emerging threats of biological warfare, the emerging threats of terrorism, these metaphors are driving a lot of what the reaction is to cloning even though I do not think those are the appropriate metaphors. There are things I think we need to be thinking about, but I do not think those are what they are.

So the science that was exciting about cloning was for scientists, understanding what you could do to get genes to turn back on and understanding a lot about the properties of DNA in adult cells, that people had assumed once they had sent out their final messages to make specialized cells and organs, they had done their job, they would never recreate a creature again. And yet for Dolly and the mice that were produced in Hawaii and the report that come from Japan about cows, it looks that some cells, not maybe all adult cells, but in some cells you can get them to turn back on and govern development of a new organism. So that is the exciting science.

Well, what I have tried to say to you is the ethical objections go way outside what makes that all of interest and excitement within the scientific community. Their worries and some ways in which the culture is painting fears because of history, legacy of misuse and misapplication of say knowledge in nuclear physics and just worries more particularly about where is genetics taking us anyway? Should we be immortal? Is it arrogant

What Is Wrong With Human Cloning?

to kind of engineer ourselves? Should we use others, genetically engineer them to our purposes? That is the body parts business and so on. These sorts of worries combined with the history that produced this nut factor worry and the Harkinism view that we cannot stop anything so it is all going to go off the rails, they are, I think, not so much and inappropriately linked up to cloning. I do not think cloning has to carry the weight. There are certainly issues to be talked about with genetic engineering. That is for sure. But I do not think cloning is there. And I will tip my hand about human cloning. I said, "What's wrong with it?" I am going to tell you something's wrong with it in a minute, but we're going to take a voyage off to pet land here. But before I tell you about pets and before I tell you some things I think might be wrong although not so wrong as to ban it, just things to think about or things to be worried about with human cloning, I will say this. I believe that there will be a human clone. I hope there's no public radio here because then they'll start coming to me and I will have to go around saying, "And I am going to make it in my basement". I am sure some day, someone will clone a human being. I actually think that will be moderately interesting and fairly a matter of relative reproductive indifference to what human beings are doing. I do not think a lot of people are going to want to reproduce asexually. Most people find it more alluring to mix their gametes with a partner in the passion of sexuality. I think making something in a dish will not be all that attractive to most people age say, sixteen to forty. There may be some who say they cannot reproduce by any other means other than to clone themselves if they have fertility problems or perhaps are gay or maybe very old. But I do not think that is going to turn out to be a majority way to reproduce and I think partly due to human nature and certain drives and impulses wired into us, our tendency will be to still mate and exchange gametes and take the genetic lottery in some ways and see what happens.

Cloning, copying ourselves, literally copying your genes to send them on to somebody else, I do not think is going to be a very big activity for humans. I mean, it is going to be a really big activity for animals.

The Ethics of Technological Reproduction, 1998

One way to put this simply is if you think about your pets, and I am heading here, most of us love our animals literally for their bodies. My son has a hamster. I have got cats. We've got dogs. We've got animals coming up the wazoo in my house. I usually try to admire and love or engage with people for their minds. I tend to favor interest in animals for their bodies. The further away they become from pet status, the more my interest in their bodies grows. Dolly looks to me like lamp chops walking around. Maybe a blanket. And for a large part of humanity not convinced of the moral standing of the animals, they use animals and exploit them for their bodies. Cloning is very good when you're trying to replicate bodies. It is not very good when you're trying to replicate minds. And so I suspect for another reason, human cloning as a reproductive act is not going to turn out to be as attractive once people understand what they can and cannot really do with it.

If you ask me what the future will bring, I will tell you a few human clones for odd purposes that will, of course, be the subject of intense fascination perhaps in the media. But the future as genetically engineering ourselves and whether that is a good or bad thing to do, to enhance ourselves, improve ourselves, change our genes. Who actually would really want to send on to future generations their asthma, diabetes, depression, and baldness, all of which you send on with the clone? It is cruel. Who really wants to be you again? That rotten, defective body and flawed recessive genes, bad diseases, terrible.

Better, you should genetically engineer your children. The goal, morally, is to do better by your children, improve them, try to make their lives better, give them more abilities and capacities, but that is going to require genetic engineering, not some kind of vanity license plate reproduction. So I do not think cloning actually is going to have much of a big future. I could be wrong. But I think in the animal world it will.

Let's spend a second looking at animals just to see if we can tease out maybe from that case example what some of the things are that might be wrong about cloning humans or animals. One of the things that people sometimes say about human cloning is, "Well, no one should interfere with it or ban it because people have a fundamental right to reproduce and they should be able to reproduce without interference from anyone ever." We do not encounter this issue with animals. We rarely recognize a fundamental right to reproduce of animals actually unless they are deer in our parks and then we will not do anything to interfere with them. But normally we spay them and neuter them and do other things to them. This deer crack I am making is because where I live in Philadelphia, the deer are eating the park to oblivion but no one is willing to neuter them, kill them, or do anything to them. They actually have established a fundamental right to reproduction. But short of the deer--it is a Bambi factor problem. We do not recognize any fundamental right of animals to reproduce. So we can put aside what sometimes distorts this debate about the rights and wrongs of cloning although I am going to come back to it about do humans have a fundamental right to reproduce. So we can say that animals generally do not. So that opens the door up. Why would we think about cloning animals, cloning our pets in particular?

Let me tell you a couple of things that people have said on the Internet that I have pulled down. There's a place called Canine Cryobank which offers pet cloning but what they are promising is that they will store cells from Fido or Fluffy and when cloning techniques are perfected, you'll be able to get Fido or Fluffy back. There's another Internet site called Genetipet. It is a company in towns in Washington near Seattle actually. They sell a kit for extracting blood from your pet to be sent to their frozen storage facility. Costs you 200 dollars to do that and 200 dollars to store a little bit of your pet. Their advertising says, "Our idea is basically this. Your pet is gone but only in a sense. Not really. He's not totally gone if we still have his blood and his DNA. If we do not save your pet's DNA now, no amount of money will be able to bring him or her back once the DNA is lost. If scientists are able to create higher life forms through genetic engineering, then we are ready. We have the material stored here and ready to go. If it does not happen, what have you lost? Money. But that is the risk."

The Ethics of Technological Reproduction, 1998

Those of us who are pet lovers really could have them back again. So that is Genetipet. And then there's the Misiplicity project. This is the Texas millionaire I mentioned before who is now ponied up or promised to pony up $2.3 million to a group of Texas A&M led by Mark Westhuesen, very competent animal biologist veterinarian, to undertake the work to clone their pet. Their pet, Missy, is a Collie/Husky mix that they got at the pound, is now 11, they love the dog very much. I am not going to go into the detail of their website, but basically what they are saying is they love their dog and they want to see their dog restored to them and they would like to have Missy cloned because they love her so much. They love her bark. They love her behavior. They love her cute little idiosyncrasies. The way she brings her bones in and the slippers in and the whole thing. That that is their dream.

Well, what's wrong with this? Why should anybody object if someone wants to bring Missy or Fluffy or whoever back? Obviously one thing wrong with it is what was wrong with those early objections to human cloning. These people are all of the opinion and in fact being told in part by places like Genetipet that they are going to restore their pet if they do this, that their pet will be back. That is very unlikely. The pet is not going to come back. Something that looks like the pet may come back. And I would even go so far, being a believer in genetics that an animal may come back with dispositions, behaviors that resemble many of the things that their pet once had. But strange as it may seem, one of the reasons that people love their pets is exactly what was said on the Missy site. Their little idiosyncrasies, little habits, their little nuances, it is their individuality that they like. They do not fall in love with a generic cat. They do not fall in love with a generic dog. They like the little tricks and stunts that their--I mean, if I ask my son why he likes his hamster, which is the stupidest thing I have ever seen in my life, he will tell me that it quivers in a certain way and squeaks when he comes and does all this stuff. I do not know. I mean, I think it is all accidental contingent behavior, but I cannot break this news to him. But he loves the little idiosyncrasies of this thing, Nuget, the hamster. And that is exactly what he identifies with. He's not identifying with dispositions and the soft-wiring propensities and the general propensity to hoard and chew on little seeds and store things and run forever in endless circles in the little plastic rotating cylinder. He loves his nuances. But the nuances are what you're not going to get back in cloning because it is training and environment and development that is going to have to shape and produce them. If Missy comes back or his clone somehow, she won't have lived a few years in the pound and all the little things that she learned and all the little peccadilloes that she has are going to have to be reproduced somehow. But can they be because they cannot recreate the past that brought those things to bear. Maybe they can. I am actually somewhat skeptical that they are going to be able to feel that Missy has come back to them given the way she's going to behave. The very things that we might think are trivial and slight differences from the point of view from dog behavior, 95 percent of her behavior being the same, it is the five percent that made them fall in love with her. And they won't get that back. That is the part that is shaped by other factors and forces.

So I believe in part that one reason that it is bad to clone something is if you dream not so much of immortality, that is too strong, but if you believe somehow you're going to get back what you've lost, you cannot bring back what you've lost because you cannot put the same genes in the same river of environment twice, so to speak. Time changes. Those factors change. It would be very tough to recreate all those variables. And if we really do admire and engage one another as people as well as our pets for the small differences and the little nuances and the funny little habits and the little traits, those will be the hardest of all to get back. We will know right away that it is not the same dog because even though she does bring our slippers, she zigzags this way when she does it as opposed to zigzagging that way when she did it. Why? I do not know but that is not the same dog. It is a pretty close copy. Reminds me a lot of old Missy, but it is not Missy.

The Ethics of Technological Reproduction, 1998

And so one reason to be nervous or worried about cloning pets or people I think that comes out of the animal case may be that we hope or we dream that somehow we're going to be able to replicate what is lost. But I think what we know about genetics, what we know about behavior, what we know about what makes us identify with one another as individuals is precisely what cloning cannot bring us. So we risk some disappointment.

Another odd fact about cloning and why you might not think it is a good idea for animals is, weirdly enough, it may make them more disposable. It may make them more of a production so that if I said--well, put aside the details of cloning. Is it safe? Will the animals age right? You might say another reason to be nervous about pet cloning is precisely what makes Missy fun is that there aren't other dogs like her. But what if you really could reproduce her? And what if you get pretty close to a lot of the same behavioral and temperamental and physical attributes? Would you in fact have cheapened her value by making her something that you can create? Now I am here to tell you, I have been to puppy mills. I know what it means to mass produce animals for laboratory experiments and other purposes. I know that we do that already so to speak. We have as close to cloning in many arenas of animal production as you would ever want to see. Almost none of those animals wind up being pets. They have no individuality. It is their production line apparatus that makes it hard to relate to them. It probably tells us something about a problem in human cloning. Here's what I'd say the problem is.

The danger of human cloning, when you think about what might be wrong about cheapening pets because you can mass produce them and almost turn them into throw away items, you can get another one sort of like that. Do not worry about it. The first one did not work out. We will make you another one. When you move that into the people arena, you do not want to find people's individuality challenged or compromised because they feel somehow that their uniqueness is not so unique. That their feeling of individuality is threatened. Actually, I think that is what its issue--what people are trying to express when they object to cloning. In

What Is Wrong With Human Cloning?

a society that is obsessed with individuality and individualism, that is us, more than any other society on earth, the prospect of having many copies is terrifying because we love our individuality, even if it is only 99 percent copying because I am still making some room for the environment and developmental differences. Even if I was a complete genetic reductionist, which I am not, but I am a strong believer in a lot of power in genetics making us who we are, I still believe that it frightens us to think that we might make ourselves less unique, less special because we are copyable.

And so that is the message that you can see about what really might be frightening people, particularly in individualistic Western societies about cloning. It is not so much that nuts will come around and--well, I mean, it is a fear like that. But what they are trying to say is, "I do not want to be devalued. I like my specialness. Do not take away what was different about me. Do not tell me anybody can make me again and again and again."

Which leads me to a third kind of worry. This does not come from pets. The two points I made do come out of the pet--thinking about pets and why you might or might not want to clone them. They might disappoint you and you might cheapen their value if you could actually do it, but the other reason I think human cloning is suspect has absolutely nothing to do with anything about danger to others or threats to the rest of us. What's gotten lost in the ethics of human cloning discussion is the question that I think is at the core of this. And these two points about losing individuality and finding yourself perhaps bothered that you couldn't bring back what you had lost, a disappointment, point me toward the issue, is it in anybody's interest to be made as a clone?

That, I think, is a very interesting question. And it is gotten almost no attention in all these debates. Why would not it be in your interest to be made as a clone? I am going to give you three things to think about. I do not think any one of them overwhelms the argument to say, "Well, we would never clone anyone then." But I think they are things to think about. In all of reproductive technology, I have to sneer now and say,

The Ethics of Technological Reproduction, 1998

when we talk about reproductive technology, what we tend to do is say, "If the parents want it, if the woman wants it, if the man wants it, then it should just be done and that is the end of it and we will have no laws and no one will get in the way." Remember I mentioned that fundamental right to reproduce? Stay out of my face and do not tell me anything. Well, the truth is that there is a reason to be concerned about new technologies for making people, whether it is test tube babies or cloning because you do want to ask, "Is that going to be good for the person who's made in this way? Will it put them in any position where they are burdened or saddled?" I will give you a simple example.

I have had women at University of Pennsylvania who have asked that we take sperm out of their husband who died unexpectedly. And some of you know I have been writing about this and published some studies about post-mortem sperm procurement. One of the terrible issues about doing something like this is is it good to make someone who has no dad? Is it good to honor somebody's wish to make a person after the dad is dead when in fact the mom may be acting out of guilt or emotional trauma? The man's died unexpectedly. She wants the sperm taken. Does she know what she's doing? Is she going to feel the same way about this a year or two years or four years from now? What if you take the sperm and make the baby and the mom remarries and does not want a reminder of the former husband? It is a new life. Things have changed. So there are things that you need to think about. I will give you the ultimate case. Soon we're going to be getting adept, it started, at freezing eggs. Should we ever make babies from dead parents when mom and dad are both dead and we pull the egg and the sperm out and fertilize them and make something later? Do you need anybody's permission or you just do it?

When we ask questions about reproductive technology, the interest of the parties who want to use it are very important. But what we tend to look away from is what does it do to the person who is made this way? And that is what I want you to be thinking about with human cloning. And I have been trying to push there from the pet examples.

What Is Wrong With Human Cloning?

The three other points I want you to think about is this first. Why might it not be a good idea to be a human clone? Because if you are the copy of someone you are the involuntary subject to the most systematic genetic test ever done. You will know all of the things that are under genetic control or predisposition that will happen to you except you will know them by watching them unfold in the person from whom you are cloned. We argue a little bit these days about things like, "What kind of counseling would we supply to someone if they knew they were at risk of Huntington's disease?" And we thought about a genetic test or BRCA1 and two testing for breast cancer. And I think most of us would agree that we shouldn't force someone to have a test for Huntington's disease or breast cancer if they do not want it. They should choose to know. Clones will not choose. They will know they are bald at thirty. They are impotent at forty. They are ridden with stomach cancer at fifty. They are depressed. Is not this a morbid life? Who is this clone parent? Who do we make them from? But they are going to know a great deal about what will await them, what will happen to them, what their future holds because it is going to be written in terms of a biological program that is unfolding 20, 30, 40, 50 years ahead of them. That is a problem. It may not be an overwhelming problem as a reason not to make a human clone, but it is a problem.

You might put it this way. The philosopher Joel Feinberg once wrote many years ago, "Children are owed an open future. You should be able to chart your course as to what you want to be." If you have all this genetic information thrust upon you because of the way you were made, it may limit who you can be because you cannot be as free knowing what you know about how you are going to look, what you will be like, what will happen to you in many ways because of this forerunner. Twins do not have this problem. They age simultaneously. Clones will have to look forward. You might call it the Dorian Gray problem. You are going to see yourself age. No matter what you do, you are going to know these facts and fates that await you.

The Ethics of Technological Reproduction, 1998

The second issue I want you to think about is, is it a good idea if you are a human clone and made in this way, from the point of view of your interest to look like somebody else exactly who has had a life in front of you? And this again relates to the question of the psycho-social emotional burden. Let me give you an example by describing as the Woody Allen syndrome. Some of you know that Woody Allen married his adopted daughter. Some of you thought that might have been weird. Why? Because normally we think that it is a bad idea to mix parenting with sexual affection for marriage purposes, that you should not mix the roles. Now he is not biologically related to the woman that he is now married, who he helped to raise. So it is not a question of incest. There's something else going on about roles. If I make a clone of my wife because I love her dearly and now the clone grows up, what is happening in my relationship to my daughter? I am looking at the person I fell in love with. I am looking at the person I had all kinds of feelings about except she's now 30 years younger than her clone mom. And how do my psycho-social emotional reactions go as I try to deal with this person who is becoming somebody else that I had all kinds of feelings about but here they come again in this bodily-shapen form that I am very familiar with but in fact might have all sorts of older feelings about because this is the person from long past--my appearance, not the same person. I have already explained it is not re-creation. But many things are going to be triggered if you will, psychologically, biologically, emotionally by seeing a particular appearance and presentation.

That is at one extreme. Clones would face many of those challenges as well if I made a clone and I was just single and the clone person came here and stood here. People would say, "Oh, I bet you're interested in bio-ethics, huh?" Well, actually, no, I am not. Now a lot of us have to deal with the legacy of our parents and the legacy of our fathers and what they wanted us to be and explain why we're not architects or lawyers or engineers or plumbers or whatever their dream was or baseball players. It is one thing to deal with a legacy that is psychological. It is another thing to deal with a legacy that is complete appearance imitation. Much tougher to fend it off. Much tougher to carry the burdens. So that might be a problem for a clone. It may not be in your interest to have to lug around the weight of someone appearance-wise in a society very sensitive to that that went before you. I am not saying it is overwhelming. I am not saying it is a reason to ban it. I am just saying it is something that we have to be thinking about when we ask, "What are the reasons you would want to clone someone? And is that worth the potential cost to their psychological or their, if you will, individual options and choices for what they might become?"

Probably the other type of reason to worry about human cloning, and I saved this to last because I did not want you to obsess about it is, it is not clear that it is safe. Now safety has been the thing that national commissions have worried about and safety has been the thing that probably has driven more bans of cloning than anything else I know. It is not safe. In medicine if you had done an experiment where you had successfully cloned one sheep, 20 mice, even though the mice reproduced, and two apparent cow clones, you would not start clinical human trials. Well, you might in certain institutions, but you would be wrong to do that. That would not be--you would not be right to do that. We do not know what age Dolly is aging at. We have no idea what her dispositions are to disease and disorder. We do not know what really has been created and it is going to take a while to study that, to get a handle on that. You certainly may make an argument that it would be prudent to have a moratorium on human cloning for a few years just to see about safety and risk. What's the aging process? Will Dolly drop dead as a seven year old animal, the cells from which she came, or a new animal that is just lugging along some oddball genetic misinformation that is not going to harm her? I have no idea. I am certainly willing to defer to experts who study this and think about this. But it has to be shown before you would get anywhere near human beings.

Having said that, that to me is an argument for a moratorium, not a ban. That is an argument for waiting, proceeding with caution and

The Ethics of Technological Reproduction, 1998

prudence. The other arguments I tried to present to you today are closer to arguments about why you might say it might not be a good idea to do it. It might not be a good idea to do it. Does it threaten our individuality? Does it make us feel somehow that we have to live up to somebody else's future? Are we lugging baggage through life that we do not want because we know many things that are going to await us? Are we finding ourselves being reacted to and responding to people in ways that we do not like because we look and appear so similar to those who went before us? In that sense, it seems to me--there's a fundamental question about, is it in our interest to be a clone? Is it in the best interest of a person to be made in this way?

My own view is there is not anything fundamentally essentially wrong with human cloning. My own view is too, that the discussion about human cloning to date has gone off the rails with the kinds of objections that have greeted it. To recap to you, the nut factor worry, the Harkinism, we cannot control it. It is going to crush us, kill us, run us over, something. We will exploit people using it in terms of turning them into our tissue farms and so forth. None of this, I think, is what we need to be worried about with human cloning. I have hinted to you that I do not think human cloning is going to turn out to be all that much of interest, so the debate will be, if you will--and the way I think we ought to think about it and the way I'd like you to think about it, should we allow people to exercise the option of human cloning knowing that the psychological emotional best interest arguments and what they have to overcome? Could they be overcome? Should we ask people to subject themselves to an assessment? Counseling? A review?

Well, that gets us to the final comment I want to make. People have said, "Well, we cannot do that because no one can interfere with anybody's right to reproduce." The one thing I want you to understand as you leave here today, if you get nothing else out, a right to reproduce comes in two shapes. Philosophers like to talk about two kinds of rights. There are positive rights and negative rights. The easiest way for me to explain to you why there is a limit on reproductive rights is for me to point out to you--well, you know, I have been thinking that one of the things I might want to do after this lecture, I will be pretty tense, I think I'd like to exercise my right to reproduce. And I have been looking at the women in the audience and I have got some in mind that I am going to tell them I want my right to reproduce. And I am going to claim it. You guys can try this in bars and things. It does not work very well.

Clearly, something is odd about saying that you have a right to reproduce that is unlimited, that is unbounded. It is true that there is a right to reproduce recognized morally and legally, in fact, both in United Nations documents and in certain American laws about the right to be left alone and not interfered with when you are reproducing. That is a privacy zone if you want to think of it that way. It has nothing to do with the entitlement to reproduction. The state does not supply you with girlfriends. I cannot get a mate. I cannot run around saying, "Well, I really want to reproduce now." I have tried that. Nothing happens.

So you do not have a positive right. You have a negative right to reproduction. It is perfectly legitimate if we choose to do so, to ask people who want to use technological means and assistance to facilitate reproduction, to submit to some sort of review or deliberation about why. Why do they choose to do this? We can do this on two grounds. There is no entitlement to a technological assistance in reproduction. If you are lucky enough to be fertile you can go to the bedroom with a willing mate and make all the babies you like. If you are unlucky enough to be infertile, you need adoption. You need IVF. You may need cloning, but in this era we feel that it is appropriate for society to step in and say, "Before we pay for that or before we make this available to you, if we want to, we can restrict who can use this and why." We might say, "If you're 80 years old, we do not make orphans." We haven't. I think we should. We could. We might say, "It is not good to make children from two dead parents." We might even say, "Not good to make people when the gametes from which we are getting the people, there has been no permission." If I were to run around here and take samples of all your cells after you had left and find Richard Seed and his clone company and make copies of all of you, you might feel offended saying, "I should have the right to control my reproduction. You should not have the right to reproduce me without my permission." Of course, cloning would not really--to work would give me the option of reproducing you by getting a piece of your Kleenex. We would just go out and say, "Oh, I have got the DNA. I can make Art whenever I want. Sneeze again, Art. We will have another 20."

So there's clearly something wrong about saying this whole discussion is off the rails because we have a fundamental right to reproduce. It is a negative right. It is a right to be left alone. When technological assistance is required, when entitlement or empowerment is required to reproduce, society can--it hasn't chosen to do much of this, but it could set limits, ask for justification. What I have tried to do today is to convince you that it is not clearly in the best interest of a person to be made as a clone. So it would be reasonable to perhaps set some steps out that people would have to overcome before they would be allowed to do it. I am not saying they could not. But the psychological, emotional, and individuality worries about the best interest of the to-be-cloned person seem to me to be appropriate reasons to limit access to technological assistance in this area. Again, not that you could not meet it. Not that there are not ways for you to say, "I can handle it. I know I am not going to get emotionally entangled the way you are talking about it. I can respect the individuality. Do not worry. I can deal with all this." I can imagine someone meeting the arguments, but they must be met. They should be met. And I hope, in fact, that we do not listen to Tom Harkin in that we begin to craft policies that will allow them to be met in the years to come.

Thanks.

No Place to Hide: Threats to Confidentiality and Privacy in Medicine, 1999

Paul S. Appelbaum, M.D., Professor of Psychiatry, Medicine, Law, Columbia University

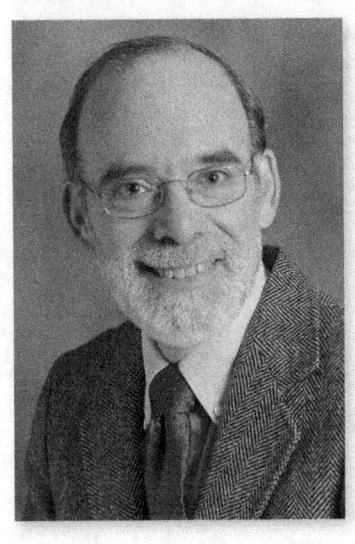

Phil, thank you very much for that introduction. It is a pleasure and an honor to be this year's Waggoner lecturer. I am delighted to join you. There is, in fact, a connection between my talk this morning which focused on informed consent issues in research settings and my talk here this afternoon which focuses on issues of confidentiality in the medical setting. And the connection is simply this, that in research we have taken it as a matter of policy that patients, potential research subjects, will be given the opportunity to make their own decisions about whether or not to participate in research, that they will control the situation. They will make the determinations regarding what happens to them, even regarding what happens to their information and whether or not it should be employed in research settings. In general medicine and psychiatry in particular, we have generally taken the same approach with regard to who has control over patients' medical record information. The answer to that question has been the patient who gets to determine where the information goes, who gets to use it and whether or not it is employed for research purposes, administrative purposes or to other ends.

We are, however, on the verge of what could be, a major change, a revolution you might say in the way in which medical record information is handled and in the answer to the question, who has control over the information that is collected about patients' medical situations. And it is that potential revolution that is really, in a number of ways, the subject of my presentation to you here this afternoon.

Confidentiality has, as many of you know, always been a cornerstone of psychiatric treatment in particular, but medical treatment in general. You all know the words of the Hippocratic Oath, which depending on which translation you use, that the practitioner will not speak of that which should not be spoken of to other men. That is, what the practitioner, what the physician learns in contacts with his or her patient will remain with the physician and not be further disseminated. Psychiatry in particular won a major victory two years ago in the U.S.--I guess it is now three years ago in the U.S. Supreme Court decision in Jaffee versus Redmond which declared a psychotherapist/patient privilege to exist. In the federal courts, Justice Stevens writing for the unanimous majority of the court, noted that effective psychotherapy depends upon an atmosphere of confidence and trust, and therefore the mere possibility of disclosure of confidential communications may impede development of the relationship necessary for successful treatment. And you could probably substitute psychiatry for psychotherapy and probably medicine in general for psychotherapy and still have a valid statement regarding the importance of confidentiality.

Despite these words, however, threats to the confidentiality of medical treatment seem to be coming at us from every direction. And you do not have to go far to find them. For example, I have an article here that came from the Washington Post not very long ago. It's a story written by a reporter who was walking down the street headed to his house when he found papers blowing down the street, an unusual occurrence

Threats to Confidentiality and Privacy in Medicine, 1999

in his suburban Maryland neighborhood. He stopped to pick one up and discovered it was part of a medical record and he gathered more of them and sort of Hansel and Gretel like traced the trail back to where they were coming from. And there was a large dumpster outside a house that was being renovated from which these records were being blown out by the wind. He took a pile of them home, looked at them more closely and discovered that they were, in fact, psychiatric records including patients' names, diagnosis, problems that they were having in treatment, and the like including one ironic note describing a particular youngster thought to be a suicide risk who was described as, "very concerned about people seeing him as crazy and knowing that he was in psychiatric treatment." Well, the reporter dug into the story a little bit and discovered that the house that was being renovated used to belong to a psychiatrist. Psychiatrist had retired, moved across the river to Virginia and somehow the records left in the house made their way into the dumpster and were being blown across the street. He called the psychiatrist, tracked him down in Virginia. The man said, "Oh, I have no idea how this could happen. I destroyed all my records, of course, when I retired from treatment. It must be that one of my employees stole the records and that's how they ended up in the dumpster." Well, if the employee stole the records, he or she stole them and then left them in the same house and it all seems rather improbable. It seems like one of those instances where it was all too easy for a practitioner to ignore the question of patient confidentiality and to not give a second thought to what would happen to the records that he had accumulated over a lifetime of rendering clinical care.

So the threat that your medical record may be blowing down the street one day is a clear and obvious threat. But other threats to our medical record confidentiality are lesser known and they stem from activities that have been going on in Washington that have gotten us very close to the point of essentially overturning centuries of tradition with regard to the control of information that derives from the delivery of medical care and may lead us in just a few months into a very different world, a new order, if you will, in which medical record information is no longer controlled by patients but controlled by the government instead. And I will describe a little later to you exactly what the dimensions of that change might be.

Now since I can't possibly provide a comprehensive overview of all the issues related to the current status of confidentiality, my goals today are a little bit more modest. I'd like to review with you three of the major forces that are threatening confidentiality. Today, computerization of medical records, the creation of medical record or medical information databanks, and access to records by managed care companies and these are probably all issues with which you've had experience. And then I would like to update you on the current legislative initiatives and tell you a little bit about where things stand because they change day to day. But this is a critical time, really. Whatever you believe about the importance of confidentiality or the importance of access, what goes on in Washington in the next four to six months is probably going to shape a generation, the next generation of how we deal with medical record information. It may shape the next hundred years of how we deal with such information.

So let's start with a look at the issue of computerization which is really what's driving a lot of the current situation. What is going on in the world now of medical record computerization? Well, many medical entities are considering adopting computerized records and some already have. And in the last day I have talked with people here at the university and discovered that you are really in the lead as far as these developments are concerned having developed both a computerized medical record system and made some special provisions which we'll talk about in a broader context with regard to psychiatric records per se.

An example of the debate that is likely to ensue when these efforts are not done well came from Massachusetts in the last three years where one of our leading health plans, then called the Harvard Community Health Plan, now known as Harvard Pilgrim Healthcare, a non-profit HMO at one point affiliated with Harvard, now quite independent and the largest HMO in the state went to a computerized medical record system giving relatively little thought to the question of what information would be included in that system and deciding that everything would be included in that system including information that some people might consider to be particularly sensitive, particularly in this case medical-- I'm sorry, psychiatric record information. The Boston Globe picked up the story and revealed to its readers that this million plus member system with tens of thousands of people in its employ and literally thousands of physician and non-physician caregivers had created a system where from any clinic or affiliated physician's office, anybody with a password could punch in a patient's medical record number and see their entire medical record, whether or not that person was involved in their care and no matter how sensitive the information was, and the Globe focused in particular on psychiatric record information because there is an intuitive sense I think that most people have that that is particularly sensitive. That is the kind of medical information that perhaps along with information about sexual transmitted diseases, abortion, and perhaps still cancer with the stigma that that carries, people would very much not like to have bandied around.

In the face of a public outcry, Harvard Community Health backed down and went to a complete segregation of its psychiatric and medical records and took their psychiatric records offline and made it back into a paper record system which they continue with to this day. And they are running two separate parallel medical record systems as a result and they have spent enormous effort trying to contain the fallout from their initial move. So clearly there are dangers both for the entities that are moving to computerized records and to patients themselves in the process.

Where's the push coming from for computerization? Why do we see one entity after another adopting a computerized medical record? Well, there are, to be sure, powerful forces behind this move. In a very influential 1992 Institute of Medicine report, computerized medical records were endorsed as the future of medical record keeping. It was, although this may be hard to remember now, part of the Clinton healthcare plan of blessed memory and some aspects of it were adopted in little known provisions of a bill called the Kennedy-Kassebaum Health Insurance Portability Act which I'll discuss in just a moment. It has been the focus of intense lobbying by the information industry, which is eager to facilitate this. Hardware companies, software companies, data management companies all see enormous profits to be made in this process of conversion to computerized medical records. Nobody forgets that Ross Perot's money came from being the man who had the contract to computerize the Medicare billing and payment system. And there are more millions or billions to be made as the nation moves towards a computerized medical record system.

Now to be sure, it's not just money that's at stake here. There are valid arguments made for the good that can come from increased computerization. And I presume it was arguments that, like these, that led to the adoption of a computerized system here. Computerization, it is argued, probably rightly, will increase the availability of information in ways that are beneficial to patients, at other sites in a system if a patient turns up, people who turn up in emergency rooms, when care is shifted to new providers or even people who turn up in an emergency room across the country and need rapid access to information about a patient's medical situation. It as well provides an increased ability to detect patterns of care, patterns of presentation and response, patterns of use or misuse of medical interventions. There's greater efficiency of record management. At some point, our medical record rooms, if we keep using paper records, will get bigger than our hospitals and the hospital will be, especially given the current trend toward downsizing in patient beds, will be a little wing off the back of the medical records facility. Clearly at some point we need a way of being more efficient about how we keep our records. And it is argued as well, and again legitimately, that there will likely be cost savings from the increased ability to track utilization in a system and potentially on a regional or national basis.

Well, you might ask, if computerization can be so helpful, and it probably can be, why should we be concerned about it? And I think the answer can be illustrated by another case that happened in my backyard in Boston at the Beth Israel Hospital, one of the major Harvard teaching hospitals, in which a man who worked at the facility, a janitor or somebody in the building staff, got access to their computerized medical record system and sent a very personalized, sexualized letter to a woman whose medical record he pulled up at random there. She was appropriately outraged. He was appropriately fired but it helped to demonstrate just how vulnerable people are. Now even with paper records there's always the opportunity for that kind of intrusion. Witness the story I started with about the records blowing down the suburban Maryland street. But the ease of such invasions of privacy and their potential scope are increased enormously when records are computerized. Records can be scanned remotely. You don't have to be in the medical record room where it's easy to catch you while you're doing it. It is easy to search by patient name, diagnosis, age, or for particularly embarrassing diagnostic data. There was a well known incident that occurred in Florida where a man was reported in a bar with a computer diskette in his pocket, one of those three and a half inch diskettes, bragging to his friends that before they went out on their next date they ought to check with him because he had the list of everybody in Florida who was HIV positive. And in fact, he did. The Department of Public Health kept that record. He worked for that agency. He somehow got access to that list and ultimately it came to light. He was picked up and the information was confiscated. But it does, again, illustrate just how easy it is to pass information around in this new information age. And you can imagine pedophiles or rapists or other offenders making great and illegitimate and unfortunate use of access to databases of that sort.

Moreover, as record systems are linked together, the risk multiplies. It is not just one hospital now. Now we have hospital systems. HMO's cover millions of patients often across many states. And if you look at national, for example, in mental health care, behavioral health management companies, the managed care organizations that control essentially the delivery of mental healthcare in this country today, the largest of them delivers them care or controls the delivery of care to more than 60 million people at this point. And although their data systems are not completely linked and integrated yet, you can certainly see the potential for that to happen.

Moreover, in addition to these actual risks from breach of confidentiality, there's also the perception issue. When patients learn of computerization, they may become reluctant to reveal important information to us, information that we rely on to make accurate diagnoses and provide appropriate treatment. And not just in systems that are already computerized. The lack of trust that may result can generalize to all medical and psychiatric care systems.

Just last month I picked up another article from the Washington Post and interestingly--I mean, if you're interested in this area, the leading sources of information are our daily newspapers. The scholarly literature has not caught up yet in any systematic way and there is very little careful empirical study of risk to confidentiality. It is the Washington Post, New York Times, your local paper as well that are more likely to carry these kinds of stories. Let me just read to you the lead of a story in last month's Washington Post. The headline is, "Long Reach into Patients' Privacy; New uses of data illustrate potential benefits and hazards." Two months ago, a 42-year-old woman named Mimi walked into her pharmacy in Fairfield, Connecticut to pick up a refill of the medicine she had taken for years for her migraine headaches and stormed out with a headache larger than she'd ever imagined. She could not get a refill, her druggist told her, because a company that manages pharmacy benefits for her managed care company had decided she was taking too many kinds of medication. Mimi, who herself is a mother and part-time psychotherapist called two of her doctors, only to discover that the company had written a letter to each of them listing every medication she was taking for asthma, joint pain and allergies, along with the migraines. And she responded in the following way. And she said, "I felt violated because the company did all this behind my back. It made--it looked like they were insinuating I was a drug addict." And the article goes on to talk about the impact that that experience had on her trust in the security of her medical record data. I suspect most of us do not know sitting here today whether the companies that insure us or manage our care or the pharmacies at which we have our prescriptions filled are part of these extensive medical information databases and whether there is somewhere a file that sits on each of us with all our medications, all of our diagnoses and all of the information about the care we're getting. And the evidence suggests that that is true to a much greater extent than any of us imagine at the moment.

Well, what can we do about it? What should we do about it? I don't think we can stop computerization of medical records in general, and I am not sure we should. The pressures for cost saving and the other advantages of computerization are really too strong. But we do need to decide how we deal with computerization and whether there are some kinds of information that we ought not to computerize or ought to protect in special ways. The question that Harvard Community Healthcare didn't ask itself before it put all its records online. It may be, for example, and I would maintain as a psychiatrist that in fact is that psychiatric records, per se, should be dealt with differently. Now not all of my colleagues in psychiatry even would agree with that. Many psychiatrists value the integration of psychiatric and general medical care and fear that treating psychiatric records differently will impede that process and by segregating psychiatric information off on one side will reduce the quality of that care.

Now others point out that compromising information can be found throughout a patient's medical record. Are you HIV positive? Did you ever have a sexually transmitted disease? Have you a history of substance abuse? Were you once suspected of child abuse when you brought your son or daughter into an emergency room? I can tell you from experience our oldest was one of these kids who was breaking a bone every other month. And after the fourth or fifth broken digit, toe, arm, or whatever, we got very unusual looks from the emergency room personnel when we brought him in for the next one. Well, is that in his medical record as well? And some of my colleagues are perhaps appropriately concerned that singling out psychiatry or any other area of medicine for special treatment will lead to greater stigmatization of that area and of those patients.

Granting the legitimacy of those arguments, I do think nonetheless that psychiatric records still need special protection as other sorts of information in those records may as well. There are, after all, some kinds of information that are still more likely to contain sensitive information, more likely to be stigmatizing, and more likely to dissuade patients from seeking care if they think that information is insecure. And I understand that here at the University of Michigan you have taken the step of segregating, partitioning, if you will, your psychiatric record information from the general medical record. And the system that has been described to me seems to me to make a great deal of sense. We are now just moving into computerized records at the University of Massachusetts and are doing the same thing. I would actually like to move to a much more sophisticated system than our technical people tell me is possible at the moment. Rather than having one firewall and all the psychiatric information on one side and the general medical information on the other, with anybody in psychiatry able to access any of the psychiatric records, I would like to create special access to each patient's record to those people who need to see that record. And the rest of our seventy-odd psychiatrists who have no business looking at that record need not have access to it. I think that the potential for doing that exists. Technically it is certainly feasible. We just need the software written and these programs that are being developed on a commercial basis constructed to take those kinds of needs into account.

Moreover, I would suggest that there are other things we should be doing as we moved into this world of computerized medical records. I think patients should always be told whether or not computerized records are being used. There are some patients who may elect to seek care elsewhere. And that seems to me to be their right and they cannot exercise that right unless they have knowledge of the situation. They may also elect not to reveal certain information. Now the medical profession tends to react adversely to that prospect. We have a belief imbued in our medical training that we have the right to know everything about our patients and patients who withhold information from us are bad patients in some way. But I doubt if there are any of us in this room, and I will include myself here, who have ever fully disclosed everything we could to our caregivers. I think we all have used discretion at times regarding what we have or have not communicated. And I think if we do so knowledgably, that is appropriate. That is, if we are willing to trade off some measure of care for a greater degree of confidentiality, that seems to me to be a reasonable option for us to have.

Some organizations have been willing to give patients the right to opt out of computerization and retain paper records for certain purposes. And if systems can be constructed that way, again, at least at this point where we don't yet have the kinds of computerized record system safe guards that we might want to have, that is not an unreasonable option either.

We need to develop more experience with partition of sensitive information and I suggest to you there are a number of ways we could do it. We could partition records based on the nature of the caregiver, psychiatrist versus not, the nature of the treatment, substance abuse treatment versus other, the nature of the disorder, HIV positive versus other, the type of information, suspected child abuse versus something else. Technology in this case should actually help us in achieving that kind of fine grain differentiation among various kinds of medical record information. We don't know yet which of these approaches will work best and we are at the stage where experimentation is needed. And clearly appropriate security measures need to be developed. We were talking yesterday, when we were talking about the Michigan system about audit trails, which I understand are built into the system, you can track everybody who has ever had access to the record. And that is fine but if you talk to technical people, what they will tell you is audit trails only take you so far. Somebody has to look at the audit trail to determine whether unauthorized access has occurred, and if you have got 100,000 records in your system, that's hard to do on a systematic basis. Moreover, the person who is looking has to know whether or not the access that is documented there was appropriate or inappropriate and that implies a fair degree of knowledge about who should or should not be going into any particular record. It is not as simple a solution as it sounds. It may be something of a deterrent to unauthorized access, but it is not a great system for people who are dipping into records without proper authorization.

Above all, I would suggest to you that as a profession we need to be vigilant about these developments. The software exists for medical record computerization. It is being marketed aggressively. HMO's, clinics, hospital systems, even individual practices in the long run will have a strong incentive to move over to computerized records and if we do not pay attention to the implications for privacy, we will wake up one morning and discover that neither our patients' privacy nor our own privacy when we are patients is well protected.

The next level of concern here after computerization of records at an individual location is the assignment of these record systems into regional or national databanks. What would something like this look like? They would be regional or national depositories of data concerning all medical services and presumably would be linked with individual identifiers so that the information that you generate when you see your OB/GYN for your annual pap smear could be linked with the information that comes from your primary care physician who treats your allergies and asthma.

Interestingly, the Clinton plan, that's almost five years ago now, proposed required reporting of every medical contact that took place, whether or not you paid for it out of pocket or it was covered by the

Threats to Confidentiality and Privacy in Medicine, 1999

Clinton plan insurance component. Even if you didn't want that information to be tracked, you had no option to withhold the information from the system. It's an astonishing provision in many ways. It's the ultimate big brother as far as medical records are concerned, but to my amazement, the entire aggressive campaign against the Clinton health plan--Harry and Louise on TV discussing how the future would be bleak if the Clinton plan were adopted never mentioned the issue of medical records privacy. This was a non-issue although it was there in broad daylight and certainly played no role in the defeat of the Clinton plan.

With the defeat of that plan, the impetus for the creation of these databanks ebbed just slightly but the forces--the proponents of it have regrouped and are moving forward again. Again, there is a similar coalition, software, hardware data management companies, this time supported by managed care companies and researchers who literally drool over the prospect of access to such data, huge banks of data involving medical care of all of us around the country. Think of the outcomes research. Think of the epidemiological studies that could be done.

But this really is big brother. For data to be useful, they'll have to be linked individually over time. Someone will have the key. There literally will be no place to hide. And if reporting is mandatory, even patients who pay out of pocket in an effort to protect their privacy will not be able to do so.

Where do things stand now? Well, this is sort of interesting and in a way illustrates the stealth way in which these issues have moved forward in Washington. Several years ago you will recall that a measure passed Congress called the Kennedy-Kassebaum Health Insurance Portability and Accountability Act, HIPAA for short. HIPAA was best known for providing some small measure of parody for psychiatric treatment and also for insuring the so-called portability of health care insurance, if you lost a job and were moving to a new job and it limited the use of pre-existing condition restrictions on health insurance provision. But buried in the Kennedy-Kassebaum bill was a measure provision dealing with so-called administrative simplification. Now I will tell you that although administrative simplification sounds a lot like motherhood and it is difficult to be against it, how many of us are for administrative complexity after all? In fact, it's a code word for computerization of medical record information. The administrative simplification provisions required within 18 months of adoption of the bill, which has long since passed, the secretary of HHS had to come up with standards for electronic transmission of information, including claims or in counter information, billing and payment information. It didn't require electronic transmission, but if electronic transmission were used and HMO's and insurers increasingly are looking for claims to be submitted by modem, they would all have to conform to a single standard.

Moreover, within 12 months of adoption, the secretary of HHS had to propose recommendations with regard to privacy to Congress, including how a national plan for a unique identifier system could be implemented. The unique identifier meant that each of us would be assigned a number as the lawyers in this debate say from sperm to worm that would be with us forever and would be the number under which all of our medical record information would be compiled. You could not escape scrutiny of your medical encounters.

Now just over a year ago, a year ago August when the national commission on Vital and Health Statistics started holding public hearings on this issue in Chicago, there was finally, although this had been enacted in law two years before that, a huge outcry regarding national unique identifiers. And a one year moratorium was passed in Congress on any further action and Vice President Gore on behalf of the administration announced that they were putting a hold on any further development. But there is no legal impediment at this point to further movement on unique identifiers and it has always struck me as unusual that so few people know about this issue. There are, after all, people in Montana who are scanning the skies looking for black helicopters sent by the United Nations as the lead force to take over the country for a one-world government who believe that there are signals on the back of all road traffic signs directing the United Nation troops where to go. And yet these people are oblivious to the real threats to individual privacy in this country such as the creation of a unique identifier system that would encompass all medical record information.

Well, why a unique identifier? Why uniform data transmission? Why should the government care why data is sent? Well, there is only one purpose in creating a unified standard and that is once it exists, data from different systems can be merged into national or large regional databanks. And since there will be little purpose to having such databanks unless all data are included, the provisions on electronic transmission may well become mandatory as they were in the Clinton proposal.

What should we in medicine be doing about this? Well, this is going to take a major effort if we are truly concerned. I am truly concerned about it. But it must be coupled with public education. There is a general tendency for people to be infatuated with computers and cyberspace and to see developments there as generally positive, or at least, irresistible. We need to convince people if we think that medical care will be harmed by such a threat to privacy that not everything that can be done with computers should be done. And I would suggest that as soon as an action like this is taken becomes general knowledge and the first leak occurs, we are going to see patients' medical information just dry up and people just simply are not going to reveal to their physicians anything they think might be embarrassing. And physicians are not going to put it in the medical records and therefore the utility of these records for tracking care or doing research will be vitiated as well.

Let me skip over in some regards the managed care company issues. You know what is going on there. Companies are demanding extraordinary access to actual medical records. They are not accepting summaries. We have no idea where these records go or what is done with either the physical record or the information once it lands in the managed care company's lap nor are there any regulations for the most part governing,

No Place to Hide:

certainly no national regulations governing what is done with that information and is a matter for legislative attention. But because I want to save some time for your questions and comments because you may well disagree with my concerns here, I want to tell you a little bit about the current legislative efforts that are going on in Washington.

For the last several years, essentially since the collapse of the Clinton plan in 1994, legislation has been introduced every year in every congress by a number of major players on medical records confidentiality. And they are usually labeled something like, "Patient Medical Confidentiality Rights Bill," or "Medical Record Confidentiality Act of 1999." In fact, what these bills often do--in fact, typically do is remove many of the protections of medical record confidentiality that have traditionally existed and they might better be called Medical Record Access Bill of 1999 because they are being written and promoted in an effort to increase and facilitate access by all kinds of people to medical record information. Let me give you some examples.

A typical bill of the numerous bills--there are about three in the House--I'm sorry, four in the House and three in the Senate right now is the Jeffords bills. Senator Jeffords is chair of the subcommittee of the Senate Labor, Health, and Pensions committee that has jurisdiction over this legislation. Senator Jeffords is from Vermont and is a moderate Republican. The Jeffords bill would do, among other things, the following. First it would remove effective patient control of medical record information. It would no longer be the case that patients would have to release information from their records or it could not be released. In fact, the bill would require employers' health plans and providers to obtain blanket releases at the time of enrollment to a health plan as a condition of entering the health plan which would allow disclosure to take place for purposes of treatment, payment, or health care operations.

Now, consider what some of these things mean. Treatment, right now you determine whether your medical record information is transferred from, for example, your psychiatrist to your primary care physician or to your dermatologist for that matter. And if you think your dermatologist needs to know that you are taking lithium because you are bipolar, which he or she might in order to give you good care for your rash, well then you authorize the release of that information. If you think it is irrelevant to the tinea that you have between your toes, then you might not want to release that information. Under the Jeffords bill and all of its Republican-sponsored colleagues in the Senate right now, you would no longer have that choice. Information that was deemed relevant to care would be available to all of your caregivers whether or not you authorized its disclosure.

And what about healthcare operations? Well, that is a very vaguely defined term that is included in all of the Republican bills. Remember Republicans are in the majority in both houses right now and so it is their legislation that gets the primary focus because it is most likely to move through Congress. They would allow information to be released for a wide variety of purposes that in some way relate to the functioning of the insurer, the managed care company or other entities that are responsible for providing or managing your benefits, for example, pharmaceutical benefit management companies. Now this raises the prospect again of an episode similar to what occurred on the east coast last year when patients began receiving letters in the mail urging them to change from one medication to another for the condition that they had. And some patients began wondering, "Well, how on earth does the pharmaceutical company that sent me this letter know what my condition is or what medication I'm taking?" It turned out that CVS, a large--I don't know if you have CVS out here. It's a large pharmacy chain up and down the east coast sold that information which it had in its computers. Now whenever you go into a chain pharmacy, there is a computer. They enter in all of your prescription information. Sometimes it is very convenient because they have your pharmacy benefit information there as well and they know what your co-pay is or whether it is free or whether you have to pay the full price. But that all goes into a data bank. And

CVS decided that it could mine those data and sold it to drug companies that were interested in persuading consumers--patient consumers that they do better with one drug rather than another. And the privacy issues were completely, completely neglected. Well, the outcry ensued. It was inevitable and CVS said, "Oh, we're sorry. We'll never do it again." But in fact, much of this congressional legislation would appear to permit such actions to be taken as a matter of course.

The Jeffords bill would also allow parents access to minors' records--all minors' records. No more saying to parents, "Look, if you want me to treat your son or daughter for their problems, I need to have some confidential relationship with them. We'll talk to you when it's appropriate, but basically you have to trust that I am going to be treating your son or daughter appropriately." Researchers would get almost unlimited access whether or not you wanted them to have it. And in the initial version the police, when the records were likely to contain relevant information regardless of state laws, controlling their access to that information could just ask for it. The latest version of the Jeffords bill now requires a warrant, but Senator Bennett's bill--Senator Bennett is a Republican from Utah, still has no warrant requirement and is, in fact, the bill that has been endorsed most strongly by the Association of American Medical Colleges because it most easily and most completely makes medical record information available for research purposes. And the AAMC, which in some respects should be representing us, has chosen to focus on one interest here which is the interest of researchers and getting access to data and completely neglected the interest of caregivers and patients in maintaining some control over that medical record information.

Moreover the Jeffords bill and all of the Republican measures, in fact, preempt all state laws on medical record privacy. The Jeffords bill preempts them going forward. The Bennett bill just preempts everything that exists right now.

Some of the bills in the House and Senate now are a little better than Jeffords. Some are a little worse. The best bills from a privacy perspective are the Democratic bills that echo each other that are submitted in the Senate by Senators Kennedy and Leahy and in the House by Markey and Condit. But there is no possibility that the Democratic bills will move in a Republican Congress.

I would suggest that if one looks at this from the viewpoint of a medical practitioner that there ought to be several principles that guide this legislation if we're going to have national legislation and that those principles are not hard to discern. If we want patients to come clean with us and tell us the information we need to make diagnoses and provide treatment, we ought to generally allow patients to control access and disclosure. And that has always been the case. Exceptions to that rule which need to exist in some circumstances should be very narrowly defined. Identifiable information should be released only when non-identifiable information is inadequate for the purpose, and this is something that the congressional bills completely fail to address. Somehow the legislators on Capitol Hill just don't get it that for many of these purposes you can use non-identifiable data. I've testified at three different Congressional hearings on this privacy legislation and it comes as news to the senators and representatives each time that that ought to be possible as a general rule.

When you need to release identifiable information, it should be the least amount of data needed to achieve the goal at hand. And states should be allowed to experiment with higher levels of protection. National legislation should be a floor on patient protection, not a ceiling. Given that technology is moving as rapidly as it is and how difficult and how long it takes to get legislation passed in Congress, we're much better off allowing the states some flexibility here so they can experiment with more rapid adaptations to changing circumstances.

Well, where do things stand right now? Because of the difficulty of dealing with these issues, Congress has been stalemated. And though they set themselves a deadline of August to complete work on a bill, they have not done so. The statute that they passed--actually, it is HIPAA again, the Health Insurance Portability and Accountability Act actually empowers the Department of Health and Human Services to set its own binding standards. HHS is now at work and unless Congress either passes a bill in the next couple of months, and there may be renewed pressure to do that because Congress would much rather do it itself than allow HHS to set the standards. But if Congress either doesn't pass a bill or extend the deadline, we will have new guidelines governing all medical record information in the country and it will be promulgated by HHS.

Now having met with Secretary Shalala and with the president's chief medical advisor, health advisor Chris Jennings, I can tell you that there is no greater sensitivity towards issues of medical record confidentiality at that level than there is in the Republican side of Congress. The focus is on cost. There is a belief in HHS, which after all oversees a large amount of federal entitlement dollars, that more availability of information will lead to greater potential for reducing costs by identifying patterns of expenditure that could be pressured to contract.

I would suggest, in closing that however you feel about these issues, we are at a time that will set the pattern for the next generation at least, century perhaps and maybe even millennium for how medical records are being dealt with. And it is too important for us all not to pay careful attention and to weigh in. And the next couple of months are likely to be a critical time for your senators, representatives, and even the president given that the executive branch is now at work on this to hear from you how you feel about these issues.

Integrity in Scientific Publications: Implications for Research, 2000

Catherine D. DeAngelis, M.D. Editor, Journal of the American Medical Association, and Professor of Pediatrics, Johns Hopkins University School of Medicine

THE CHANGING PROFESSION OF MEDICINE

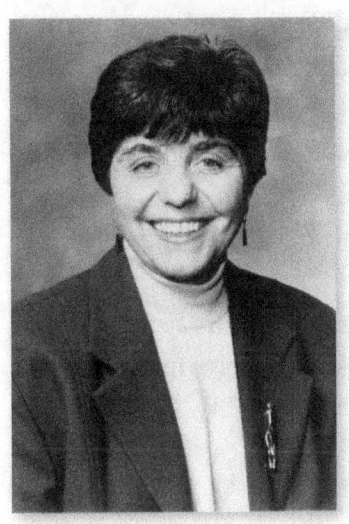

There were two guys on a train in Italy. The first guy turned to the second and asked, "Whatsa you name"

2nd Guy My name isa Giuseppi Pasquelini. Whatsa you name

1st Guy My name isa Giuseppi Pasquelini too. Where you from?

2nd Guy I'ma from Palermo. Where you from?

1st Guy Ima from Palermo, too. How you spell you name?

2nd Guy takes out a pen and paper and makes an "X" on it and asks, how you spella you name?

1st Guy takes out a gold pen and paper and makes 2 X's on it.

2nd Guy Hey, you Giuseppi Pasquelini, Ima Giuseppi Pasquelini, you froma Palermo and Ima from Palermo. How coma you get 2 X and I get only one X

Integrity in Scientific Publications:

1st Guy (pointing to the first X) Ahhh Ima Giuseppi Pasquelini (and pointed to the second X) Emma D.

Now I certainly am not making fun of my ancestors but the story makes an important point (in addition to 2 X's being better than one X). That point is that an "emma D" or M.D. signifies extra importance and privilege. In other words, people generally admire, respect, and trust the doctor (or physician) simply by virtue of someone being one. Now that extra respect, admiration and trust must be reciprocated with integrity and respect for the patient.

I used to wonder why "Primum non nocere"---first do no harm... rather than first do good is the basic tenet of Medicine. After way too many years of experience as a clinician, clinical scientist, educator, administrator, and editor, I realize the wisdom of this tenet. If physicians involved in patient care, either directly or indirectly, can honestly know at the end of their professional careers that indeed they were not involved in the deliberate harm of patients, they have been successful. Doing good is wonderful and can be accomplished if we follow the basic rule of curing when we can but caring always. Caring is essential but potential or actual curing can be fraught with danger for harm. This is what must be guarded against.

Medical investigators, authors, reviewers and editors have a special requirement to do no harm because their work can involve many patients beyond those for whom they accept direct responsibility. Published articles are read by many clinicians and they, in turn, care for many patients; hence the greater responsibility.

For example, many physicians, clinical investigators, and others put great emphasis on journals IF, that is the Impact Factor. I believe the far more important IF is the journal's Integrity Factor. One major necessity to insuring the integrity factor is to control conflicts of interests (COI). I say control, rather than eliminate, because some COIs are essentially inevitable and ubiquitous and are certainly nothing new. As far back as 1850 the Webster Dictionary defined COI's as, "Conflicts between the

Implications for Research, 2000

private interests and the official responsibilities of a person in a position of trust." The key point is that the individual involved is in a position of trust- - -that is, people trust that what the involved person says, writes or publishes, is the truth, at least so far as can be determined or written with cautions stated if any doubt or questions remain.

COIs may be perceived or real, potential or actual, inconsequential or harmful. Obviously, those that actually cause harm are the major problem. Investigators or authors can be involved in COIs for career advancement, peer recognition, competing research interests, competition for research grants, garnering high profile publications, intellectual biases or passions or (the most egregious) financial reasons Editors can be involved in COIs to improve the impact factor of their journal, increase subscriptions, eliminate or decrease hostility or harassment or increase financial profitability.

A financial COI is a paid affiliation or financial involvement (other than a grant earned through competition) with any entity that that has an interest in the subject or materials in a study. As is evident from many published medical articles, such COIs are increasing. According to pub med, the number of published articles on COI increased from a few through the late 1980's to over 500 over the past few years and continues to increase. There are many reasons for this increase. First of all, for-profit pharmaceutical and medical devise companies have placed more emphasis and resources on the business and marketing departments rather than the scientific and new product departments. This is evident by the decreasing number of new drugs in the pipeline. Second, the medical profession has had more emphasis placed on the business aspects of patient care. The intrusion of insurance companies and health maintenance organizations into the physician-patient relationship has had profound deleterious effects.

More physicians are now working for institutions or companies and are rewarded for seeing more patients in less time and generating more laboratories, radiological and other fees. The increase in malpractice suits, whether actual or perceived, has lead physicians to practice defensive medicine, that is ordering more tests and treating more possible or potential problems to decrease the likelihood of being sued. All these factors have created a somewhat cynical atmosphere among many physicians, some of whom are retiring early.

Another factor that has affected the practice of medicine is the desire for having a decent home and social life. The day of the private practitioner who was on call 24/7 or even taking call every second or third day and weekend is coming to an end. House calls are out of the question for many reasons as is caring for private patients in the hospital. Almost every hospital now employs hospitalists or residents to care for hospitalized patients and ER specialists to cover the emergency rooms, each for a specific number of hours.

Finally, the relative reimbursement to primary care physicians as compared to specialists has made it difficult if not impossible for graduating medical students to choose primary care as a career path. This is especially true when the increased burden of $100,000 or more in loans is considered. Nurse practitioners have taken on a great deal of primary care, but they are not trained to care for many of the problems seen by primary care physicians, especially those who care for the elderly and those with chronic illnesses. I say that as someone who is a strong proponent of nurse practitioners. However, they simply cannot provide the same level of care as physicians. Further, the aging population with so many patients living well into their 80's has made for a real problem to get proper care to all.

So where does this distressing scenario leave us? Well, in general, medicine is still a great and most noble of all professions. The medical profession is a vocation, a calling physicians have answered to care for those who are ill. There is simply no other way to view medicine without denigrating the profession. So we must remember this and consider that we have an MD and not an MDeity, and therefore cannot be expected to be treated like gods and that we cannot always cure. However the MD does provide us with all we need to care and many opportunities to care. That extra "X" I spoke about in the beginning of this talk provides us with a privilege that we must reciprocate by doing the best we can while not becoming conflicted or cynical and thereby professionally put our own interests above those of our patients. We cannot accept gifts from for profit organizations who provide them only as a means to get us to prescribe their more expensive drugs when other less expensive drugs work just as well or to order unnecessary tests to satisfy the business end of practice or to do all the other things that denigrate the trust patients put in us. In other words, we must first do no harm.

Ethical Considerations in Research on Human Subjects: A Time for Change... Again, 2001

Harold T. Shapiro, President Emeritus University of Michigan and Princeton University, Professor of Economics and International Affairs, Princeton University

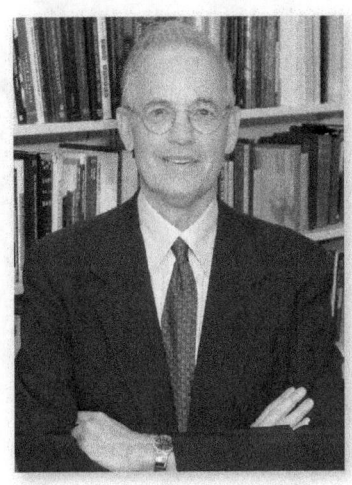

Research using human subjects will continue to play an important role as part of a great humanitarian effort to understand ourselves better and to relieve distress and disease.

To use human beings as subjects in medical experiments – or any type of research – is a special privilege which carries with it special ethical responsibilities

Preface

Let me begin by noting how delighted I am to be back at the University of Michigan Medical Center and especially to deliver the sixth annual Raymond Waggoner Lecture. Unfortunately, I was not a personal friend or close colleague of Dr. Waggoner, but I certainly knew a lot about him and the many contributions he made to the Department of Psychiatry, to the Medical School, and The University of Michigan. It is, therefore, an honor for me to have been awarded this

Ethical Considerations in Research on Human Subjects:

lectureship and in some very small way to connect my name to his and, even more indirectly, to the distinguished history of this Department and the University of Michigan Medical School.

Finally by way of prefatory remarks, I want to say a few words about the Medical Center. I have many friends here and I think often about many of them and all they have done and continue to do for the Medical Center and the University. At this particular moment, however, I recall especially those efforts to revitalize the medical center that began over two decades ago and continues to this day. As I think back on those initial struggles I am amazed and enormously gratified by what has been accomplished over this period through the leadership of the current faculty, staff, and administration of the Center and the University. All of us who care deeply about the University, about the welfare of patients and our ethical obligation to push forward the bio-medical frontier, have accumulated a significant debt to all levels of today's leadership in the Medical Center and the University. I hope you will consider my presence here this afternoon as a small down payment on my share of this obligation.

I. Introduction

This annual lectureship has as its focus ethics and values in medicine and in a few moments I will speak directly on one aspect of this rich, diverse and important area. Indeed, there are so many aspects of ethics and values in medicine that it is often difficult to locate the right balance among our various ethical obligations in particular circumstances. This is not because physicians, or other health care professionals cannot be bothered to struggle with moral issues, but because they operate within a highly contextualized and deeply uncertain environment where ethical behavior requires complex moral calculations/considerations. Moreover, at any moment in time there are often competing ethical demands that leave us with difficult, even tragic, moral choices. In addition, there are a lot of ethical issues in medical practice and biomedical research because these activities directly impact the interests of others. Moreover, since the ethical issues that do arise require practical implementation, one has to find ways to cross the chasm that often separates moral theories and ethical practices. Indeed, one of the chief burdens of my remarks this afternoon is that health care professionals engaged in human subjects research cannot escape the moral anxieties that characterize everyone that thinks deeply about behaving in an ethical fashion.

This is certainly the case for investigators involved in research using human subjects since few endeavors have the <u>potential</u> to present more strikingly the tension that can arise between individual and society interests than does medical research involving human subjects. The problems and moral choices you face are not simple ones and usually raise competing interests. It is understandable, for example, that as we strive to meet our ethical responsibilities to future generations of pushing forward the scientific and clinical frontier, that we may lose sight of other ethical imperatives or, more likely, simply not give them sufficient weight. In this latter respect I think one of the most important ethical lessons of the recent decades is that assigning relative weights to competing moral demands in human subject research is not a matter that can be left to one group, say, physicians, or policy makers, or religious leaders, or human subjects themselves. Rather it must result from a process of social negotiation where all those whose interests are affected have some standing in the deliberations.

This is especially the case now because commercial interests have become deeply embedded in all aspects of biomedical science. Indeed, biomedical science has become a vast commercial activity. This may or may not be a good development, but for many researchers it certainly generates a new and expanded portfolio of actual or perceived conflicts of interest. As a result, the public no longer considers individual self-regulation adequate. In fact, however, it was always difficult to imagine that given the multitude of pressures that physician/scientists work

Ethical Considerations in Research on Human Subjects:

under that they could adequately address the ethical implications of their own work. In my view it has always been unreasonable and unfair to leave all the ethical decision making to the moral sensitivities of the individual medical investigator. Given the various pressures investigators work under, we protect neither subject nor investigator by having a system devoid of meaningful third party oversight.

The ethical considerations involved in medical experiments that involve human subjects is hardly a new topic, but I have chosen to speak about it because I think it is time for some important changes in attitude and regulation/oversight in this arena. I will begin by reminding ourselves of the historical legacy we share in this area (including the status quo) and move on to suggest what changes in attitude, ethical commitments, and principles are necessary to serve more fully, both the advancement of medical science and the protection of human subjects. It is my own strong belief that good ethics can not only mean good science, but is essential to sustain the strong public support upon which all aspects of the bio-medical enterprise are dependent. My emphasis will be on the beginning and the "end" of the ongoing narrative connecting investigators and human subjects, namely, the historical legacy we share in this arena and what I propose for the future.

By way of introduction I want to suggest that there are four key issues relating to our ethical responsibilities to human subjects participating in medical experimentation that arise over and over again. The first is how to most effectively balance the interests of the human subject and those of science and future patients. The second is whether and in what manner the conduct of the investigator should be monitored and/or controlled by third parties. The third is what special arrangements are justified for what may be considered vulnerable populations. Finally there is the issue of how one insures that the experiment is well designed scientifically. This latter concern is one that relates to all research, but it has very special moral salience when human subjects are involved. In my view all the various controversies in the area of medical experiments using human subjects swirl around attempts to deal with some combination of these four issues. The current regulations, however inadequate and unloved, are an attempt to address these questions in a manner that will protect both investigator and subject. Let me now sketch the general contours of our historical legacy on these matters.

II. The Historical Legacy

Although formal medical experiments were either rare or nonexistent in the ancient or medieval world, the historical record does contain some evidence of using slaves, criminals (not quite persons in the moral sense), or even patients for this purpose. By the eighteenth century, however, there are numerous recorded incidents or orphans and/or slaves being used as "human guinea pigs." The term "human guinea pig" was coined somewhat later by George Bernard Shaw, but the use of these particular populations did reflect our lack of full respect for them and our failure to see them as worthy of full moral respect. In one of the most famous clinical trials in this period, however, we see a rather different approach when Edward Jenner vaccinated both his son and another healthy child with cowpox. Even as late as the eighteenth century, however, formal medical experiments were still few in number and, thus, when Thomas Percival published his justly famous "Medical Ethics" in 1803 he has very little to say regarding medical experiments using human subjects.

However, when Claude Bernard, the French physiologist, published his "Introduction to the Study of Experimental Medicine" a half-century later, he was already sensitive to some of the ethical issues involved. He seemed to have believed that since Christian morality required one not to harm their neighbor, medical investigators would, as an ethical matter, need to restrict their pool of human subjects to those that might benefit from the experimental intervention. On the other hand, he and others at the time had no problem doing medical experiments on condemned criminals since, the argument went, no additional harm could come to

Ethical Considerations in Research on Human Subjects:

them. Earlier William Beaumont a self-described "humble inquirer after truth" had done a whole series of experiments on one Alexsis St. Martin who was bound to Beaumont by a formal indenture. It was not until the end of the nineteenth century, however, that the healthy adult volunteer became an important participant in medical experiments. One of the first of these experiments was the justly famous experiments headed by Walter Reed dealing with the origin of yellow fever.

Whatever the ethical problems may have been during these earlier periods, the rise in experimental medical science that began in earnest in the nineteenth century has transformed both medical practice and medical science. Indeed, one must conclude that the resulting developments in our understanding of human biology, disease and the more effective clinical modalities that have resulted must be considered both an enormous scientific accomplishment and a significant humanitarian achievement. In the last two centuries we have witnessed extraordinary declines in mortality due, not only to better nutrition and improved economic circumstances, but to a combination of public health measures and a large number of new clinical modalities that have enabled us to overcome what previously were often fatal conditions.

Nevertheless, the historical record also reveals that in the general enthusiasm to develop new and more effective clinical modalities some investigators, with or without consent, deliberately infected human subjects, often drawn from what today we would call vulnerable groups, to test various theories. The record shows that as the need for medical experiments grew, many physicians and others treated institutionalized infants, dying patients, and mentally impaired individuals as not quite persons in the moral sense. Moreover, indigent patients in hospitals were often treated in a similar fashion. Indeed, during the last half of the nineteenth century indigent patients and their advocates became increasingly concerned that they were often the unwitting subjects of medical experiments, and the objects of unwanted dissection after death.

Clearly these "vulnerable" individuals were thought of as not quite eligible for the moral consideration we would feel obliged to extend to those who were, in our judgment, full persons in the moral sense. They were, our practices suggested, not entitled to the same rights and respect that others enjoyed. While some of these experiments produced great benefits for succeeding generations and society as a whole, they often involved overlooking the rights and welfare of the human subjects involved.

These matters did not go unnoticed by the medical profession. Ever since the rise in experimental medical science in the latter half of the nineteenth century, some members of the medical profession were quite aware of these tensions and of the variety of ethical issues raised by the use of human beings in medical experiments. William Osler, for example, suggested that one way to mediate this tension was to insist that animal experimentation be carried out first and that patients should only be involved if a direct benefit to them was likely to follow. Of particular concern to Osler and many other physicians was the preservation of what he termed "the sacred cord which binds physician to patient." With respect to healthy subjects, Osler, and many others, thought that some sort of consent should be the key requirement.

Given the long history of medicine, and the fact that doctors have always experimented in the treatment of their patients, it may seem surprising to some that the moral tension, or uncertainty regarding whose interests were being served, as between the investigator and subject has come to the fore only relatively recently. The "late" arrival of this issue is, of course, the result of two principal factors. The first is the relatively recent rise of what we would recognize as scientific medicine, and therefore, the whole issue of medical research ethics. The second set of factors, however, is less well appreciated, and I want to take a few moments to focus on it.

These are the new cultural commitments associated with the rise of democratic and pluralistic liberal societies. Most importantly the values underlying the development of these liberal societies brought renewed emphasis and commitment to notions of individual freedom, responsibility, and autonomy. Moreover, these very same cultural commitments released the latent talents of many individuals to try out a wide variety of experiments, not only in science, but with all of society's institutions. That is, the same forces that were responsible for directing so much human creativity and effort towards scientific activity also caused us to refine our notions regarding the integrity, autonomy, and value of each individual, and our ethical responsibilities to every individual whose interests are significantly impacted by our actions. Perhaps it should come as no surprise, therefore, that sooner or later the demands of science would come into conflict or tension with our evolving moral sensibilities.

In any case, it is important to remember, therefore, that the two principal cultural commitments of modern times, namely, the active pursuit of our mastery over nature – now including human nature – and the construction of a cultural framework that places a high value on accommodating the multiplicity of individual interests that naturally arise from the wide diversity of individual circumstances, beliefs, and historical contexts, can come into tension with each other. That is, these two great commitments of modern times can, in some circumstances, become competing interests. Unfortunately, medical experiments using human subjects are one example where such a tension may arise, since any scientific activity, no matter how worthy, that undermines the dignity of individuals or devalues them as autonomous moral agents, now creates what one may call a cultural contraction.

We should, however, not despair. There is nothing very unusual about such a cultural contradiction. Often we find ourselves in situations in which there is no way of acting that can satisfy all the ethical requirements to which we are committed. Existing realities often force hard, even tragic, moral choices. Moreover, in a morally pluralistic society such as ours, there are bound to be ethical conflicts that are not due to such unworthy characteristics as selfishness, prejudice, ignorance, or poor reasoning. In such circumstances our best strategies are to acknowledge the difficulty and to devise plans that enable us to minimize the negative impact on the interests of others of our inability to meet all of our ethical responsibilities. Indeed, existing regulations governing research using human subjects, however bothersome, irksome, and bureaucratic they may seem, need to be understood also as an attempt to manage just such a complex ethical situation.

For reasons that are perhaps understandable, during the nineteenth and first half of the twentieth century reconciling the needs and rights of patients and other human subjects with the growing demands of worthy medical research was not easily accomplished. In particular, consent was a complicated, murky, and often ambiguous feature of medical experimentation until quite recently. Indeed, it is quite understandable given the clinical environment during the late-nineteenth and early twentieth centuries that many well-motivated physicians/investigators saw little wrong with direct or indirect coercion to gain some form of consent. In particular, since benevolent deception and nondisclosure was the clinical norm it was almost "natural" to carry this attitude over to the issue of consent to serve as a subject in a medical experiment. In this respect it is useful to recall that Thomas Percival's 1803 work on medical ethics, which remained very influential through the first half of the twentieth century, argued that a patient's right to the truth could be "suspended and even annihilated" in certain circumstances.

Nevertheless, the apparent lack of sympathy for experimental subjects and the clinical detachment with which physicians described experiments on human beings remained a recurrent theme of the debate through at least the middle of the twentieth century. Many of those concerned with the abuse of human subjects continued to associate medical experimentation with the excessive claims of investigators, reckless innovation, quackery and, most importantly, as a new threat to the moral order.

Ethical Considerations in Research on Human Subjects:

The particular focus of the critics of medical experimentation at that time was on what they believed to be the dubious ethical acceptability of non-therapeutic experiments and on their insistence on the ethical necessity of the written consent of the subjects. The debate, however, often became polemical with groups concerned with animal rights warning over and over again that what we allow today regarding the use of non-human animals in scientific experiments we will allow tomorrow with respect to humans. Indeed, term "human guinea pig" was introduced to make clear the notion that experiments involving the mistreatment of non-human animals was sure to be followed by experiments involving the mistreatment of humans.

For the leaders of the medical profession as a whole, however, especially the elite university-based investigators, any interference with the use of animals for research and teaching threatened the therapeutic promises of scientific medicine. Moreover, on the legislative front, legislators were apparently convinced that any regulation would retard medical progress and inhibit the development of badly needed new clinical modalities. As far as I can tell outside of certain tabloids and the interest of animal rights groups there was little public concern about the entire issue. Both the public and the Congress perceived little difference between the physician's moral responsibilities when acting as an investigator or when fulfilling their role as a clinician. No one wished to regulate medical practice, and there seemed to be little distinction in most people's minds between the need for oversight in research and the need for such oversight in clinical practice.

As a result, clinical investigators lacked any formal guidelines until the 1940s when the AMA amended their professional codes to require (in a rather vague way) voluntary consent of the subject and prior animal testing. There were, however, no means of oversight or enforcement suggested. Paradoxically, it was Germany (in 1900) that first developed a code of ethics for research protocols that involved experimenting on human subjects. The general theme of this early code was to restrict

A Time for Change... Again, 2001

the pool of human subjects to competent adults who could give fully informed consent. At the same time I must note that there were continuing reports of abuses in Germany through the first three decades of the twentieth century, and new regulations had to be issued in 1931!

Despite the ethical lapses that characterized certain medical experiments during the first five decades of the twentieth century, it did become generally accepted that one should try to avoid unnecessary risks and that voluntary participation was a preferred feature of participation in research protocols. Unfortunately little attention was paid to this latter issue in the case of vulnerable subjects, and oversight responsibilities were left solely to the moral integrity of the investigator and his/her moral discretion in the implementation of whatever informal guidelines existed.

During World War II, any growing qualms about the inappropriate use of vulnerable populations gave way to patriotic constructions of ethical priorities. Indeed, the lessons that medical researchers may have learned during this period was that ends certainly did justify the means. Abstract moral issues like consent were superseded by a genuine sense of urgency to find clinical modalities needed by the armed forces.

In the two decades that followed World War II and preceded Henry Beecher's exposé of ethical lapses within the American medical research establishment there was an enormous expansion of human experimentation in medical research, but the broad attitudes towards the ethical imperatives faced by clinical investigators remained basically unchanged despite the cessation of hostilities. In short, the two key principles of consent and voluntary informed participation were often disregarded.

Even as the National Institute of Health (NIH) began its enormous expansion, the Clinical Center did little to inform patients to be alert to, for example, the investigator's possible conflicts of interest or to question the researcher closely about the protocol. Instead, they invoked or relied upon the ethos of the traditional doctor/patient relationship and essentially asked human subjects to trust the doctor who was the one most likely to be able to balance the costs and benefits of a particular

Ethical Considerations in Research on Human Subjects:

protocol. As a result, the Clinical Center set neither formal requirements to protect human subjects nor clear standards for investigators to follow in their protocols.

Further, as the money flowed out of the NIH into the nation's hospitals and laboratories, little attention was paid to the rights and welfare of the human research subjects. While investigators were more and more conscious of their ethical responsibilities to subjects, it was the wisdom and beneficence of physicians that continued to be relied on. In fact many researchers demonstrated little interest in the ethics of research during this period. Research ethics was considered, perhaps, an unnecessary obstacle to progress, and many investigators during these early decades following World War II let themselves slide into nontherapeutic experiments without any form of consent.

In retrospect, it is somewhat surprising that these attitudes persisted despite the Nuremberg trials and the behavior tolerated in many wartime experiments in the U.S. In fact, neither the horrors described at the Nuremberg trial of the infamous Nazi doctors, nor the ethical principles that emerged from it (i.e., the Nuremberg Code) had a significant impact on the American research establishment. The reaction seemed to be that only Nazis needed such regulation and in any case the real problem was the Government (in this case the Nazi government) which had interfered with the medical research agenda. Ironically, only the Department of Defense made the Nuremberg Code the ruling policy for medical experiments using human subjects in the area of atomic, biological, and/or chemical warfare. The problem was that the policy was classified as "Top Secret" and hardly anyone had access to it or knowledge of it. To most Americans, however, Nuremberg addressed madness, not medicine. Indeed, as late as the 1960s and even after the Thalidomide controversy there was still very little sentiment in Congress to adopt any regulations for the protection of human subjects.

As I noted above, Congress seemed incapable of differentiating either experimentation from therapy or investigators from physicians. To

A Time for Change... Again, 2001

put the matter another way, lawmakers seemed unable to distinguish subjects from patients, or the examining room from the laboratory. In essence, the ethos of the examining room was extended to the laboratory and the trust extended to the physician as healer extended to the physician as investigator. As a result the understandable wish to avoid regulating clinical practice led to a great reluctance to regulate in any way experiments using human subjects. Therefore, investigators ran their protocols free of external ethical oversight. The autonomy they enjoyed in conducting human experiments was limited only by their individual consciences which, as it turned out, was not always sufficient to avoid serious ethical lapses.

All this began to change in the mid-1960s with, perhaps, the publication of Henry Beecher's article in the New England Journal of Medicine. The ethical lapses that were documented, there and subsequently elsewhere, drew our attention to what should have been the quite obvious tension that could arise within clinical trials between the general good and the rights and welfare of the individual subject between the role of the physician as "healer" and the role of the physician as investigator.

In my judgment, the various revelations regarding abuse of human subjects that began to receive renewed attention in the mid-sixties might have had limited impact on behavior if so much authority and influence with respect to medical research were not concentrated in the NIH and the FDA, organizations that were very sensitive to congressional pressures and public opinion. The most important change in attitude that took place at that time was the public acknowledgement that an inherent conflict of interest arose in the interaction of the investigator and the subject. It became clear that the bedrock principle of medical ethics – that the physician or other health care professional acted only to promote the well being of the patient – did not necessarily hold in the context of research protocols. Instead, and inherent conflict of interest might be expected to cloud the ethical judgment of even very thoughtful investigators.

Ethical Considerations in Research on Human Subjects:

As a result of both this enhanced sensitivity and continued revelations of ethical lapses, two similar but distinct systems of decentralized oversight were established. One was established by the FDA (for protocols supporting a submission to the FDA) and one by the NIH (for protocols they sponsored). Both of these systems mandated both voluntary informed consent and independent review to ensure a balance of risks and benefits.

From the mid-sixties onward, therefore, the idea that human subject protection required oversight by a disinterested party gradually replaced our complete dependence on the conflicted moral sensibilities of investigators and their staff. Progress in this area, however, proceeded in stutter-step fashion. It took the work of the National Commission for the Protection of Human Subjects of Biomedical and Behavioral Research (referred to as the National Commission), which only began its work in 1974, and the subsequent President's Commission for the Study of Ethical Problems in Medicine and Biomedical and Behavioral Research (referred to as the President's Commission), appointed in 1974, to construct a coherent, if limited, framework for the protection of human subjects.

The National Commission produced The Belmont Report which articulated the underlying set of principles to support a system of oversight in this arena and a focus on the two key protections needed, namely, informed consent and independent review of proposed protocols. It was the President's Commission, however, that produced the operational guidelines that came to form the basis of the Common Rule (which now governs almost all federally-sponsored human subject research) and the FDA regulations and gave much overdue attention to the protection of vulnerable groups. I should note, however, that it took almost ten years to get the Common Rule adopted by the key federal agencies although the NIH and the FDA moved considerably faster. Thus, it took over four decades from the Nuremberg trials to the effective adoption of a system of oversight and review that attempted to meet the challenge of both protecting human subjects and supporting the continued advancement of medical science.

III. Looking Ahead

I do not want to spend anytime this afternoon outlining the detailed regulations that now govern human subject research. They are well summarized in the Common Rule, its various subsections and the analogous regulations of the FDA. While these regulations may not be loved, they are relatively well known by both IRB members and the community of investigators. Whether successful or not, they are intended to help us all avoid ethically unacceptable research by providing for informed consent and independent review of the balance of costs and benefits. They require that both prospective subjects and a committee of independent peers to conclude that the risks involved are appropriate in view of the potential benefits and provide special protection for vulnerable groups. Moreover, the system is decentralized in the sense that each community of investigators establishes a mechanism to meet the requirements of the Common Rule and/or of the analogous FDA regulations. What, therefore, are the limitations of the current regulations, and why is it time to modify them once again? Let me now turn my attention to those shortcomings that must be addressed if we are to sustain the effectiveness and credibility of the systems.

First, the current system has inadequate coverage in the sense that all human subjects do not fall under the protection of either the Common Rule or the FDA regulations. If neither federal funds nor FDA requirements are involved, there is no system of oversight at all. This leaves an unknown number of investigators and subjects unprotected.

Second, given the vast enterprise that clinical research has become, both IRBs and those involved in system oversight are too overburdened to fulfill their role effectively. Moreover, the typical response to this heavy and under-appreciated workload has been to focus on fulfilling the various bureaucratic requirements rather than on the substantive requirements of their oversight responsibilities. In many ways this is an iatrogenic or self-inflicted problem since nothing prevents an individual institution, or the federal government, from providing greater support for IRBs and those charged with overall system oversight. Simply put, our system of decentralized review is seriously under-resources. No one should be surprised that ethical lapses, even at the most distinguished centers of medical research, continue to occur. Until all partners in the medical research enterprise devote more resources to this effort, no human subject can be assured of appropriate protection. In the long run, failure to address this issue will begin to undermine public support for the entire enterprise.

Third, the critical process of informed consent has become a rather legalistic document-oriented event rather than a serious process of sustaining a meaningful level of understanding between the human subject and the investigating team.

Fourth, even those areas that are covered by existing regulations, there are no single uniform set of requirements or a single source of authoritative guidance to turn to.

Fifth, the current system is so difficult to change that it is unable to adapt to the changing realities of medical science. For example, it deals in a very cumbersome and inefficient way with the increasingly important multicenter trials.

Sixth, the current system ignores the fact that the integrity of a decentralized system depends on the education and training of all those involved on the research enterprise at the local level. Nothing can substitute for the enhanced ethical sensitivity of all those participating in human subject research from the most senior investigator to all other members of the research team. They must not only have a working knowledge of the oversight system, but a clear understanding of the source of their own ethical responsibilities and when they should look for additional guidance. It is my view that no one should become part of a research team unless they have been trained and certified, as appropriate to their

A Time for Change... Again, 2001

responsibilities, in these areas. Such training is not difficult, and both training and certification could easily be made available on the Web.

Seventh, there ought to be a system of compensation for those human subjects that are injured as a result of their participation. While this principle is pretty straightforward, there are many practical difficulties in implementing such a proposal. It is often very difficult to determine if an injury is research-related, and it is not obvious how one should fairly finance such a system. Perhaps compensation could be financed in a manner similar to Federal Deposit Insurance.

Eighth, the entire system and process needs to be more publicly accountable, especially at the local level. There are a number of ways to achieve this. Let me suggest a few. The number of "outside" members of the IRB could be increased. When particular protocols are being considered, especially if they involve more than minimal risk, mechanisms to consult with members of the group most directly impacted should be considered. Such consultations might even improve the experimental design. Alternatively, each IRB could produce a publicly available annual report that described the general nature of its efforts and highlighted the most "interesting," or even the most problematic protocols. Such a report could even provide information on the protocols that were not approved. A different approach to accountability would be to install an audit system of some type that annually would examine a sample of protocols to determine if all appropriate steps had been followed both in the approval and implementation process. I have always thought that a good system of audit could substitute for the constantly increasing number of bureaucratic requirements. Moreover, it would highlight our often overlooked responsibility to monitor the implementation of protocols not just their initiation.

Ninth, we need to reconsider our notions of what we consider vulnerable populations. Although vulnerable individuals need additional protection in research, they should not be arbitrarily excluded from research alone. Generally speaking we consider vulnerable people as those more open to harm (e.g., children), or more subject to coercion (e.g.,

Ethical Considerations in Research on Human Subjects:

institutionalized persons). It is important to understand that it is not their group designation that exposes them to injury or coercion, but rather their situation that can be exploited by ethically unacceptable research. I believe our approach in this arena should not be either to exploit these groups, or to exclude them as subjects, but to search for research designs where members of these groups are not unnecessarily harmed.

Tenth, we need some help from the medical profession to understand somewhat better how we should characterize that "gray zone" that exists somewhere between clinical practice and medical research where innovative and untested medical innovations are being tried out. If a formal research protocol is not involved current regulations do not apply. Further, even if a formal research protocol is involved, if federal funds and/or the FDA are not involved, current regulations do not apply. Nevertheless, in this "gray area" it is uncontested that we have ethical obligations to those patients and/or human subjects that are participants. We need to understand better whether any third party oversight and/or new professional guidelines are needed in this area. We need more forthright discussion and/or guidance on this issue.

Whether or not all these changes are made it is essential that we find a way to provide a far more expeditious review path for a large number of protocols. In particular, we need to define a far more expeditious and less burdensome review path for those protocols that involve only minimal risk. In the same spirit we must find ways to relieve both investigators and IRBs from the review of trivial changes in protocols that are always necessary in the implementation stage of any research trial. To fail to do so simply works to undermine the credibility of the current system which spends too much effort fulfilling bureaucratic requirements and too little providing meaningful protection of human subjects. Simply put, we need to do a better job of matching the level of protection and review to the level of risk involved.

The ability to do this, however, depends on the training of the investigator and those with authority to expedite or exempt a particular study

A Time for Change... Again, 2001

from review. Education that helps researchers to anticipate and work towards minimizing risks can also greatly expedite the review process. Only by focusing our attention on those studies with a meaningful level of risk or where vulnerable populations are involved can we be assured that the system will deliver substantive protections where needed and not relapse into a bureaucratic maze. It would be much easier to accomplish this badly needed reform, however, if the spirit of the suggestions I have made particularly those dealing with education, certification, and audit were adopted.

No one is more enthusiastic than I am of the continuing potential of medical science, or more appreciative than I am of the great advances announced almost daily regarding advances on the scientific frontier, or more optimistic about what will be accomplished in the years ahead. However, I think it is in the self interest of all those working on this great endeavor to demonstrate to all how much we value and respect those individuals who agree to serve as human subjects especially in risky experiments. Historically, when doctors themselves agreed to serve in this capacity they were rightly thought of as heroes. Now, therefore, we should return the favor by treating those who agree to participate in our experiments as both heroes and partners in an exciting and morally rewarding joint enterprise.

Epilogue[1]

A great deal has changed in the two decades that have passed since I had the honor of presenting the sixth Raymond W. Waggoner lecture in 2001. Even then twenty years of experience with the Common Rule and the dramatically evolving scientific frontier generated a critical need to re-examine and adapt our approach to human subject protection. Indeed I concluded my 2001 lecture with some modest suggestions regarding needed changes and a more dynamically adaptive system. Since then developments on the scientific frontier both in bio-medicine

---

1 Added December 2011

and information technologies have not only impacted research design in biomedicine but in large swaths of the humanities and social sciences. Moreover the relationship between biomedicine and the social sciences and humanities has deepened and has been aided not only by intriguing developments in the humanities and social sciences themselves, but by the rapid development of particular technologies and suffused in particular by the growing importance of a wide spectrum of new information technologies. It is now widely appreciated that we have a vastly altered research environment that requires the adaptation/expansion of the Common Rule and a reconsideration of some of its requirements. What is required is an amended Common Rule that in the context of our new environment both improves the effectiveness and efficiency of the system while simultaneously enhancing human subject protection.

In the decade 1885-1995 there were no less than twenty government reports or reports commissioned by the government on various aspects of our system for protecting human subjects with most of these recommending an expansion of coverage and/or a more dynamic and adaptive system. In 2003 a report from the Institute of Medicine called for an expansion of Common Rule protections to all human subjects, better risk-adjusted safety monitoring, addressing financial conflicts of interest, continuing review and adaptation of the system, and acknowledging that the IRBs were most importantly representatives of the interests of the human subjects. In the same year a Government Accounting Office [GAO] report on human subject protection in the Veterans Administration medical centers focused on the need for monitoring and oversight, adverse events reporting, and the appropriate training and support for investigators and IRBs.

While change and adaptation of the Common Rule was needed in 2001 it has now become critical that needed changes be seriously addressed and on July 26th 2011 the U.S. Department of Health and Human Services (HHS) in coordination with the Office of Science and Technology Policy (OSTP) published an advanced notice of

A Time for Change... Again, 2001

proposed rulemaking (ANPRM) regarding changes in the Common Rule.

The foci of the proposed changes in the Common Rule are a set of issues surrounding informed consent, new risk-based protections, new data security and information protection standards, data necessary for system oversight, extension of federal regulations, and harmonizing and clarifying both regulatory requirements and agency guidance.

In the arena of informed consent (including for the use of bio-specimens) the new proposals aim at simplifying forms and broadening the bases for some sort of expedited review and waiver of consent. The emphasis here is on both simplification and the view of consent as a process that is more understandable to human subjects.

With respect to the collection and protection of data the ANPRM proposes mandatory data security and information protection practices that would apply to all potentially identifiable information. These proposals aim at aligning the Common Rule with HIPPA privacy regulations and are especially relevant when dealing with very large data bases. In essence data security would become a necessary condition for research to proceed.

Given the growing importance of multi-site studies the ANPRM contains proposals to streamline the various approval processes. In particular these new proposals suggest a single IRB approval for many of such studies (international trials and FDA-regulated devices still need local IRB approval). Moreover the ANPRM also proposes the redeployment of IRB resources toward higher risk research by changes in the definition of excused, expedited, and exempt categories of human subject research.

These new proposals also require a more systematic approach to the collection and analysis of data regarding adverse events, the collection of data necessary to continually enhance the effectiveness and efficiency of the system as the scientific frontier moves and finally initiatives to clarify and hopefully harmonize regulations and agency guidance. Finally

Ethical Considerations in Research on Human Subjects:

ANPRM proposes an important but limited expansion of activities covered by the Common Rule.

While this is not the place to launch a full scale evaluation of these new proposals it is perhaps useful to note some of the issues that have been raised. Perhaps the most serious concerns have come from scholars in the humanities and social sciences who are concerned that their access to vast quantities of previously published secondary data might be at risk. In particular they are concerned that the proposed new regulations would not allow them access to identifiable *non-health* related data. For the behavioral and social sciences the secondary analysis of data is critical and they fear the application of the new rules as proposed would prevent access to such data without re-consent etc. Not surprisingly there is also great concern about the lack of clarity in the proposals regarding the requirements for qualifying expedited, excused or exempt status and/or continuing review. In the context of such concerns and others it is important to note that these are proposals and that reactions from the affected communities have been requested. Most importantly HHS has asked for community input on a number of key issues such as when research use of data originally collected for non-research purposes require consent. Are HIPPA standards regarding identifiable and de-identified health related information appropriate for research studies? Should one ever be allowed to re-identify data? Should IRBs be charged with dealing with financial conflicts of interest?

These and other concerns are an important part of an on-going dialog aimed at improving the Common Rule in view of our experience, our values and the changing profile of the scholarly and technological frontier. The important lesson is the most obvious one namely that if our system is to protect the interests of human subjects as well as to promote the development of important new knowledge the system will have to be as adaptive as our evolving values and scholarly interests. It seems to me that this requires two elements that have been missing to date. First would be an on-going evaluation of the system both with regard to compliance and with respect to effectiveness. In this respect I have always been in favor of some sort of randomized audits of IRB operations where the audit report would be publically available. Second would be an institutionalized commitment to constantly update the Common Rule to reflect the evolving values and aspirations of the society in the context of a rapidly expanding scientific frontier.

"Care Without Coverage: Too Little, Too Late" A Report On The Institute Of Medicine Committee On Uninsurance, 2002

Mary Sue Coleman, PhD, President University of Michigan; Professor of Biological Chemistry, University of Michigan Medical School

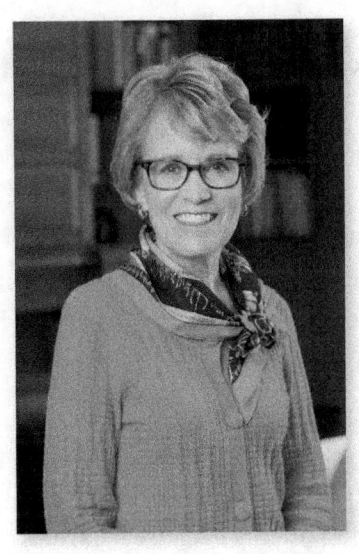

Many of us have grown up with and always assumed we would enjoy quality health care. This is especially true in a state like Michigan, where health care coverage—for workers and retirees—historically has been an integral part of employee compensation packages in the auto industry, in higher education, in the pharmaceutical industry, and in many other sectors of our economy.

The University of Michigan's leadership role in promoting insurance as a vehicle for safeguarding the public's health goes back many years, and we should be rightly proud of this tradition. In the 1940s, Professor Nathan Sinai in the Department of Health Management and Policy developed a voluntary health insurance plan that became the prototype for Blue Shield. Dr. Sinai was a member of the Carnegie-funded Committee on the Costs of Medical Care in the late 1920s and an early advocate of prepaid group practice—a forerunner to the HMO. His colleague, Professor Sy Axelrod, studied voluntary health insurance plans, launched the Bureau of Public Health Economics in

"Care Without Coverage: Too Little, Too Late"

1943, and contributed to President Truman's efforts to implement a comprehensive health insurance plan in 1950.

Today, Michigan residents obtain benefit from excellent community-based hospitals and, of course, the University of Michigan Health System, which consistently ranks among the nation's top 10. The first university-owned medical facility in the United States, the U-M Health System is known for many other "firsts," including the nation's first Department of Dermatology and the first human genetics program. It is home to a top-ranked medical school, the nation's first comprehensive Depression Center, and is a leader in proteomics and applied genetics research. Its clinical specialists in virtually every discipline of medicine are simply among the best in the world.

But access to clinical care like that afforded to most of us in this room is unaffordable or unavailable to far too many of our fellow citizens. In this country, it is the harsh reality that about 40 million Americans—including some 8.5 million children—are without health insurance. Very recent Census Bureau data put the number now at over 41 million. Being without health insurance often implies a drastic decline in one's quality of life and, in the worst of cases, premature death. With rising health care costs and increasing numbers of employees being asked to pay more of their health care costs, there is little relief in sight.

If we doubted whether any of this affects us here, The *Ann Arbor News* recently reported that Hope Medical Clinic in Ypsilanti, for the first time in its 20-year history, is turning away new adult patients because it cannot meet the increasing demand for free medical care to uninsured children and adults. All newspapers in the region have recently reported that the numbers of medically uninsured are growing in Michigan.

Our nation's patchwork of employment-based and publicly funded medical insurance is fraying, leaving all of us—individuals, families, our communities, and our nation—vulnerable.

As co-chair of the Institute of Medicine's Committee on the Consequences of Uninsurance, I have had the opportunity to examine

A Report On The Institute Of Medicine Committee On Uninsurance, 2002

the labyrinth of uninsurance in depth, and can only conclude that the U.S. health care distribution system, as we know it, belies our nation's reputation and character as a fair and compassionate society. Let me explain the purpose of the committee's work, the manner in which it is being conducted, and the results that lead our committee to our conclusions.

The Institute of Medicine (IOM) periodically undertakes studies related to American health care and public policy. The Committee on the Consequences of Uninsurance is a sustained effort by the IOM to inform the public debate about this pressing and persistent challenge. We are very fortunate that the Robert Wood Johnson Foundation has similar interests and has provided funding for our work, the results of which will be released in six reports spanning about three years.

The 16-member IOM committee brings a breadth of expertise (See Figure 1) encompassing the fields of clinical medicine, epidemiology, public health, nursing, health and labor economics, strategic corporation planning, academic health care, and provision of care to those without coverage and other populations at risk. Each of the six reports was also crafted with the assistance of subcommittees, specific for each topic. We held two workshops early in our deliberations and invited public comment. Staff at the IOM has kept the aggressive study and publication schedule on time. The entire project is under the guidance of Janet Corrigan, director of the Board on Health Care Services. Wilhelmine Miller and Diane Wolman have worked tirelessly on the drafting of each report. Normal external peer review processes were utilized, as is customary with IOM studies.

Our three-year study has two objectives: To assess and consolidate evidence about health, economic, and social consequences of uninsurance, and to raise awareness and improve understanding by both the general public and policy-makers.

In addition to providing baseline information to assess the consequences of uninsurance, we have sought to identify strengths and limitations of existing data, evaluate the evidence relating health insurance and

"Care Without Coverage: Too Little, Too Late"

access to care, explain the dynamics of health insurance coverage, and describe the uninsured population and those most likely to be uninsured.

We have systemically reviewed the vast research literature on the composition and demographics of the uninsured and on health outcomes as a function of insurance status. As IOM committee members, we felt compelled to undertake this serious vetting and culling process so that when we went to the public, there would be no doubt regarding the validity of the data. Subcommittee members conducted unbiased, systematic literature searches to identify studies, employed explicit criteria evaluating the quality of the methodology, and reviewed and abstracted studies. In each report, typically in an appendix, the reader will find a list of explicit evaluative criteria for judging the literature reviewed in that volume, as well as a specific bibliography. We focused on individuals under age 65 since the federal Medicare program provides nearly universal coverage for those 65 and older. While we understand that under-insurance is also a troubling problem, we confined our study to those lacking health insurance for at least one year. The health outcomes we evaluated were based on measures of health status and guideline-concordant care, e.g., U.S. Preventive Services Task Force standards. We also identified and evaluated important covariates of insurance status.

Our first goal, the topic of the first report, "Coverage Matters, Insurance and Health Care in 2001," was to identify the problem: Who are the uninsured? The second report, "Care Without Coverage, Too Little, Too Late," released earlier this year; focuses on whether having health insurance makes a difference in overall health status and this is the title I captured for the talk today. Our third report, "Health Insurance Is A Family Matter," published in September 2002, examines family dynamics and the impact of lacking health insurance on the whole family.

In subsequent reports, we will examine the impacts of uninsured populations on communities, the economic costs of significant populations of uninsured to society, and ultimately offer suggestions for models and criteria for health financing reforms.

A Report On The Institute Of Medicine Committee On Uninsurance, 2002

We started with the questions, who are the uninsured and how do most Americans view the problem of uninsurance? Quickly, it became apparent that as a nation we underestimate the numbers of uninsured among us; we hold misperceptions about their identity and how they lose insurance (or never gain it) and about the economic and health consequences of being uninsured. Let's start with the myths:

Myth #1

People without health insurance get the medical care they need.

Reality

Over and over, studies show that those without health insurance are less than half as likely to receive needed medical care. They are much less likely to have a physician visit within a year, have fewer visits annually, and they are more than three times as likely to lack a regular source of care. They also are less likely to receive preventive services and appropriate routine care for chronic conditions than those with insurance.

Myth #2

The number of Americans without health insurance is not large and has not been growing.

Reality

The Census Bureau estimates 38 million to 42 million people in the United States lacked health insurance coverage in 1999 (See Figure 2). That is about 15 percent of the total population of 274 million persons and 17 percent of the population under 65. Unfortunately, this intractable problem has persisted for many years.

Myth #3

Most people without health insurance decline coverage offered in the workplace because they are young and healthy and don't think they need it.

Reality

Young adults are more likely to be uninsured mostly because they are ineligible for workplace coverage. Only 3 million workers between 18 and 44 are uninsured because they decline workplace health insurance.

"Care Without Coverage: Too Little, Too Late"

Eleven million workers between 18 and 44 are uninsured because their employer does not offer them coverage.

Myth #4

Most of the uninsured do not work, or they live in families where no one works.

Reality

More than 80 percent of uninsured children and adults under the age of 65 live in working families (See Figure 3). Even members of families with two full-time wage earners have almost a one-in-ten chance of being uninsured.

Myth #5

Recent immigrants account for the increase in the number of uninsured persons.

Reality

Immigrants who have come to the United States within four years comprise a relatively small proportion of the general population (See Figure 4). Non-citizens represent less than one in five uninsured persons.

Let me summarize for you the principal ways that people living in this country gain or lose insurance coverage:

Employment-based insurance is by far the most common type of coverage available. Workers purchase coverage when it is offered, as well as additional coverage for family members if they can afford it. Work-based plans are more likely to cover the entire family than other types of insurance. Marriage increases a family's chances of having employment-based health insurance. But because of the predominance of employment-based coverage in the U.S., families who have enjoyed excellent health insurance coverage for years may suddenly lose this safety net when a working parent changes jobs, is laid off, dies, or divorces. Life transitions such as changing jobs or retiring can put such coverage at risk, whether it is employment-based or public coverage, since eligibility is often based on family income.

A Report On The Institute Of Medicine Committee On Uninsurance, 2002

Money may not buy love, happiness, or good health, but there is a strong correlation between family income and having health insurance. Ninety percent of families with incomes of more than 200 percent of the federal poverty level are able to insure all family members. This contrasts with lower-income families, of which only 59 percent are able to obtain insurance for the whole family. In reality, if your family is headed by a single parent, or you recently emigrated to the U.S., or you are a member of a racial or ethnic minority group, your family is less likely to have insurance for some or all family members.

Perhaps most disturbing, it would require almost 40 percent of the yearly income of a family of four with an income at the federal poverty level to purchase an average employment-based health insurance premium for family coverage in 2000.

So, who are the uninsured? They are likely to have at least one wage earner in the family, earn less than 200 percent of the federal poverty baseline, and lack a college education. They also are likely to be self-employed, employed by a small firm of fewer than 100 workers, or work in the wholesale and retail trade, agriculture, forestry, fishing, mining, and construction sectors. In terms of life stage, the uninsured are most likely to be adults and young adults, unmarried, and members of families that include children. It is also true that the probability of being uninsured varies vastly by geographic region (See Figure 5). The highest proportions of medically uninsured are found in the mid-South and Southwestern states, with occasional high ratios in other areas such as Florida, Alaska, and California.

Having described the face of the uninsured in America, our next task was to evaluate the literature about the health consequences of uninsurance, because establishing this causal link is critical to shaping public policy and gaining support for widespread health care financing. For this aspect of the project, we evaluated the best-designed research studies about the health of working age adults (18 through 64) with and without health insurance. As this audience well understands, such research is challenging because controlled longitudinal trials are not feasible. However, to be selected by the IOM committee, the studies had to encompass two factors: 1) an individual's health insurance status as an independent variable or "predictor" and 2) the effect of insurance status on one or more health-related outcomes. The complete definitions of insurance status and entire bibliography may be found in the published report.

Let me give you the "punch line" first:

> The committee finds a consistent and statistically significant relationship between health insurance coverage and health outcomes for adults.
>
> Coverage is associated with having a regular source of care, which promotes continuity of care, and with greater use of appropriate health services. The ultimate result is improved health outcomes.

We concluded that health insurance is associated with better health outcomes for adults and with their receipt of appropriate care across a range of preventive, chronic, and acute care services. Adults without health insurance coverage die sooner and experience greater declines in health status over time than do adults with continuous coverage.

Now to some specific findings:

> Adults with chronic conditions and those in late middle age are the most likely to realize improved health outcomes as a result of gaining health insurance coverage because of their high probability of needing health care services.
>
> In particular, population groups that tend to lack stable health insurance coverage have worse health status and would benefit from increased health insurance coverage.
>
> Longitudinal studies over one to four years document relatively greater decreases in general health status measures for uninsured adults and for those who lost insurance coverage during the period studied than for those who enjoyed continuous coverage. Over

two years, major declines in health status were reported by 22 percent of continuously uninsured adults, 16 percent of intermittently uninsured, and just 8 percent of continuously insured adults.

Longitudinal, well-controlled studies of mortality reveal a higher risk of dying prematurely for those who were uninsured at the beginning of the study than for those who initially had private coverage. In fact, over a 13- to 17-year follow-up period, adults initially uninsured had a 25 percent greater risk of dying prematurely than did adults with private insurance. Over a two- to five-year follow-up period, black men and white women who were uninsured had a 50 percent greater risk of dying prematurely than their insured counterparts, and uninsured white men had a 20 percent higher risk. For reasons we do not understand, the risk for black women did not differ by insurance status.

Uninsured adults are less likely than adults with any kind of health coverage to receive timely preventive and screening services. We found that health insurance that covers preventive and screening services is likely to result in more appropriate use of these services, and that it would likely reduce racial and ethnic disparities among those receiving preventive and screening services.

Because of delays in diagnosis, uninsured persons with breast, cervical, colorectal, prostate cancer, and melanoma generally are in poorer health and are more likely to die prematurely than persons with insurance. Tragically, uninsured women diagnosed with breast cancer have a 30 percent to 50 percent higher risk of dying than women with private insurance. Uninsured women are more likely to receive a late-stage diagnosis of cervical cancer than are women with any kind of insurance, and uninsured patients with colorectal cancer have a 50 percent to 60 percent higher mortality rate.

A number of studies evaluated chronic diseases and the impact of insurance status. Those living with chronic diseases—diabetes, cardiovascular disease, end-stage renal disease, HIV infection, and mental illness—are less likely to receive appropriate care to manage their health conditions than those who have health insurance.

Twenty-five percent of adults with diabetes who are uninsured for at least a year had not had a routine exam within the past two years, compared with 5 percent of those who had insurance. Adults with diabetes who are without insurance are less likely to receive recommended services such as foot exams or dilated eye exams.

Lacking health insurance for longer periods can lead to uncontrolled blood sugar levels, which, over time, put diabetics at risk for additional chronic disease and disability.

Uninsured adults with hypertension or high blood cholesterol have diminished access to care, are less likely to be screened, are less likely to take prescription medication if diagnosed, and experience worse health outcomes. Not surprisingly, adults with hypertension who lost health coverage had poorer blood pressure control than those who remained insured. And if you are without insurance and have a heart attack, you are less likely to be admitted to a hospital that performs angiography or revascularization procedures. You also are less likely to receive these diagnostic and treatment procedures and are more likely to die in the short term.

Among adults with HIV, having health insurance has shown to reduce the risk of dying within a six-month period by 71 percent to 85 percent. Uninsured adults with HIV infection are less likely to receive highly effective medications that have been shown to improve survival and die sooner than HIV-infected adults with coverage.

Adults with health insurance that covers any mental health treatment are more likely to receive mental health services and

A Report On The Institute Of Medicine Committee On Uninsurance, 2002

care consistent with clinical practice guidelines than are those without any health insurance or with insurance that does not cover mental health conditions.

Uninsured patients who are hospitalized are likely to receive fewer services when admitted and to experience substandard care and injury when admitted than are insured patients. Perhaps most disturbing, they also are more likely to die in the hospital. In one statewide study, uninsured victims of auto crashes had a 37 percent higher mortality rate than insured crash victims, controlling extensively for personal injury and hospital characteristics.

Health insurance that provides for adequate physician panels and that includes preventive services, prescription drugs, and mental health care is more likely to facilitate the receipt of appropriate care than insurance than does not have these features. Broad-based health insurance strategies across the entire uninsured population would be more likely to produce the benefits of enhanced health and life expectancy than would health insurance aimed only at the seriously ill.

Our committee has concluded that providing insurance would result in improved health, including greater life expectancy. Increased rates of health insurance coverage would especially improve the health of those in the poorest health and those most disadvantaged in terms of access to care.

We believe several policy implications may be drawn from these findings:

    Empirical evidence affirms that having health insurance results in better health outcomes

    Continuity of coverage appears to account for some of the health benefits of insurance

    Scope of benefits is related to receipt of appropriate care

    Insurance coverage that begins only after an illness is diagnosed will not achieve all of the potential positive impacts on health

"Care Without Coverage: Too Little, Too Late"

The way our health insurance distribution system is configured is part of the problem. Although most of us live in families, insurance goes to individuals. For example, publicly financed health insurance programs tend to cover individuals—poor children or pregnant women—rather than the family. However, our nation's well-being depends, in part, on providing conditions for families to successfully raise the next generation of Americans.

In the third report, the Committee examined the wide range of consequences to families having one or more uninsured members. What we concluded is that the physical, psychosocial, and financial health and well-being of the whole family can be adversely affected if even one member lacks health insurance. And the number of families in this situation is large. One out of every five American families has at least one member who has been uninsured throughout the previous year. This means that roughly 58 million individuals are either uninsured themselves or live with a family member who is uninsured.

Many family transitions affect insurance coverage. Children typically lose coverage under their parents' policies when they reach age 19. The death of a spouse who had family coverage through work can mean loss of insurance for the surviving family members. A spouse who retires at age 65 may immediately qualify for Medicare, but a younger spouse and other dependents may be left with no coverage.

We know that serious health problems and large medical bills can shake a family's financial foundation. Families with no members insured during the year are more than twice as likely as families with all members insured all year to have medical expenses that exceed 10 percent of their income. Two-thirds of working-age adults with high medical bills resort to borrowing from family or friends. Twenty-five percent obtain a loan or mortgage to cover medical expenses, and some families declare bankruptcy, putting their credit rating and financial future in jeopardy. Medical expenses are a factor in almost half of all personal bankruptcy filings.

A Report On The Institute Of Medicine Committee On Uninsurance, 2002

We have found that families without insurance use health services very selectively. They may delay or forego treatment or preventive care to reduce short-term costs, to the point of jeopardizing their long-term health. Children who are without health insurance fare much worse in the health care system than those privileged children whose parents do have insurance. Because a child's early development depends on the health and well-being of his or her parents, parental coverage is extremely important. We have found that parents who understand and use health services appropriately themselves are more likely to seek care for their children. Unfortunately, the nine million uninsured parents in the United States are more likely to be in poor physical or mental health and have greater difficulty obtaining care than parents who have health insurance. They also are more likely to lack a regular source of care than parents with private insurance and to forego needed care, not just for themselves, but also for their children.

Children without health care coverage are more likely to receive no or delayed care, placing them at greater risk of hospitalization for such conditions as asthma that could be treated less expensively on an outpatient basis. Children who are not treated for such common childhood conditions as ear infections and iron deficiency anemia may suffer consequences that affect their language development, long-term school performance, and success in life.

The impact can be even more severe on children with serious illnesses and disabilities who require more medical care than average children. One out of every nine children with special needs is uninsured; these children are less likely to have a usual source of care, less likely to have seen a doctor in the previous year, and less likely to get needed prescriptions, medical, mental health, dental, or vision care than their peers with insurance.

And, if a child requires hospitalization, those without insurance typically fare much worse than children who have private insurance. For example, uninsured infants with coarctation of the aorta, a birth defect

"Care Without Coverage: Too Little, Too Late"

in the major artery from the heart, are more likely to die than children with the same condition who do have private insurance.

In the United States, where prenatal visits early in the pregnancy and continuing through delivery are the standard of care, the effect of being born without health insurance starts in the womb. Uninsured women and their newborns receive, on average, less prenatal care and fewer expensive services such as cesarean sections. They also are more likely to have poor outcomes, including greater likelihood of maternal complications, infant death, and low birth weight. On the continuum of care, publicly insured women receive less care than women with private insurance but more care than the uninsured.

Let me reiterate our conclusions from the study of impact of health insurance coverage on families:

> First, the current hodgepodge of employment-based and public insurance leaves gaps in coverage for many families. These gaps occur both over time and across the members of the family.
>
> Second, uninsured families—that is, families with at least one member who was uninsured throughout the entire previous year—often cannot afford major health bills or insurance premiums and therefore avoid seeking care.
>
> Third, pregnant women, newborns, and children without health insurance have worse access to care, receive fewer services, and often have poorer health outcomes, and
>
> Fourth, children whose parents do not have health insurance coverage are less likely to be insured and less likely to receive appropriate health care, regardless of the child's eligibility for coverage.

There are a number of policy implications that have emerged from this last report. We now know that a family's financial stability can be jeopardized by having even one uninsured member. We know that if a family is uninsured through work or public benefits that the costs of insurance and medical bills are more than most families can afford. We

A Report On The Institute Of Medicine Committee On Uninsurance, 2002

know that when public insurance programs cover parents, their children are far more likely to be enrolled. And we know that uninsured children experience poorer access to care and worse health than those with insurance coverage.

When we consider all three reports, what have we learned? Being uninsured usually is not a choice. Health insurance does contribute to improved health. The lack of health insurance, even for a single individual in a family, can adversely affect the entire family.

Will Americans demand a fairer and more efficient system of health insurance? It has been almost a decade since we closely examined the issue of health insurance in the United States, and the situation has deteriorated during a time of great national prosperity. As more people become aware of how intractable the current system is and how vulnerable it leaves us at all levels of society, I believe that we will muster the collective will to change. We must.

I think that many of the solutions will come from the academy as faculty study and provide the analysis we need to make the right decisions. At the University of Michigan, we have many faculty working on ethical and policy issues related to health care.

Dr. Susan Goold (from our department of Internal Medicine) and her colleagues at the National Institutes of Health are among those looking at ethical issues and the uninsured. They have developed a game about health insurance called CHAT, the acronym for Choosing Healthplans All Together. The object of the game is to develop an imaginary group health insurance plan. Throughout the simulation, participants have to make tradeoffs between competing needs for limited resources. CHAT presents the challenge of a full array of possible health care options, but limited resources. Nine to 15 players play through four rounds, deciding what to include and to eliminate from their health insurance plans. They can choose from more than a dozen types of services—dental care, hospital care, mental health, drug coverage, and long-term care—at three levels of coverage (basic, medium, or high) and then test their

"Care Without Coverage: Too Little, Too Late"

choices by drawing "Health Event" cards determined by the spin of a roulette wheel. The goal is to help people better understand health insurance and to help health insurance policy-makers better understand the health care priorities of ordinary people.

When Dr. Goold and her colleagues used CHAT in a study of more than 200 uninsured individuals from clinical and community settings in central North Carolina, they found that groups of low-income uninsured individuals are able to identify acceptable benefit packages that are comparable in cost but differ in benefit design from managed-care contracts offered to many U.S. employees today. Dr. Goold says that with adequate time and information, the public is willing and able to engage in allocation of finite resources.

Health economist Catherine McLaughlin (from our School of Public Health) and her colleagues at the Michigan-based Economic Research Initiative on the Uninsured (ERIU) are contributing to the uninsurance debate with research and by helping policy-makers better understand the interplay between labor force dynamics, health insurance coverage, and markets in general. Now in its second year of a three-year, $9 million grant from the Robert Wood Johnson Foundation, ERIU's goal is to diversify the pool of experts who study health insurance coverage trends, to ask new questions about the issue of the uninsured, and to bring new perspectives to the field. In fact, Hans Kuttner, Senior Research Associate from ERIU, has been a consultant to our IOM study.

For example, a recent ERIU-funded analysis of people in their 50s and early 60s revealed that while 90 percent were insured at some point in time, 22 percent were without coverage at some time between 1992 and 1998. Professor McLaughlin notes that a five- to six-month coverage gap for this population can impose serious financial burdens and jeopardize timely treatments. ERIU estimates that 40 percent of all workers were without private coverage at some point during 1996 and 1998. More than half of the gaps were because of a job change.

A Report On The Institute Of Medicine Committee On Uninsurance, 2002

Many of you are familiar with the Consolidated Omnibus Budget Reconciliation Act (COBRA), which was created at the federal level to cover unemployed workers in transition from one job to the next. However, we are learning that fewer employees are eligible for COBRA than is commonly believed. The Urban Institute estimates only 57 percent of non-elderly workers and their adult dependents are potentially eligible for COBRA. Also, the COBRA take-up rate is fairly low, which is not surprising, given that the premium is often a fairly high percent of income. Unemployed workers would face average annual premium costs of $2,700 for an individual plan and $7,000 for a family plan based on average employer plan costs in 2001, according to the study by Professor McLaughlin and Sarah Crow, a Ford School of Public Policy alumna and research associate at ERIU.

Health economist Michael Chernew (from Public Health, Internal Medicine, and LSA), another ERIU associate, has been studying the creation and use of health plan "report cards"—performance-based evaluations of health insurance plans—and how such an evaluation system would impact employers and consumers when choosing plans. He also is studying the determinants of rising health-care expenditures and the extent to which rising health care premiums cause coverage rates to decline.

Although the statistics and the capricious nature of not having health insurance are discouraging, I believe that, armed with accurate information and thoughtful analysis, we will find better, more workable solutions.

Thank you for allowing me to share with you some of my concerns about the state of health insurance in America. I hope that you will stay tuned for our committee's subsequent reports. What I urge all of you to do is to alert me to individuals on this campus who might be interested in suggesting new public policies for our final report on the uninsured in America.

I leave you with one last thought from Goethe. It has been a guiding principle for all of us serving on the Committee on the Consequences of Uninsurance: "Knowing is not enough; we must apply. Willing is not enough; we must do."

Ageless Bodies, Happy Souls: Biotechnology and the Pursuit of Perfection, 2003

Leon R. Kass, M.D., Ph.D., Hertog Fellow in Social Thought, American Enterprise Institute, Washington, D. C.

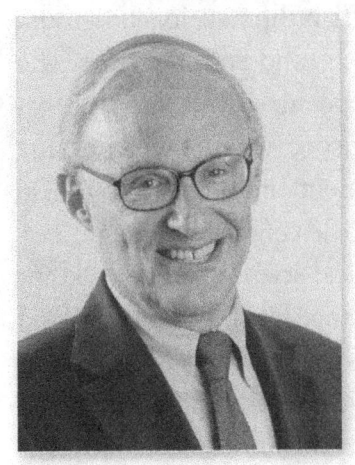

Thank you very much, Dr. Margolis. Thank you ladies and gentlemen for your attention this afternoon. It is a great pleasure to be here at the Medical School at the University of Michigan and a great honor to be invited to give the Waggoner Memorial Lecture. I too am honored by the presence of the Waggoner family and have very much enjoyed meeting you these last two days. I spent the last hour sort of collecting my thoughts before coming down here in Dr. Greden's conference room staring the portrait of Dr. Waggoner in the face and trying to see what lay behind that wise appearance and that marvelous smile. I wish I had known him. I am honored at least in this small way to be connected.

The talk I'm going to give is a kind of overview of the topic of beyond therapy, which in fact has been a concern of the President's Council on Bioethics for about a year and a half and was just issued last month in a report published by the Council called, *Beyond Therapy – Biotechnology and the Pursuit of Happiness.* Slightly different from the pursuit of perfection, but not actually unrelated. Two commercial houses have in fact produced it -it's now in bookstores. This one from Harper Collins. This is much better than what you are going to hear from me today. Regard this talk as a kind of introduction to the subject. The things that are in the report are much more carefully and thoroughly done, but this is I think to whet your appetite to the subject and to at least try to persuade you there is something here worth thinking about.

As nearly everyone appreciates, we live near the beginning of the Golden Age of biomedical science and technology. For the most part we should be mightily glad that we do. We and our friends and loved ones are many times over the beneficiaries of its cures for disease, prolongation of life, and amelioration of suffering, psychic and somatic.

We should be deeply grateful for the gifts of human ingenuity and for the devoted efforts of scientists, physicians, and entrepreneurs who have used these gifts to make those benefits possible. And mindful that modern biology is just entering puberty, we suspect we ain't seen nothing yet. Yet not withstanding these blessings, present and projected, we also have seen more than enough to make us a little concerned. For we recognize the powers made possible by biomedical science can be used for non-therapeutic purposes serving ends that range from the frivolous and disquieting to the offensive and perdicious. These powers are available as instruments of bioterrorism. For example, genetically engineered drug resistant bacteria or drugs that would obliterate memory. Where as agents of social control, for example, drugs that tame rowdies and dissenters or fertility blockers for welfare recipients. Or as means of trying to improve or perfect our bodies and minds and those of our children. For example, genetically engineered super muscles or drugs to improve memory.

Anticipating possible threats to our security, freedom, and even our very humanity, many people are increasingly worried about where biotechnology may be taking us. We are concerned not only about what other people might do to us, but also what we might do to ourselves. We are concerned that our society might be harmed and that we ourselves might be diminished indeed in ways that could undermine the highest and richest possibilities of human life.

Biotechnology and the Pursuit of Perfection, 2003

In this lecture I want to discuss only the last and most seductive of these disquieting prospects, the use of biotechnical powers to pursue perfection, both the body and of mind. I do so partly because I think this is the most neglected topic in public bioethics. Yet it is, I believe, the deepest source of public anxiety represented in concerns about man playing God or about the brave new world or about a post-human future. It raises weighty questions about the ends and goals of the biomedical enterprise, the nature and meaning of human flourishing and the intrinsic threat of the humanization or the promise of super humanization. It compels attention to what it means to be a human being and to be active as a human being. And it gets us beyond our narrow preoccupation with the life issues of abortion or embryo destruction, important though they are. To deal with what is genuinely novel and worrisome in biotechnical advance. Not the old crude power to kill the creature made in God's image, but the science-based sophisticated powers to remake him after our own fantasies.

What exactly are the powers that I am talking about? What sorts of ends are they likely to serve? How soon are they available? They are powers that affect the capacities and activities of the human body; powers that affect the capacities and activities of the mind or soul; and, powers that affect the shape of the human life cycle at both ends and in between. We already have powers to prevent fertility and to promote it. To initiate life in the laboratory, to screen our genes, both as adults and as embryos, and to select or reject nascent life based on genetic criteria. To insert new genes into various parts of the adult body and someday soon, also into gametes and embryos. To enhance muscle performance and endurance, to replace body parts with natural or mechanical organs, and perhaps soon to wire ourselves using computer chips implanted into the body and brain. To alter memory, mood, temperament and attention through psychoactive drugs, and to prolong, not just the average, but also the maximum life expectancy.

The technologies for altering our native capacities are mainly those of genetic screening and genetic engineering, drugs, especially psychotropic ones and the ability to replace body parts or to insert novel ones. The availability of some of these capacities using these techniques has been demonstrated only with animals, but others are already in use in human beings.

Now it should bear emphasis that these powers have not been developed for the purpose of producing perfect or post human beings. They have been produced largely for the purpose of preventing and curing disease or reversing disabilities. Even the bizarre prospect of machine brain interaction and implanted nano-technological devices, starts with therapeutic efforts to enable the blind to see and the deaf to hear. Yet, the dual use aspects of most of these powers encouraged by the incredible human urge toward improvement and the commercial interests that see market opportunities for non-therapeutic uses means that we must not be lulled to sleep by the fact that the originators of these new powers were no friends to brave new world. Once here, techniques and powers can produce desires where none existed before and things often go where no one ever intended.

How to organize our reflections. We should resist the temptation to begin with the new techniques themselves or even with the capacities for intervention that they make possible. To do so runs the risk of losing the human import and significance of the undertakings. Better to begin with the human desires and goals that these powers and techniques are destined to serve; better children, superior performance, ageless bodies, happy souls, a more peaceful and cooperative society, etcetera. These are, by the way, the principles of organization in the Council's report with four chapters on the first four of those items.

In this talk I want to leave aside the production or the pursuit of optimum children or superior performance or better citizens to concentrate on the strictly personal goals of self-improvement. To those efforts, to preserve and augment the vitality of the body and to enhance the happiness of the soul. These goals are arguably the least controversial, the most continuous with the aims of modern medicine and psychiatry for better health and peace of mind, and the most attractive to most potential consumers, probably indeed, to most of us.

It is perhaps worth remembering that it was these goals now in the realm of possibility that animated the great founders of modern science, Francis Bacon and Rene Descartes. Flawlessly healthy bodies, unconflicted and contented souls and freedom from the infirmities of age perhaps indefinitely. Here then are some of the technological innovations that in varying degrees can serve the purposes. With respect to the pursuit of ageless bodies, we can already replace worn out parts with organ transplantation, and we look forward to the prospect of regenerative medicine where decayed tissues are replaced with new ones produced from stem cells. We can improve upon normal and healthy parts, for example, via precise genetic modification of muscles through injections of growth factor genes that keep the transformed muscles whole, vigorous, and free of age related decline. These powers, by the way have already been used to produce Mighty Mouse and Super Rat and they are soon going to be clinically tested for the treatment of muscular dystrophy and muscular weakness in the elderly, but as Dr. Sweeney at Pennsylvania who is doing this research, reported to us also of interest immediately, the football and wrestling coaches and to the hoards of people presumably who spent two hours daily pumping iron and sculpting their bodies.

Most radically, we can try to retard or stop the entire process of biological senescence. We should keep in mind recent discoveries in the genetics of aging that have shown how the maximum--a maximum lifespan of worms and flies can be increased two and three-fold by alterations in a single gene. A gene now known to be present also in mammals. With respect to the pursuit of happy souls, we can eliminate psychic distress. We can produce states of trance euphoria. We can engineer more permanent conditions of good cheer, optimism, self-esteem, and contentment. We should therefore keep in mind, and this is a field in its infancy, drugs now available that if administered promptly at the time of memory formation, may blunt markedly the painful emotional content of newly formed memories of traumatic events; the so-called memory blunders, a remedy which is being pursued to try to prevent post traumatic stress disorder. We should keep in mind second, the simple euphoria's like Ecstasy, the forerunner of Huxley soma widely used on college campuses. And finally, the powerful, yet seemingly safe antidepressant and mood brightening drugs like Prozac, wonderful for the treatment of major depression and other psychiatric disorders, but that are also capable in some people who don't have clinical disease, of utterly changing their outlook on life from that of Eeyore to that of Mary Poppins.

The analysis proceeds in five parts. The first part of which is called, Problems of Description, Limitations of the Therapy Enhancement Distinction. People who have tried to address our topic, have usually approached it through a distinction between therapy and enhancement. Therapy, the treatment of individuals with known diseases or disabilities, enhancement the directed uses of biotechnical power to alter by direct intervention, not diseased processes, but the normal workings of the human body and psyche.

Those who first introduced this distinction hoped by this means to distinguish between the acceptable and the dubious or unacceptable uses of biotechnical technology. Therapy is always ethically fine. Enhancement is, at least, prima facie, ethically suspect. Gene therapy for cystic fibrosis or Prozac for psychotic depression is fine. Insertion of genes to enhance intelligence or steroids for Olympic athlete is not. Health providers and insurance companies, by the way, have at least for now bought into this distinction paying for treatment of disease but not for enhancements.

This distinction is perfectly useful as a point of departure. Everybody distinguishes between restoring to normal and going beyond the normal. But if you look at it more closely, it proves finally inadequate for the moral analysis. Enhancement even as a term is highly problematic. Does it mean more or better? And if better, by what standards? Can both improve memory and selective erasure of memory, both by enhancements? If enhancement is defined as an opposition to therapy, one faces further difficulties with the definition of healthy and impaired, normal and abnormal, and hence, super normal, especially in the area of behavioral and psychic functions and activities. Some psychiatric diagnoses are notoriously vague. The boundary between shyness and social anxiety disorder, the boundary between spiritedness and some forms of hyperactivity disorder, between mark independence and oppositional disorder.

Furthermore, in many human qualities, from height to IQ that distribute themselves normally over a normal distribution curve, does the average also function as a norm or is the norm itself appropriately subject to alteration? Is it therapy to give growth hormone to a genetic dwarf, but not to an equally short fellow who is just unhappy to be short? And if the short are brought up to the average, the average now having become short will have precedent for a claim to growth hormone injections. This by the way has just been approved by the FDA earlier this year.

Needless arguments, therefore, about whether something, whether or not something is or is not an enhancement gets in the way of the more proper question. What are the good and bad uses of biotechnical power? What makes a good use good or even just acceptable? It does not follow from the fact that a drug is being taken solely to satisfy ones desires that it is objectionable. In conversely certain interventions to restore a normal functioning, for example, to enable post-menopausal women to bear children or 60 year old men to keep playing professional ice hockey, might well be seen to be dubious uses of biotechnical power. The moral meaning and assessment are unlikely to be settled by the term enhancement anymore than they are by the nature of the technological intervention itself.

My last observation points to the deepest reason why the distinction between healing and enhancing is going to be finally insufficient, both in theory and in practice. For the human sole whose healing is sought or accomplished by biomedical technology, is finite and frail, medicine or no medicine. The healthy body declines and its parts wear out. The

Ageless Bodies, Happy Souls:

sound mind slows down and has trouble remembering things. The soul has aspirations beyond what even a healthy body can realize and it becomes weary from frustration. Even at its finest--sorry, even at its fittest, the fatigue able and limited human body rarely carries out flawlessly, even the ordinary desires of the soul. Moreover there is wide variation in the natural gifts with which each of us is endowed. Some are born with perfect pitch. Others are born tone deaf. Some have flypaper memories; others forget immediately what they have just learned. As it is with talents, so too with the desires and temperaments. Some crave immortal fame; others, merely comfortable preservation. Some are sanguine; others, phlegmatic, still others bilious or melancholic. When nature deals her cards, some receive only from the bottom of the deck.

Conversely, it is often the most gifted and ambitious who most resent their limitations. Achilles was willing to destroy everything around him so little could he stomach that he was but a heel short of immortality. As a result of these infirmities, human beings have long dreamed of overcoming limitations of body and soul, in particularly, the limitations of body decay, psychic distress, and the frustration of human aspiration. Dreams of human perfection and the terrible consequences of pursuing it are the themes of Greek tragedy as well as by the way, The Birthmark by Nathanial Hawthorne, the short story with which the President's Council of Bioethics began its work.

Until now these dreams have been pure fantasies and those who pursued them came crashing down in disaster, but the stupendous successes over the past century in all areas of technology and especially in medicine, have revived the ancient dream of human perfection. Like Achilles, the major beneficiaries of modern medicine are less content than they are worried well and we regard our remaining limitations with less equanimity to the point that dreams of getting rid of them all together become turned into moral imperatives. For these reasons, thanks to biomedical technology, people will be increasingly tempted to realize these dreams, at least to some extent. Ageless and ever vigorous bodies, happy or at least never unhappy souls, and excellent human achievement with diminished effort or toil.

Why should anybody be worried about these prospects? What could be wrong with efforts to try to improve upon human nature to try to help, with the help of biomedical technology, to gain ageless bodies and happy souls?

In Part two I begin with some familiar sources of concern. Not surprisingly, the objections usually raised to the beyond therapy used of biomedical technologies reflect the dominant values of modern America, health, equality, and liberty.

First, health issues of safety and bodily harm. In our health-obsessed culture, the first reason given to worry about any new biotechnical intervention is safety and that is true also here. Athletes who take steroids will later suffer premature heart disease. College students who take Ecstasy will damage dopamine receptors in their basal ganglia and suffer early Parkinson's disease. To generalize, no biological agent used for the purpose of self-perfection will ever be entirely safe. This is good conservative medical sense. Anything powerful enough to enhance system A is likely to be powerful enough to harm system B. Yet many good things in life are filled with risks and free people if properly informed, they choose to run them if they care enough about what is to be gained thereby.

If the interventions are showed to be highly dangerous, many people will later if not sooner avoid them and the FDA and/or tort liability will constrain many a legitimate purveyor. It surely makes sense as an ethical matter that one should not risk basic health pursuing a condition of better than well. But on the other hand if the interventions work well and are indeed highly desired, people may freely accept and tradeoff even considerable risk of later bodily harm. But in any case, the big issues have nothing to do with safety. As in the case of cloning children, the real questions concern what to think about the perfected powers assuming that they might be safely used.

Second, then equality, issues of unfairness and distributed justice. An obvious objection to the use of personal enhancers by participants in competitive activities is that they give those who use them an unfair advantage. Blood doping or steroids in athletes, stimulants in students taking the SATs. Still even if everyone had equal access to brain implants or genetic improvement of muscle strength or mind enhancing drugs, a deeper disquiet that would still remain. Besides, not all activities of life are competitive. It would matter to me if she said she loves me only me because she is high on erotogenine, some new brain stimulant that mimics perfectly the feeling of falling in love. It matters to me when I go to a class that the people with whom I am conversing, are not drugged out of their right minds.

The distributive justice question is less easily set aside than the unfairness question, especially if there are systematic disparities between who will and will not have access to the powers of biotechnical improvement. The case can be made yet more powerful to the extent that we regard the expenditures of money and energy on such niceties as a misallocation of limited resources in a world in which the basic health needs of millions go unaddressed.

As a public policy matter, this is surely an important consideration. But once again, the equality of access does not remove our disquiet to the thing itself. And it is to say at the least, paradoxical in discussions of dehumanizing dangers of say eugenic choice, when people complain that the poor will be denied equal access to the danger. The food is contaminated, but why are my portions so small? Check it out. Yes, Huxley's brave new world runs on a deplorable and impermeably rigid class system. But would you want to live in that world if offered the chance to enjoy it as an Alpha, a member of the privileged class? Even an elite can be dehumanized. Even an elite can dehumanize itself. The central matter is not the equality of access, but the goodness or badness of the thing being offered.

Third, questions of liberty; questions of freedom and coercion overt and subtle. This comes closer to the mark especially with uses of biotechnical power exercised by some people over other people, whether for social control, say in the pacification of a classroom of Tom Sawyer's or for their own punitive improvement, say with genetic selection of the sex or sexual orientation of a child to be. The problem will of course be much worse in tyrannical regimes, but there are always dangers of desperatism within families as parents already work their wills on their children with insufficient regard to a child's independence, needs, or childly wellbeing. To the extent that even partial control over genotype, say to take a relatively innocent example, musician parents selecting a child with perfect pitch. To the extent that even this partial control adds to existing social instruments of parental control and its risks of despotic rule, this matter will need to be attended to. And one of the arguments, I think against human cloning among other reasons, it is the charge of the genetic despotism of one generation over the next that this would make possible.

There are also more subtle limitations of freedom, say through peer pressure. What is permitted and widely used may become mandatory. If most children are receiving memory enhancement or stimulant drugs, failure to provide them for your child might be seen as a form of child neglect. If all the defensive linemen are on steroids, you risk mayhem if you go against them chemically pure. At a point subtler still, some critics complain that as with cosmetic surgery, Botox and breast implants, the enhancement technologies of the future will likely to be used in slavish adherence to certain socially defined and merely fashionable notions of excellence or improvement, very likely shallow, almost certainly conformist.

This special kind of restriction of freedom, let us call it the problem of conformity or homogenization, is I believe, rather serious. We are right to worry that the self selected non-therapeutic uses of new powers, especially were they to become widespread, will be put in the service of the most common human desires, moving us towards still greater homogenization of human society. Perhaps raising the floor, but greatly lowering the ceiling of human possibility and reducing the likelihood of genuine freedom, individuality, and greatness. Indeed, such homogenization may be the most important society-wide concern if we consider the aggregated effects of the likely individual choices for biotechnical self-improvement each of which might be defended or at least not objected to on a case by case basis, but the problem of what the economists call, negative externalities. For example, it would be difficult to object to a personal choice for a life extending technology that would extend the users life by three healthy decades. Or a mood brightened way of life that would make the individual more cheerful and untroubled by the world around him. Yet, the aggregated social affects of such choices widely made could lead to the tragedy of the commons where genuine and sought for satisfactions for individuals might be nullified or worse owing to the social consequences of granting them to everyone. And I myself will make such an argument toward the end with respect to the choice for ageless bodies. As Aldous Huxley suggested in Brave New World, "Biotechnical powers to produce contemptment in accordance with democratic tastes threaten the character of human striving and diminish the possibility of human excellence." In his world, the best thing to be hoped for was the preservation of pockets of difference as on the islands to which excellent were sent with the desire for high achievement has not been entirely submerged in the culture of the last man.

But once again important though, this surely is as a social political issue, it does not settle the question regarding individuals. What if anything can we say to justify or disquiet over the individual uses of performance enhancing genetic engineering or mood brightening drugs for reasons other than medical necessity. For even the safe equally available non-coerced and non-faddish uses of these technologies for self-improvement raise ethical questions; questions that I think go to the heart of the matter. The disquiet must have something to do with the essence of the activity itself. The use of technological means to intervene in the human body and mind, not to ameliorate disease, but to change and improve their normal workings. Why if at all are we bothered by the voluntary self-administration of agents that would change our bodies or alter our minds? What is disquieting about our attempts to improve upon human nature, even our own particular instances of it?

It is very difficult to put this disquiet into words. Initial repugnance's are hard to translate into sound and moral arguments. We are probably repelled by the idea of drugs that would erase our memories or that change our personalities or that interventions that would enable 70 year olds to bear children or play professional sports or to engage in some wilder imaginings of mechanical implants that might enable men to nurse infants or computer body hookups that would enable us to download the Oxford English Dictionary. But is there any wisdom in this repugnance? Taken one person at a time with a properly prepared set of conditions and qualifications, it is going to be very hard to say what is wrong with any biotechnical intervention that could give us more ageless bodies or make it possible to live more happily. If there is a case to be made against these activities, for individuals, we sense that it might have something to do with what is natural, or what is humanly dignified, or what is the attitude that is properly respectful of what is naturally and humanly dignified? I will try to come with these essential causes of concern for three directions. The goodness of the ends, the fitness of the means, and the meaning of the over arching attitudes seeking to master control and even transform one's given nature.

Three human goods will figure prominently in the discussions: Modesty and humility about what we know and can do to our selves, the meaning of aging and the life cycle and the nature of human activity and human flourishing and the importance of exercising the first and seeking the second through fitting means. Here I can only hope to open the questions starting first with the matter of the proper attitude.

Part three, Hubris or Humility. Respect for the Given. A common man on the street reaction to these prospects is the complaint of man playing God. An educated fellow who knows Greek Tragedy complains rather of hubris. Sometimes the charge means the sheer prideful presumption of trying to alter what God has ordained or nature has produced or what should, for whatever reason, not be fiddled with. Sometimes the charge means not so much usurping God-like powers, but doing so in the absence of God-like knowledge. The mere playing at being God, the Hubris of acting within sufficient wisdom. Now the case for respecting Mother Nature has been successfully made by environmentalists. They urge upon us a cautionary principle regarding our intervention in all of nature usually by the way, with the inexplicable exception of our own nature. Go slowly, you can ruin everything. The point is well taken. The human body and mind highly complex and delicately balanced as a result of ions of gradual and exacting evolution almost certainly is a risk from any ill-considered attempt at improvement. There is not only the matter of unintended consequences already noted, but also the question about the unqualified goodness of our goals, something to which I will return.

A very interesting version of the Hubris objection has been offered by one of my colleagues, Michael Sandel, in a working paper he prepared for the Council. What is wrong with biotechnological efforts and enhancement and recreating ourselves, is what Sandel calls, "Hyper-agency, a promethean aspiration to remake nature including human nature to serve our purposes and to satisfy our desires." The difficulty, Sandel suggests, seems to be both cognitive and moral. "The failure properly to appreciate and respect the giftedness of the world." I quote him. "To acknowledge the giftedness of life is to recognize that our talents and powers are not wholly of our own doing or even fully ours, despite the efforts we expand to develop and to exercise them. It is also to recognize that not everything in the world is open to any use we may desire or devise. An appreciation of the giftedness of life constrains the promethean project and conduces to a certain humility. It is in part a religious sensibility, but its resonance reaches beyond religion."

As a critique of the promethean attitude of the enhancers, Sandel's suggestion is on target. On the side of manipulator appreciating that the given world as well as his natural powers to alter it, are not of his own making, could induce an attitude of modesty, restraint, and humility. But the giftedness of nature also includes smallpox and malaria, cancer and Alzheimer disease, decline and decay. And to repeat, nature is not equally generous with her gifts, even to human beings, the most gifted of her creatures.

Modesty board of gratitude for the world's giftedness may enable us to recognize that not everything in the world is open to any use we may desire or devise, but it will not by itself, teach us which things can be fiddled with and which should be left inviolate. The mere giftedness of things cannot tell us which gifts are to be accepted as is, which are to be improved through use or training, which are to be housebroken through self-command and medication, and which oppose like the plague.

The word given has two meanings, the second of which Sandel's account omits. Given does mean bestowed as a gift, but given as in mathematical proofs means something granted, something definitely fixed and specifies. Most of the given bestowed of nature have their species specific given natures. They are each and all of the given sort. Cockroaches and human beings are equally bestowed, but differently natured. To turn a man into a cockroach would be dehumanizing. To try to turn him into more than a man might be so as well. To avoid this therefore, we need more than a generalized appreciation for nature's gifts. We need a particular regard and respect for the special gifts that belong to our own given nature.

In short, only if there is a human giveness that is also good and worth respecting, either as we find it or as it could be perfected without ceasing to be itself does the given serve as a positive guide for choosing what to alter and what to leave alone. Only if there is something precious in the given beyond the mere fact of its giftedness, does what is given serve as a source of restraint against efforts that would hubristically degrade it.

Coming then to the human biotechnical engineering, only if there is something inherently good or dignified about say, natural procreation human finitude, the human life cycle, and human erotic longing and striving. Only if there is something inherently good or dignified about the ways in which we engage the world as spectators and appreciators, teachers and learners, leaders and followers, agents and bakers, lovers and friends, parents and children, and as seekers of our own special excellence and flourishing, in whatever areas to which we are called, only then can we begin to see why those aspects of nature need to be defended.

I move then from this hubristic attitude of the powerful designer to look at the proposed improvements as they impinge upon the nature of the ones being improved. But the question of human nature and human dignity in mind, I move to the question of the means and then to the ends.

Part four, Unnatural Means. The Dignity of Human Activity. How do and how should the excellent ones become excellent? This is a notorious question made famous by Plato's Meno at the start of the dialogue baring his name. "Can you tell me Socrates, whether human excellence is teachable, or is it not teachable, but be it to be acquired by practice or training? Or is it neither acquired by practice nor by learning, but does it originate in human beings by nature or in some other way." Teaching and learning practice and training, sources in our power. Natural gift or divine dispensation, sources not in our power. Until only yesterday, these exhausted the sometimes competing, sometimes complimentary alternatives for acquiring human excellence perfecting our natural gifts by our own efforts. But perhaps no longer. Biotechnology now may be able to do nature one better, even to the point of requiring no teaching and less training or practice to permit an improved nature to sign forth. The insertion of the growth factor gene into the muscles of rats and likes, bulks them up and keeps them strong and sound without the need for nearly as much exertion. Drugs to improve memory, alertness, and amiability could greatly relieve the need for exertion to acquire these powers leaving time and effort for better things.

Some people not thinking very hard will object to these means because they are artificial, unnatural. But the manmade origin of the means cannot be the problem. Beginning with the needle in the fig leaf, man has from the start been the animal that uses art to improve his lot. Supplementing healthy diet, rest, and exercise, ordinary medicine makes extensive use of artificial means from drugs to surgery to mechanical implants. If the use of artificial means is absolutely welcome in the activity of healing, it cannot be there unnaturalness alone that upsets us when they are used to make people better than well.

Yet in those areas of human life in which excellence is until now been achieved only by discipline and effort, the attainment of those achievement by means of drugs, genetic engineering, or implanted devices looks to many people to be cheating or cheap. We believe or until yesterday, believed that people should work hard for their achievements. Nothing good comes easily. Even if one prefers the grace of the natural athlete whose performance that deceptably appears to be effortless, we admire those who overcome obstacles and struggle to try to achieve the excellence of the former who serves at the object of the latter's aspiration and effort and the standard for his success or failure.

This matter of character, the merit of discipline and dedicated striving, though not the deepest basis of one's objection to biological shortcuts, is surely pertinent. For character is not only the source of our deeds, but also their product. People whose destructive behavior is remedied by pacifying drugs rather than by their own efforts are not learning self-control. If anything they are learning to think it is unnecessary. People who take pills to block out from memory the painful or hateful aspects of a new experience will not learn how to deal with suffering or sorrow. A drug to induce fearlessness does not produce courage. Yet, things are not so simple, hardly because there are non-therapeutic interventions that may assist us in the pursuit of excellence without cheapening its attainment partly because so many of life's excellences have nothing to do with competition or adversity. Drugs that decrease drowsiness or increase alertness, sharpen memory or reduce distraction, they actually help people pursue their natural goals of learning or painting or performing their duties. Drugs to steady the hand of a neurosurgeon or to prevent sweaty palms in a concert pianist can't be regarded as cheating, for they are not the source of the excellent activity or achievement. And for people dealt a meager hand in the dispensing of nature's gifts, it should not be called cheating or cheap, if biotechnology could assist them in becoming better equipped whether in body or in mind.

Even steroids for the perveriable 97 pound weakling helps him get to the point where through his own effort and training, he can go head to head with the naturally better endowed.

Nevertheless, there is one sense where the issue of naturalness of means matters. It lies not in the fact that the assisting drugs and devices are artifacts, but in their relation to the nature of human activity. Here in my opinion, is one of the more profound ways in which the use of at least some of these biotechnological means of seeking perfection, those that would work on the brain, come under grave suspicion as a possible violation or deformation of the deep character of natural human activity. In most of our efforts in self-improvement either by practice or training or study, we sense the relation between our doings and the resulting improvement between the means used and the ends sought. There is an experiential and intelligible connection between means and ends. We can see how confronting fearful things might eventually enable us to cope with our fears. We can see how curbing our appetites produce self-command. The capacity to be improved is improved by using it. The deed to be perfected is perfected by doing it. Human education ordinarily proceeds by speech or symbolic deeds whose meanings are at least in principle directly accessible to those upon whom they work. Even where the human being is largely patient to the formative action, say in receiving praise and blame, a reward and punishment, both the teacher and the student can understand both the content of the means used and the relation to the conduct of the activity that they are meant to improve.

The further efforts of self-improvement spurred by praise and blame, will clearly be the students own doing.

In contract, biomedical interventions act directly on the human body and mind to bring about their affects on a subject who is not merely

Biotechnology and the Pursuit of Perfection, 2003

passive, but who plays no role at all. In addition, he can at best feel their affects without understanding their meaning in human terms. Thus, a drug that brightened our mood would alter us without our understanding how and why it did so. Where as a mood brightened as a fitting response to the arrival of a loved one or an achievement in one's work, is perfectly because humanly intelligible. Not only would this be true about our states of mind, all our encounters with the world, both natural and interpersonal would be mediated, filtered, and altered. Human experience under biological interventions becomes increasingly mediated by unintelligible forces and vehicles separated from the human significance of the activity so altered. The relations between the knowing subject and his activities and between his activities and their fulfillments and pleasures are threatened with disruption. The importance of the human effort and human achievement now is properly acknowledged. The point is less the exertions of good character against hardship, but more the manifestations of an alert and self-experiencing agent making his or her deeds flow intentionally from his or her willing knowing and embodied soul.

To be sure an increasing portion of modern life is mediated life. The way we encounter space and time, the way we reach out and touch somebody by the telephone and the Internet. And one can met a case that there are changes in our souls and dehumanizing losses that accompany the great triumphs of modern technology. But so long as those technologies do not write themselves directly into our bodies and minds, we are in principle able to see them working on us and free again in principle to walk away from their use albeit sometimes with very great effort. However, once they work on us, we are as it were passive subjects of what might as well be magic. The same point--well, let me skip this and go to the end.

In a word, one of the major truples of biotechnical improvers is that they produce changes in us by disrupting the normal character of human being at work in the world. What Aristotle called the activity of the soul, which when fine and full, constitutes human flourishing. With biotechnical interventions that skip the realm of intelligible meaning, we cannot really own the transformations nor experience them as genuinely ours. And we will be at a loss to attest whether the resulting conditions and activities of our bodies and our minds are in the fullest sense our own as human.

Finally, the last section, Partial Ends, Full Flourishing. In this concluding section I want to raise briefly some questions about the ends that we have isolated for consideration, ageless bodies, happy souls. What do we think about these goals? Would their attainment in fact improve or perfect our lives as human beings? These are very big questions too long to be properly treated here, but let this be an opening.

The case for ageless bodies seems at first glance to look pretty good. The prevention of decay, decline, and disability, the avoidance of blindness, deafness, and ability, the elimination of feebleness, frailty, and fatigue, all seem to be conducive to living fully as a human being at the top of ones powers of having as they say, a good quality of life from beginning to end. We have come to expect organ transplantation for our worn out parts. We will surely welcome stem cell based therapies for regenerative medicine, reversing by replacement the damaged tissues of Parkinson's disease, spinal cord injury, and many other degenerative disorders. It is hard to see any objection to obtaining in our youth, the genetic enhancement of all of our muscles that would not only prevent the muscular feebleness of old age, but would empower us to do any physical task with much greater strength and facility throughout our lives. And should aging research deliver on its promise of not only adding extra life to years, but extra years to life, who would refuse it? And even if you might consider turning down an ageless body for yourself, would you not want it for your beloved? Why should she not remain to you as she was back then when she first stole your heart? Why should her body suffer the ravages of time?

To say no to this offer seems perverse, but let me suggest that it is not. Because this argument is so counterintuitive, we need to begin not with the individual choice for an ageless body, but to look at what an individual's life would look like in a world in which everybody made the same choice. We need to make the choice universal to see the meaning of that choice in the mirror of its becoming the norm.

What if everybody lived life to the hilt even as they approached an ever receding age of death in a body that looked and functioned, let us not be too greedy, like that of a 30 year old? Would it be good if each and all of us lived like light bulbs burning brightly from beginning to end, but then popping off without warning leaving those around us suddenly in the dark? Or is it perhaps better that there is a shape to life, everything in its due season? The shape also written as it were into the wrinkles of our bodies that live it. What would the relations between the generations be like if there never came a point at which a son surpassed his father in strength or vigor? What incentive would there be for the old to make way for the young, if the old slowed down but little and had no reason to think of retiring? If Michael could play until he was not 40, but 80. And might not even a more moderate prolongation of lifespan with vigor lead to a prolongation in the young a functional and maturity of the sort that is arguably already accompanied the great increase in average life expectancy experienced in the last century? One cannot think of enhancing the vitality of the old without retarding the maturation of the young.

I have tried elsewhere to make a rational case for the blessings of finitude in an essay called, *L'chaim and Its Limits, Why Not Immortality?* It is a chapter in my book, *Life, Liberty, and the Defense of Dignity.* I suggest there that living with our finitude is the condition for the possibility of many of the best things in human life, engagement, seriousness, a taste for beauty, a possibility of sacrifice and virtue, the ties born of procreation, the quest for meaning. Though the arguments there are made against the case for immortality they have some weight even against the modest proengation of the maximum lifespan, especially in good health that would permit us to live as if there were always tomorrow. And what I take to be the most important argument of that essay, I argue that the pursuit of perfect bodies and further life extension will deflect us from realizing more fully the aspirations to which our lives naturally point from living well rather than merely staying alive. And I argue that a concern with ones own improving agelessness is finally incompatible with accepting the need for procreation and human renewal. A world of longevity is increasingly a world inhospitable to children.

What would be needed to complete this argument about the pursuit of ageless bodies would be an attempt to say something about the goodness of the natural life cycle, roughly three multiples of a generation, a time of coming of age, a time of flourishing, ruling, and replacing of one's self, a time of savoring and understanding, but still sufficiently and intimately linked to one's descendents to care about their future and to take a guiding and supporting and sharing role. People who think about life extension think about time the way the physicists do as simply a continuum in which each part is identical. That is not live time, which is choreographed time, shape time. It has a beginning and a middle and an end and the question is whether that shape has a kind of meaning and whether adding more years to the continuum could deform that meaning. A long question, I don't have the answer.

Finally, what about as pharmacologically assisted happy souls? Painful and shameful memories are disquieting, guilty consciences disturbs sleep, low self-esteem, melancholy and world-weariness besmirch the waking hours. Why not memory blockers for the former, mood brighteners for the latter, and a good euphoriant without the risks of hangover or cirrhosis when celebratory occasions fail to be jolly. For, let us be clear, if it is imbalances of neurotransmitters, a modern equivalent for the medieval doctrine of the four humors that are responsible for our state of soul, it would be sheer priggishness to refuse the help of pharmacology for our happiness when we accepted guiltlessly to correct for an absence of insulin or thyroid hormone. An attempted answer to this question comes in three parts.

First, I would suggest that there really is something wrong with the pursuit of utter psychic tranquility with the attempt to eliminate shame, guilt, and all painful memories. Traumatic memories, shame and guilt are, it is true, psychic pains. In extreme doses, they can be crippling. Yet, they are also appropriate responses to horror, disgraceful conduct, and injustice. Once again, the point is the fitness of awareness and emotional response. Witnessing a murder should be remembered as horrible. Doing a beastly deed should trouble one's soul. Righteousness and indignation and injustice depends on being able to feel injustice's sting. An untroubled soul in a troubling world is a shrunken human being. Or fundamentally to deprive oneself of one's memory in its truthfulness also a feeling is to deprive oneself of one's own life and identity.

Second, the positive feeling states of soul, though perhaps accompaniments of human flourishing are not in fact the essence of human flourishing. Pleasure or feelings of self-esteem are not the real McCoy. They are at most but shadows divorced from the links to the underlying human activities that are the essence of flourishing. Not even the most doctrinaire hedonist wants to have the pleasures that come from playing baseball without swinging the bat or catching the ball. No music lover would be satisfied with getting from a pill the pleasure of listening to Mozart without ever hearing the music. Most people want to feel good and to feel good about themselves, but only as a result of being good, doing good, and experiencing what is fine.

Finally, there is a connection between the possibility of feeling deep unhappiness and the prospects for genuine happiness. If one cannot grieve, one has not loved and to be capable of aspiration, one must know and feel lack. As Wallace Stevens put it, "Not to have is the beginning of desire." There is in short a double-barreled error in the pursuit of ageless bodies and factitiously happy souls. Human fulfillment depends on our being creatures of need and finitude and hence beings of longings and attachments.

To sum up then, I have tried to make a case for finitude and even graceful decay of bodily powers. And I have tried to make a case for genuine human happiness with satisfaction as the bloom that graces unimpeded soul- exercising activities. The first argument resonates with

Ageless Bodies, Happy Souls:

Homeric and Hebraic intuitions; the second, with Greek philosophers. One would like to think that they might even be connectable, that the idea of genuine human flourishing is rooted in this aspiration that is born of the kind of deficiencies that come from our being limited and imperfect bodily beings.

To close then, let me suggest that a flourishing human life is not a life lived with an ageless body or untroubled soul. But rather a life lived in rhythm time mindful of times limits appreciative of each season and filled first of all with those intimate human relations that are ours only because we are born, age, replace ourselves, decline and die, and know it. It is a life of aspiration made possible by and born of experience lack of the disproportion between the transcendent longings of the soul and the limited capacities of our bodies and minds. It is a life that stretches towards some fulfillment toward which our natural human soul has been oriented and unless we extirpate the source, will always be oriented. It is a life not of better genes and enhancing chemicals, but of love and friendship, song and dance, speech and deed, working and learning, revering and worshiping. The pursuit of an ageless body is finally a distraction and a deformation. The pursuit of an untroubled and self-satisfied soul is deadly to desire. Finitude recognized Spur's aspiration. And fine aspiration acted upon, is itself the course of happiness, not the agelessness of the body nor the contentment of the soul or even the list of external achievements and accomplishments of life that fill out a curriculum vitae, but the engaged and energetic being at work of what nature uniquely gave to us is what we need to treasure and defend against the devilish promise of technological perfection.

Thank you for your attention and patience.

Academic Science and Entrepreneurship: Are the Conflicts Reconcilable? 2004

Sheldon Krimsky, Ph.D., Professor, Department of Urban and Environmental Policy and Planning, Tufts University

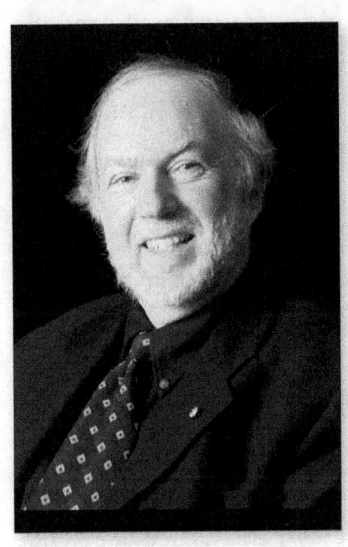

First, I want to thank Dr. Margolis and all the other wonderful hosts who have made me feel at home here at the University of Michigan. It is a distinct pleasure to be the ninth lecturer at the Waggoner Lecture and to be joining many of the other fine people who have been part of this series. I think the Waggoner family deserves some credit for their insights into understanding the importance of ethics in medicine and ethics in public life and the professions in general in supporting this series.

I'd like to start with a warning about the commercialization of academia. Thurston Devlin, students do not read him very much any more, but some of you who have been around for a few decades, may remember that name--a wonderful sociologist. He wrote, "It appears then that the intrusion of business principles in the universities goes to weaken and retard the pursuit of learning and therefore to defeat the ends for which a university is maintained." That's 1919. There were already some things going on then. Almost a hundred years ago, where the warning signs were issued about the possibility of the intrusion of commercial interest into the universities, and many of the universities were structured to try to insulate themselves from just those interests. There is nothing wrong with commercial interest. The issue is whether or not the missions of for-profit companies and the missions of universities should be elided, that is, combined in too close a fashion. That's one of the issues I will be dealing with today.

The second warning came in 1968 from James Ridgeway in a book called, *The Closed University*. In recent years professors have started a number of new kinds of companies involved in social problem solving. The idea that the university is the community of scholars is a myth. As power brokers, the professors act with one hand on the university and the other in a big corporation. They move in and out using their prestige as scholars to advance interests of the company or on the other hand using their influence with the company to help the university get research funds.

Ridgeway wrote this at a time that economics was setting up private consulting firms while holding onto academic posts. I'm going to be talking more about what is happening in the biomedical sciences and in medicine. And 1980 seems to have been a critical year. It was the year that Nature Magazine put out a special issue called the Biobusiness. But it is a year that contains many factors that influence the commercialization of the biomedical sciences. And let me explain a little of the background of that.

Late 1970s and early 1980s, there was a view by the Office of Science and Technology Policy in the United States and the Executive Branch and Congress that the U.S. was losing its competitive advantage with respect to other industrial nations. And that competitive advantage was lost not in terms of discovery, but in terms of turning discovery into marketable commercial products. So the theory was that if we could figure out a way to get the universities to move their discoveries faster into commerce, then we would be able to meet the competitive challenges that we faced from other industrial nations. And it was an interesting idea and there was a lot of public policy that was developed to

Are the Conflicts Reconcilable? 2004

foster this idea. And it was considered to be a win-win situation for all involved. That is, the university would win because there would be new streams of income coming to the university from business partnerships. The faculty would win because they would be able to increase their own funding base and perhaps even their own salaries. They would be able to get a piece of the intellectual property. The government would win because it would be able to foster technology transfer in the way that it thought would keep the United States competitive. Companies would win because they would be able to get close access to path breaking research and also get intellectual property ownership of new discoveries. So it looked like everyone was going to win. The problem was that they didn't begin to account for some of the unforeseen effects; although, some of us began to foresee some of the effects early on, the effects of too close a merger between the mission of the university and the mission of for-profit companies.

So what I have listed on the screen are some of the policies that were developed and legal issues. For example, in 1980 the Supreme Court issued a ruling called Diamond vs. Shark Reverdie, in which they ruled that life forms could be patented. What was unique about that ruling is that up until 1980, if you had a bacteria or a virus or even a cell line that you wanted to patent, it would have to be part of a process. You would have to show that the entity wanted a patent was part of a process and you would have to show the utility and the uniqueness of the process. But that nobody had total monopoly control over the organism or the cell line. They only had control over that entity as part of a process.

Actually, the organism in question that prompted that Supreme Court decision was a genetically modified bacterium that would degrade hydrocarbons that was supposed to be used in oil spills. And General Electric, which was the employer of Shark Reverdie, they were very easily given a patent for the process of the organism and the method of applying it. But where the controversy was, whether they should have a complete patent so egenerous, that is for everything possible of the organism itself for whatever other uses it might be placed and that was the big decision and the Supreme Court ruled in favor of that in 1980. As a result of that, a cascading set of events took place and the Patent and Trademark Office of the United States then began giving out patents for genetically modified animals and genetically modified bacterium of all sorts. And even genes themselves, so that our genome, sections of our genome were patented. And that means that if somebody has a patent on a segment of genomic material which we all share, that anyone else who wants to use that material, that genomic segment, has to pay licensing fees to the patent owner. This might sound strange to many of us since the human genome is not a manufactured entity. It is actually something that we all carry around. It looks like it might be a public good, but you would have to understand the logic of patenting because of the patent laws not only allow the patents for manufactured goods, but they also allow for patenting for the discovery of things. So if you discover a microorganism in the soil by some ingenious process, even though you haven't transformed the microorganism, you can take out a patent on it.

So 1980 essentially created a gold rush of entrepreneurship. I mean, imagine every university at that time, every major university was sequencing genes. I mean, molecular genetics became one of the lead areas of research at all the global universities, the world-class universities. So that means that every researcher at every university who was sequencing genes became an instant entrepreneur in a sense because every gene set they sequence, you could take out a patent for. And essentially that is what created this commercialization rush at many of the universities. I hope I've explained it simply enough.

Well, then there was the Bayh-Dole Act of 1980, also that same year. The federal government gave up all intellectual property to the university, the investigator, and their business partners from discoveries derived from federally sponsored grants. The government said, "Well, the society would be better off if we did not hold onto the intellectual property, so we will give it up." So in other words, our public funds go into

Are the Conflicts Reconcilable? 2004

grant research, somebody makes a discovery from public monies and the government says, "Well, those discoveries should be now the private property of the discoverers of the institution." And it was a good thing for universities because it was another income stream for universities and for the biotechnology industry and for molecular geneticists who could make money also on the patents of their discoveries. There was a lot of money to be made because of the Bayh-Dole Act.

Also there were revisions of the tax codes in 1980 and the development of instruments for creating incentives for companies to invest in university campuses with special tax shelters. There was also an executive order extending the Bayh-Dole Act from small businesses to industry as a whole. First it was designed to help small businesses, but then it covered all the industry. These were just a few of the new incentives for trying to create a greater proximity between commercial businesses and universities. Well, notwithstanding the optimism about the win-win situation or the triple win situation, they were beginning to see some indicators of change. Of course, there was greater corporate investment in the university research that we could expect. Overall contributions of industry-funded R&D rose from 3.5 percent in the 1970s to nearly 8 percent in 2000, so more than doubling of the industry-funded universities. And the top ten industry-funded institutions saw rapid increases in the ratio of industry to non-industry-funded R&D.

Some universities that I studied began to show a percentage of their R&D to be between 30 and 40 percent of their total R&D came from the private sector. And that begins to change the complexion and the ethos of a campus when that kind of ratio of corporate to non-corporate funding enters the university. In 1965 universities received 96 patents from academic discoveries. In 2000, universities were awarded 3,200 patents. Again, if you are an intellectual property office that is an indicator of the success of the Bayh-Dole Act. If you are concerned that these new patents are going to create all kinds of problems in the universities, then that is an indicator of other kinds of changes.

For example, there is no research exclusion for patent infringement. If you are a researcher and you want to do some work on some genetic sequence, there is no enacted exclusion for you that you can use this sequence or a transgenic animal, for example, for research. There is no exclusion for patent infringement for you even though you don't plan to commercialize any of that entity. This was clearly indicated in a case where a group of researchers at the University of Pennsylvania were using the BRCA, that is the Breast Cancer gene, BRCA1 and 2. These were two genetic sequences, which have shown to indicate a much higher risk of breast cancer. These researchers wanted to use these sequences to do some research on developing better indicators, warning signs for breast cancer. And they were told by the company that had a patent on the BRC1 and the BRC2 gene, that they could not use this genetic sequence without actually paying royalties to the company. And some of these royalties were high enough to discourage them from doing the research. So what is a university for if it cannot do research without having to pay royalties to people whom presumably own a piece of our collective knowledge? I mean, the genome, the human genome should be part of the public commons. It is something that we all can benefit from; just the knowledge of the human genome. And we are finding now that the universities have become little commercial sectors trying to protect their own intellectual property.

Increasingly universities are equity partners in professor-initiated companies creating a complex of institutional and faculty conflicts of interest. What do we mean by conflict of interest? Well, Thompson at Harvard defined a conflict of interest as a "set of conditions in which professional judgment concerning a primary interest, such as patient's welfare or the validity of research tends to be unduly influenced by a secondary interest, such as financial gain." Well, Thompson doesn't, in his definition, answer the question, "What do you mean, 'tends to influence' gives the impression of influencing, can be construed to influence, gives the appearance of conflicting roles or does influence?" These are

Are the Conflicts Reconcilable? 2004

very important in trying to weed out what the essential meaning of conflict of interest really is. And of course Thompson's definition of conflict of interest only dealt with individual conflict of interest. We have not yet framed a good definition of institutional conflict of interest and yet, as I pointed out, the institutions are very much involved in the commercialization of the discoveries coming out of those institutions.

When did conflict of interest become important in science? I have to say before 1980, you would not hear the word scientist and conflict of interest. It just was never heard in the same breath. You could not find any literature on it and there was no research on it. During the 1980s as I've indicated, the life sciences in the United States became heavily commercialized. Before that, if you were entering the field of biology, there really was not much commercial value for you to enter that field. You entered that field because of your primary interest in learning about the nature of life and building new knowledge in the field of the biological sciences or in medicine. But after recombinant DNA was discovered, it was very soon after the discovery in 1973 of taking genes from one organism and putting into another. It became very evident that we have created the possibility of manufacturing proteins and some of that has been extraordinarily useful in medicine.

One study I did, 34 percent of the articles in 14 leading science and medical journals had at least one lead author with a financial interest in the work. It was a simple question. I wanted to know at that time, and this was in the early 90s, what is the probably that if you picked out an article in a journal that the lead authors would have a--I'm not talking about conflict of interest, I'm just talking about the lead authors having a financial interest in the subject matter of the research. So as we often find it is much easier to ask questions than to answer them. It took me about two years with a collaborator from UCLA to answer this question and we answered the question for a set of objective indicators. And we found out that the answer was 34 percent. So one out of the three articles in these 14 very high profile journals had a financial interest in the work.

Academic Science and Entrepreneurship:

And I think the scientific world was rather surprised that it was so high; although, some people said, "No, I think it should be higher than that."

I remember Nature wrote an editorial about that finding and they basically said, "Well, we understand that this is happening in biomedical science, but unless the authors of this study can show that these financial interests have any impact on the outcome of the research, we will continue in not requiring any disclosure from our authors of articles." So Nature was the last holdout of all the major journals to withstand any disclosure requirements in that journal. Five years later, same editor, they came out and they said, "Well, I think we changed our minds and now we also are going to require the disclosure of author's financial interest."

A survey of 1,849 biomedical scientists indicated that 35 percent were engaged in commercial activities. So no one doubted that this was a phenomena that was really entrenched in the new biomedical arena. And there was a new ethos that was described to me by one Nobel laureate who said to me that, "Our obligation now is not only to pursue knowledge about the biological world, but to market and develop that knowledge and to transfer that knowledge." And that was a very different ethos than we had for decades before when people at universities felt that their primary and exclusive responsibility was in the production of knowledge.

Studies in the commercialization of science have appeared. A survey of life science companies reported that 92 percent sponsored academic research and of course, they were stimulated by all the federal incentive programs. The Association of University Technology managers reported that 124 of its 183 member institutions held equity in businesses that fund research performed at the same institution. That is a new phenomena where universities are now equity holders in companies that do research at their institutions. Someday, some university with those equity interests is going to be party to some litigation. It hasn't happened yet, not in any big way, but if one of the universities, for example, had some equity interests in Vioxx, those trial lawyers looking around for deep pockets, they are not only going to be looking at the pharmaceutical

Are the Conflicts Reconcilable? 2004

companies, but they will be looking at the universities where there are some deep pockets. So far, the universities have gotten away from any of these major class action suits with respect to products, but it is a real possibility given the environment that we are in.

Now, I'm going to pose the devil's advocate question as I've done in my book because I began asking myself this question. What is wrong with scientists having commercial interest? I mean, let's be self critical I said. What difference does it make from whom scientists obtain their funding to what companies they consult or in what firms they have equity? The universally held norms of scientific inquiry in pursuit of the truth make other relationships irrelevant as long as scientists are totally and uncompromisingly invested in that pursuit. A scientist who violates the cannons of his or her profession simply to satisfy a sponsor would soon become a pariah. And that is a possible way of thinking about this. I think many scientists do view that. They see things like disclosure as a form of political correctness. They may agree to it, but they do not see it as a way of enhancing scientific integrity of any sort. And if it's political correctness, then that is a very different kind of ethics than if there were some other more fundamental ethical problem associated with the mixing of commerce and science.

And that is really what I want to talk about here about the possibility of mixing commerce and science and the reasons for concern over scientist's conflict of interest. I break them up into four issues. The first is stewardship. The second is consequentialism, which is the impacts of the commercial interests and what it might do to science. The third is transparency that there is something about openness as a virtue in and of itself, and the fourth is scientific integrity, the loss of the norm of disinterestedness and the appearance of objectivity. These are four potential ethical concerns.

Let me start with the stewardship. Government conflict of interest rules are based upon the stewardship notion. Government employees are stewards of the public policies, its laws, and regulations. We require government leaders to divest themselves of their financial interests when they are in a government position. We do not trust that they will make necessarily a decision that will not be based upon their financial holdings. So Vice President Cheney, for example, has to put his holdings in the energy field into some blind trust, etcetera, etcetera. And there are legal constraints against conflicting rules in government. And there are moral grounds for conflict of interest prevention. We do not wait for the members of government to disclose. We act on a different set of principles, namely prevention.

Well, that is the stewardship model because again, government employees are stewards of the public's policies, its laws, its regulations, its lands, etcetera. So you do not want a government employee making a decision about foresting on government property when that person has an interest in the foresting industry, in the paper industry. That would be an obvious example of where this stewardship model applies. The issue is the stewardship does not fit science very well. Scientists are not stewards of the public laws and regulations. You could say that scientists are stewards of the money they get from government. It is a very restricted notion. They have to use the grant in an honorable way and in a way that meets their intentions when they write the grant proposal. But it simply does not seem to fit the stewardship model.

In Andrew Stark's book, *The Anatomy of Conflict of Interest*, he breaks conflict of interest down to three stages. There are the antecedent acts. These are the factors that condition the state of mind toward partiality. You might say even small gifts can begin to condition the mind and there is a lot of research now in social psychology because I know the AMA, for example, has a guideline that says gifts under a hundred dollars do not matter. But that is not what the social psychologists tell us in their research that small gifts can condition the state of mind toward partiality. These are the antecedent acts and then Stark says, "And the next stage are the states of mind. These are the effected sentiments, the dispositions, the proclivities conditioned by the antecedent acts." And then there is finally the behavior of partiality, the outcome behavior

Are the Conflicts Reconcilable? 2004

from altered states of minds. Stark says, "Because we cannot prevent officials from mentally taking notice of their own interests, we prohibit the act of holding certain kinds of interests in the first place." And this really does fit very well the stewardship concept of conflict of interest. That you really operate at the federal level in preventing the antecedent acts and the journalists, who have high standards, also operate at the level of antecedent acts. They will not take anything from anyone they interview. They won't take a meal. They won't take a cup of coffee. You interview somebody, you are a professional, and you do not want to have any interests at all in the people or person you are interviewing. So there are some professions that take this model very seriously.

So we go back then to if the question of stewardship is not really appropriate--well, let us take a look at consequentialism. And that is, does it make any difference to the field of science if you have financial conflicts of interest? After all, we are all invested in the integrity of science and in the quality of science, so is there any evidence that privately funded studies tend to draw a pro-industry conclusions? Is there a funding effect in science? Again, as I've said this afternoon, I do not have to argue about this in the tobacco company research because there is a rich body of evidence that the tobacco company manufactured research for 50 years and because of the litigation, because of the class action suits, it is now all online. Tens of thousands of documents that any of us can actually look at and observe to look at what was behind the class action, the memoranda and the strategies of the tobacco company to manufacture research. We will also find the same if we studied lead research. The lead industry has for many years tried to argue with highly paid researchers, some of them at prestigious universities that lead in gasoline, that lead in paint is not detrimental to human health and really doesn't affect the cognition of small children despite the growing body of research that shows that lead is highly dangerous, especially to the young growing brain.

Pesticide research, you will find the same. There are no pesticide companies that ever fund research that shows that pesticides are dangerous to human health. If anything, they try to buy up the data of research they fund so that the data will not be published. Tyrone Hays at Berkeley at the University of California actually got into a recent conflict with a company that funded his research over an herbicide and the company offered him a sizeable sum of money to buy the data so that he would not publish it. Tyrone Hays refused the money.

Of course the drug research is an area that is close to all of us. It would certainly be dishonorable to imagine that conflict of interest affected the quality of drug research, but regrettably the research that has been done shows that is in fact what is happening. So consequentialism is in fact a strong ethical factor in looking at conflict of interest in science. The outcome of the research is going to be affected. Trade secrecy has become more prevalent in universities. Surveys indicate that between 12 to 34 percent of academic researchers have been denied access to other research results. Not to their research; to the research results of others. Faculty with industry support were four times as likely to report trade secrets as other faculty. So universities have become little enclaves of proprietary information, which we thought was something that was only prevalent in the business sector. There have been studies done that indicate that where the funding comes from affects people's attitudes toward the products they are testing. This was a case I mentioned previously today about authors who have financial relationships with manufacturers of calcium channel antagonists. Those with those relationships were much less likely to be critical of the dangers of those drugs.

Marsha Angel stated at a conference in Washington, "In my two decades at the New England Journal of Medicine, it was my clear impression that papers submitted by authors with financial conflicts of interest were far more likely to be biased in both design and in interpretation." She is not the only person that has made that judgment. Other editors and some of the editors are taking a very tough stance now on conflict of interest. Another article which suggests that there is a funding effect, this was published in the *Journal of the American Medical Association*,

Are the Conflicts Reconcilable? 2004

"Strong and consistent evidence shows that industry sponsored research tends to draw a pro-industry conclusions." And the studies go on and on about that. So consequentialism is an important ethical issue. When the consequences of someone's action leads to an impairment of the knowledge that we all share, then that is a serious problem and has to be addressed. So far we really do not know how to address that problem because we just assume that scientists are operating on the norms of disinterestedness and trustworthiness and we do not know how to explain this funding effect in science.

The management of conflict of interest is left to each academic institution and there are varied policies. If you go from institution to institution, you will see a tremendous difference in the policies and after all, the institutions have a vested and self-interest in making sure that anyone who has money to bring into the institution, that that money gets brought in. So they certainly do not like to reject funding. Some institutions, for example, will not take tobacco money as a primary norm, but beyond that there are very few restrictions on funds that go in. I should say that after some problem grants, many universities will not take any contracts from private sector with restrictions on publication. And I think that is a must. There should be no restrictions on whether or not the results of research should be published.

The clinical researcher has formed a partnership with a drug company on a new AIDS vaccine. The research is institutional so has an equity interest in the vaccine. The company is funding a clinical trial on the vaccine. What ethical consideration should be considered in managing this conflict of interest? Between the investigator and the human subjects and between the institution and the human subjects? This is a hotly debated issue currently. Some institutions are saying we will not permit an investigator with a financial interest in the drug or drug device to be part of the clinical trial. And some institutions say we will not have a clinical trial at our institution if our institution has a financial interest in the drug or the drug device.

Academic Science and Entrepreneurship:

Objectivity and disinterestedness, this is an issue that is also being debated. Do you really need disinterestedness that is financial disinterestedness? Can you have objectivity and not disinterestedness? Now in the 1930s, Robin Merton, eminent sociologist of science at Columbia University discussed the norm of disinterest. This is one of four norms of scientific research. Most recently John Ziman of the United Kingdom, his view was that post-academic science disinterestedness is gone, but that you could have objectivity without disinterestedness as long as scientists were skeptical and that they keep testing their results. And probably, Ziman is correct in the long run. In the long run, science is self-correcting. But in the long run, a lot of damage can be done. We have seen that happen. So science will correct itself. Vioxx will be discovered to be a problem. But the long run means that we have lives lost or we have added fatalities or morbidity and it may not be enough to say that we can have objectivity without disinterestedness.

Ziman talked about cognitive and subjective objectivity. He bemoaned the fact that in post-academic science, we no longer have subjective objectivity; that is the perception of objectivity, but he said cognitive objectivity, which is really what we are going to learn about the physical universe, our objective knowledge will get to that even though it might take us a little bit longer. That may be okay for physics, high energy physics where there are not any human factors involved, but in medical science it's not clear that we can give up the perception of objectivity and wait for science to correct itself.

So getting back to the reasons for the concern over science's conflict of interest, consequentialism still is a very lively issue because the science can be distorted from the funding effect. Transparency openness must be around. And openness can be compromised by all the stealth science that goes on at universities these days from the protection of business interests. But then there is scientific integrity, the loss of the norm of disinterestedness and the appearance of objectivity.

That is the fourth ethical issue. What value, how do we value, the appearance of objectivity in science? How do we value the appearance of disinterestedness? That does not mean that a scientist can have a pet hypothesis or a pet theory. It does not mean that psychoanalytic psychiatrists cannot differ in their view about the mental states as, let us say, a more physiologically oriented drug oriented psychiatry. Those debates will continue and those are central to the role of science. The persuasion of scientists, their attitudes, their theories, those are out in the open and that is central to the role of science. We have to have scientists competing against one another for which of their theories and hypotheses is most robust.

But the financial interests of scientists has nothing to do with science. Good science can be carried on without significant financial interest. As a matter of fact, if my arguments are correct, the science will be better without the financial interests. And there certainly will be the appearance of objectivity. The integrity of science is the ethical reason. Perhaps even upscaling any of the other ethical reasons why we should be concerned about the commercialization of science in universities if we do not want the universities to be seen as another stakeholder, just another stakeholder. There are only a few places, a few institutions-- actually, the university is probably unique amongst American institutions. Most people who work for other institutions are not free to speak out about issues. If you work for a company, you can't just speak out freely about the company or about any other company. There is a hierarchy and you can be marginalized or even fired for public speaking on issues that affect the company's business. If you are in government, you are really not free to speak out. You will be marginalized by your agency if you are critical of what that agency is doing unless you are under oath and Congressional hearing.

In a university, by its historical precedent, by its nature, I can speak out in whatever way I want. I do not represent my university. I represent myself and it is this unique institution that gives the people at universities the special status that they have as independent. They are not beholding to the institution in which they work for their right to speak freely. But if the universities turn into small little business enterprises, then the choice of faculty and the ability of faculty to be seen as independent will be lost. Faculty who have commercial interests in universities are much less likely to serve public interest roles. So when hiring, the university may ask the question, "Who should we hire?" This person is going to be working on a potential, very valuable vaccine that will bring in umpteen millions of dollars and with intellectual property. This person is going to be working on the health effects of lead in the environment and we don't see any potential for this to bring in any intellectual property--ie you can't take out any intellectual property on lead toxicity. So who are we going to hire? And if the university makes the choice that they are only going to hire people based upon their ability to bring in intellectual property, we will lose out one of the richest contributions we have to American culture. And that is public interest science at the American universities. So that is a thought that I want to leave you with. We have to protect that as a real public value in American life.

Thank you.

When Good Men and Women Do Nothing: Where Was the Voice of Medicine at Afghanistan, Guantanamo, and Abu Ghraib? 2005

Leon Eisenberg, MD., The Maude and Lillian Professor of Social Medicine and Emeritus Professor of Psychiatry, Harvard University Medical School

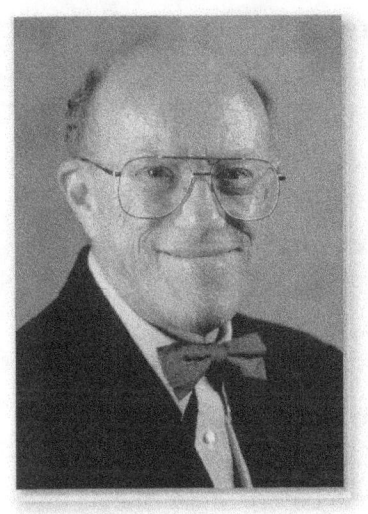

Edmund Burke, the 18th Century British statesman, is credited with having said, "The only thing necessary for the triumph of evil is that good men do nothing."

That is why the silence of military physicians at Afghanistan, Guantanamo, and Abu Ghraib is so distressing and why the failure of medical societies to condemn outright the violations of medical ethics is so appalling.

Our government has failed to acknowledge its responsibility for, and to repudiate its role in, these abuses, acts entirely foreign to the values of a democratic society and completely at odds with the traditions of our armed forces. The road to human rights violations began with President Bush's unscripted remarks calling for a "crusade", "a war on terrorism" to "rid the world of evil-doers" (Carroll 2004). Nothing is apparently impermissible in such a war: some argue that adhering to international conventions against torture ties the hands of democratic states in the fight against terrorism. Terrorists obey no

175

such constraints. Yet, in the words of Michael Ignatieff (2004): "It is the very nature of a democracy that it not only does, but should, fight with one hand tied behind its back. It is also in the nature of democracy that it prevails against its enemies precisely because it does." To the extent that we employ torture against terrorists, we have become them. The battle will be lost by joining it on those terms.

The responsibility to protest against the abuse of human rights rests with every citizen. It applies with special force to physicians who uncover abuse in the course of patient care. The physician has a duty to treat the victim **and** a duty to report the circumstances that led to the need for treatment.

It is said that, as Khrushchev took his seat after his 1956 speech to the 20th USSR Party Congress detailing Stalin's crimes, a voice called out: "And where were you, Comrade Khrushchev, when Comrade Stalin committed those atrocities?"

Khrushchev returned to the podium to ask: "Will the Comrade who put the question stand up and identify himself?"

And uneasy silence followed, Khrushchev ended the meeting by saying: "That is where I was."

Is fear the reason American doctors went along with torture in Abu Ghraib? If it is, is it an acceptable reason? I hope to persuade you that doctors should not only refuse to participate in or sanction torture, but that we are obliged to speak out against it. I will make five points:

- Torture and participation have been outlawed by the United Nations and by the United States Congress and are condemned by the ethical codes and policies of the relevant international medical bodies: the World Medical Association and the World Psychiatric Association, and by the relevant national bodies: the American Medical Association and the American Psychiatric Association.
- Despite these injunctions, there is unequivocal evidence that the U.S. military has employed torture and degrading treatment

against detainees. Some physicians in the military had to have been aware of that torture; some advised torturers how to proceed.
- The absence of a medical voice of protest is all the more distressing in view of the reservations expressed within the military itself by the Judge Advocate Generals and other officers.
- The silence of American physicians and professional organizations stands in contrast to the courage demonstrated in other countries where doctors were at far greater risk to their careers and personal freedoms.
- We must affirm that doctors serve health, not war, and give care to enemy and ally alike. In war, medical neutrality must be preserved.

The Universal Declaration of Human Rights, adopted by the UN in 1948, states that:
- "No one shall be subjected to torture or to cruel, inhuman or degrading treatment or punishment" (Article 5).
- Article II of the 1985 UN Convention Against Torture states that: "No exceptional circumstance whatsoever, whether a state of war or a threat of war, internal political instability, or any other public emergency, may be invoked as a justification for torture."
- The United Nation's Principles of Medical Ethics relevant o the Role of Health Personnel, particularly Physicians, in the Protection of Prisoners and Detainees against Torture (Resolution 37/104), was adopted by the General Assembly in 1982. The principles were prepared by the Council of International Organizations of Medical Sciences and approved by the Executive Committee of the World Health Organization. They provide that "It is a gross contravention of medical ethics, as well as an offence under applicable international instruments, for health personnel, particularly physicians, to engage, actively or passively, in acts which constitute participation in, complicity in, incitement to, or attempts to commit torture."

- The World Medical Association's Declaration of Tokyo adopted in 1975, states in its preamble that: "the utmost respect for human life is to be maintained even under threat, and no use made of any medical knowledge contrary to the laws of humanity". The declaration prohibits the physician from being "present during any procedure during which torture or any other forms of cruel, inhuman, or degrading treatment is used or threatened." It concludes with: "The World Medical Association will support… the doctor and his or her family in the face of threats or reprisals resulting from a refusal to condone the use of torture…"
- The World Psychiatric Association, in its declaration of Hawaii, adopted in 1977 and revised in 1983, insists that: "The psychiatrist must never use his professional possibilities to violate the dignity or human rights of any individual or group" and that: "Whatever the psychiatrist has been told by the patient, or has noted during examination or treatment, must be kept confidential."
- The American Medical Association's Code of Medical Ethics provides, "Physicians must oppose and must not participate in torture for any reasons." As a matter of policy, "the AMA opposes torture in any country for any reason."
- The American Psychiatric Association and the American Psychological Association issued a joint statement against torture in 1985, expressly supporting the UN Declaration and Convention Against Torture and the UN Principles of Medical Ethics relative to torture and ill-treatment.

Violations of the Geneva Conventions violate U.S. law because the Conventions were ratified by the U.S. Congress. Torture came to widespread attention when ordinary soldiers, some of whom provided pictures of themselves humiliating prisoners, posted explicit photographs on the Internet. No longer could the U.S. Defense Department deny, though it continued to minimize, covert practices including the systematic use of sleep deprivation, mock executions, painful physical restraints, prolonged isolation, hooding, sever sexual and cultural humiliation, forced nudity, use of threats and dogs to induce fear of injury or death, prolonged social isolation, threats of violence or death against detainees or their families (Physicians for Human Rights, 2005).

At various times, these acts have been explicitly authorized by U.S. commanders. An official inquiry led by Lt. Gen. Randall Schmidt, reviewing allegations by the FBI of abuse at Guantanamo, acknowledged the authorized use of sleep deprivation, long term isolation, sensory overstimulation (loud music), sexual humiliation, and military dogs against detainees (Physicians for Human Rights, 2005). FBI agents had witnessed harsh treatment of detainees at the Abu Ghraib prison in 2003. They were so troubled by what they saw that they raised the issue, both with their superiors and with the DoD, but to no avail (Lewis 2004). Army jailors in Iraq, acting at the Central Intelligence Agency's request, kept many of the detainees at Abu Ghraib off official rosters to hide them from Red Cross inspectors. The number was "in the dozens, to perhaps up to 100", according to General Kern, a senior officer who oversaw an Army inquiry (Schmitt and Jael 2004).

Miles (2004) and Bloch and Marks (2005) have documented the complicity of American military physicians in the torture of prisoners in Afghanistan, Guantanamo, and Abu Ghraib prison. "Medical personnel evaluated detainees for interrogation, monitored coercive interrogation, allowed interrogators to use medical records, falsified records and death certifications, and failed to provide basic health care" (Miles 2004). The military has notified the deaths of at least 28 detainees as confirmed or suspected homicides (Jehl 2005). Death certificates of detainees in Afghanistan and Iraq were falsified and corrected only after they were exposed. In one instance, soldiers tied a beaten detainee to the top of his cell door and gagged him. A pathologist prepared a certificate of his death stating that he died of "natural causes...during his sleep." After public disclosure, the death certificate was revised to list the death as "homicide" resulting from blunt force injuries and asphyxia. In November 2003, Iraqi Major General Mowhoush was pushed into a sleeping bag while interrogators sat on his chest. He suffocated. Attempts to resuscitate him failed; a surgeon stated that he died of natural causes. Six months later, the death certificate was revised to list homicide by asphyxia (Moffeit 2004). The record leaves no doubt that pathologists have been willing to lie to suit the purposes of the DoD.

Accounts of ill-treatment of detainees have linked health personnel, including psychiatrists and psychologists serving on "Behavioral Science Consulting Teams" ("BSCTs"), to psychologically coercive and abusive interrogations. The Schmidt report cites an instance of a psychologist who was part of a BSCT in connection with the use of a military dog in an interrogation — and who may have been under pressure to participate based on the authorization and approval of such techniques. A comprehensive investigative report in the July 11 & 18 issue of *The New Yorker*, entitled "The Experiment," provides a detailed picture of psychological coercion of detainees. Major General Geoffrey D. Miller, "who commanded the Guantanamo Bay detention center between November, 2002, and March, 2004, and who was then sent by Secretary of Defense Donald Rumsfeld to manage Abu Ghraib prison in Iraq," described the BSCTs as "essential in developing integrated interrogation strategies and assessing interrogation intelligence production." The article describes in detail several of the psychological stress techniques devised and implemented with the participation, consultation, and monitory of BSCT psychologists and psychiatrists and other health professionals.

Former interrogators at Guantanamo Bay report that military doctors aided them in refining coercive interrogations by providing advice on how to increase stress levels and exploit fears. In one case they reported that a detainee's medical files showed he had a severe phobia of the dark and suggested ways to manipulate that to induce him to cooperate. Brian Whitman, a senior Pentagon spokesperson, insists that doctors advising interrogators were not covered by ethics strictures because they were not "treating patients" but rather acting as "behavioral scientists". A recent report issued by the Surgeon General of the U.S. Army acknowledged the involvement of BSCT psychologists and psychiatrists in designing and monitoring interrogations, including help for interrogators in deciding "when to push or not push harder in pursuit of intelligence information." As part of the Taguba investigation, Colonel Thomas M. Pappas, chief of military intelligence at Abu Ghraib, provided documents showing physicians' systematic role in interrogation, including "dietary manipulation," "environmental manipulation" (raising and lowering room temperature), "sleep management" (for up to 72 hours), "isolation" (for more than 30 days). "Since late 2002, psychiatrists and psychologists [at Guantanamo] have been part of a strategy that employs extreme stress, combined with behavior-shaping rewards" in interrogations, and that medical records were made available to facilitate interrogators' efforts to exploit detainees' conditions" (Bloche and Marks 2005).

The International committee of the Red Cross (ICRC) termed these activities "tantamount to torture" and "a flagrant violation of medical ethics" (Lewis 2004). What makes this indictment of American military physicians all the more bitter is that the collaboration of physicians in torture was a hallmark of the dictatorship of Saddam Hussein, the very regime we invaded to depose.

Although we have as yet no record of protest by physicians, the Judge Advocate Generals (JAGs) for the U.S. Army, Air Force, and Marines expressed concern about the interrogation tactics being developed in the Pentagon because they not only "contravened longstanding military doctrine but would also cause widespread public outrage if they became known." The three JAGs were overruled by the General Counsel's office for the Pentagon on the grounds that the "President's inherent Constitutional authority to manage a military campaign" made a prohibition against torture "inapplicable to interrogations undertaken pursuant to his Commander-In-Chief authority" (White 2005). The JAGs did not go public.

When Good Men and Women Do Nothing:

Maj. Gen. Lester Martinez-Lopez recommended that the Defense Department stop using physicians and psychiatrists to aid interrogations, criticizing the lack of ... "policy defining the role of "behavioral science consultation teams" (referred to as "biscuit teams") which have access to medical records on the detainees. However, Lt. Gen. Kevin C. Kiley, the Army Surgeon General, acknowledging only "isolated cases" of detainee abuse involving medical personnel, refused to exclude physicians from the biscuit teams. Military physicians, according to the Pentagon, are acting as combatants, not as physicians, when they put their knowledge to use for military end. The tactics unequivocally violate the Third Geneva Convention, which rules out physical or mental torture being inflicted on prisoners of war. Dr. David Tornberg, Deputy Assistant Secretary of Defense, defended these practices on the grounds that "physicians assigned to military intelligence have no doctor-patient relationship with detainees and, in the absence of life-threatening emergency, have no obligation to offer medical aid" (Bloche and Marks 2005). Colonel Thomas M. Pappas, Chief of Military Intelligence at Abu Ghraib, emphasized that there is a systematic role for physicians in devising individualized plans for detainees. In its defense, he stated that "a physician and a psychiatrist are on-hand to monitor what we are doing", as if that assured a humane interrogation! This claim is difficult to accept at face value. The history of physician participation in torture is that they are employed to "titrate" the dose to avoid too premature a death (a dead "informant" has lost his or her value) and to revive victims who lose consciousness, with the result that their misery is prolonged.

Indeed, reservations were expressed even with the CIA. Johnm Helgerson, the CIA Inspector General, warned in a classified report that the interrogation proceedings approved by the CUIA in the wake of 9/11 "might violate provisions of the International Convention Against Torture" to which the United States is a signatory. The IG's findings were vigorously disputed" by the agency's General Counsel. The issue continues to roil the agency. (Jehl 2005).

An Army Captain, Ian Fishback, has waged an unsuccessful 17-month struggle to "get clear, consistent answers from my leadership about what constitutes lawful and humane treatment of detainees…" "I am certain," he stated, "that this confusion contributed to a wide range of abuses including death threats, beatings, broken bones, murder, exposure to elements, extreme forced physical exertion, hostage-taking, stripping, sleep deprivation and degrading treatment" (White 2005). It is altogether bizarre that the Criminal Investigation Command, rather than looking into the ubiquity of torture at Forward Operating Base Mercury in Iraq (Human Rights Watch 2005), "pressed Captain Fishback to divulge the names of the two sergeants who also gave accounts of abuse." A West Point graduate, the Captain found himself deeply troubled by the Army's response. He has been warned he may face criminal prosecution if he disobeys its "lawful order" to disclose their names. Yet he reports no regrets about having come forward because "It's the right thing to do" (Schmitt 2005 a and b). Fishback's testimony before the McCain Committee helped persuade the Senator to introduce a resolution to regulate the detention, interrogation, and treatment of prisoners held by the American military. It passed overwhelmingly in the Senate (90 to 9). The American College of Physicians, the American Psychiatric Association, and the American Psychological Association have gone on record endorsing the McCain Proposal (Hedberg et al 2005). The McCain amendment awaits final action by the House-Senate Conference Committee, a venue at which aides to Vice President Cheney are trying to gut the amendment by exempting clandestine CIA activities from its provisions (Golden and Schmitt 2005).

No doctor has seen fit to protest because "it is the right thing to do." At least there is no record of such. Perhaps some did and their protests were suppressed. But no such incident has been revealed. Court martial for revealing what this Administration decides to classify as a "military secret" is no trivial threat. Yet Article II of the United Nations 1985 Convention Against Torture states that: "An order from the Superior

Officer or a public authority may not be invoked as a justification of torture." (Article II, Number).

The claim that he was "following orders" did not exculpate Adolph Eichmann. The language of the Universal Declaration of Human Rights is unequivocal: "The doctor's fundamental role is to alleviate the distress of his or her fellow man. No motive, whether personal, collective, or political, shall prevail against this higher purpose."

The World Medical Association Tokyo Declaration demands that: "The utmost respect for human life is to be maintained, even under threat."

Have doctors ever lived up to these lofty goals? Under far more daunting circumstances, physicians and medical organizations in South Africa, Chile, and Turkey have spoken out in defense of human rights.

A courageous doctor made public the violations of medical ethics in the death of Steve Biko, a militant leader of the Black consciousness movement in South Africa (Richmond 2003). Biko was arrested in 1977 under the Terrorism Act. He was beaten so badly during prolonged interrogation in the Headquarters of the Security Police in Port Elizabeth that the security forces summoned Dr. Ivor Lang, the District Surgeon. Although Lang saw lip lacerations, bruises on the sternum, and edema of the hands and ankles and noted that Biko's speech was slurred, he wrote for the medical record: "I have found no evidence of any abnormality or pathology on the patient." The following day, accompanied by Dr. Benjamin Tucker, the Chief District Surgeon, Lang found neurological damage. On lumbar punctures, blood-stained cerebrospinal fluid was obtained. Nevertheless, Lang certified that the lumbar puncture was "normal".

A day later, Biko was in total collapse. Lang recommended transfer to a nearby provincial hospital. When the security forces refused, Tucker authorized trucking Biko in manacles 750 miles to Pretoria Central Prison without an ambulance, a medical attendant, or a referral letter. He died the following night. Lang and Tucker had provided a medical cover-up for rampant brutality and torture. They ignored their duty to Biko as their patient, a duty that should have trumped all other considerations (McLean & Jenkins 2003).

Frances Ames, Chair of the Department of Neurology at the University of Cape Town, was so disgusted by the doctors' behavior that she lodged a complaint with the South Africa Medical and Dental Council (SAMDC) charging the doctors with violating medical ethics. In the words of a former student (McCarthy 2003): "For anyone recently widowed with four sons, the responsibility of running a neurology department in a prestigious hospital would have been onerous enough. She found herself surrounded by bewildered male colleagues, too afraid to speak out against the horror that was enveloping this country for fear of having their government subsidies cut...She was confronted with open hostility by her apparently liberal colleagues...She was begged to drop the case." In the event, the SAMDC summarily rejected the complaint without convening a full hearing. Race, "state security", and politics were allowed to obfuscate the one question that mattered: did Biko receive the level of medical care that any patient was entitled to receive (McLean and Jenkins 2003)?

Dr. Ames and five physicians from the Witwatersrand University took the case to the South African Supreme Court to force the Council to hold a hearing into the conduct of the doctors. It took eight years, but the Court finally ordered the SAMDS to examine the charges (Izindaba 2003). Once the evidence was considered, the Council struck Tucker off the register and cautioned Lang. Frances Ames and two colleagues had received donations to help cover court costs (in the event they lost the Supreme Court appeal). They used those funds to initiate a Medical Faculty Ethics Committees at the University of Cape Town: Witwatersrand already had one. Wits and Capetown were "the only universities that would do so in the mid-1980s, a time of nationwide intimidation, states of emergency, and human rights violations on a grand scale" (McCarthy 2003). In June 1999, she received the Star of South

Africa from the hands of President Nelson Mandela for standing up for humanity in a time of legislated cruelty and dehumanization. "What Francis taught us through personal example was that ethics is about what happens on the ground, in our daily practice, when we are alone" — and not in lofty declarations (McCarthy 2005).

After Pinochet's military coup in 1973, doctors associated with the Vicaría de la Solidaridad, the social service and human rights arm of the Catholic Church in Santiago, were arrested, harassed, and threatened with death for providing care to "subversives". Its Medical Director, Dr. Ramiro Olivares, was held in prison for more than a year under an "anti-terrorist" statue which allowed no bail. Pinochet's functionaries usurped the governance of the Collegio Medico (the Chilean Medical Society) by appointing its officers. When the regime attempted to soften its public image in the mid-1980s by allowing members of the Collegio to choose their own officers, the democratically-elected slate initiated an investigation of doctors who had supervised the systematic torture of prisoners. The tribunal identified six and voted to expel them. Supporters of the regime organized their own medical society to accommodate the expelled physicians. Dr. Juan Luis Gonzalez, President of the Collegio Medico, and Dr. Frncisco Rivas, its Secretary General, were imprisoned for supporting a two-day general strike on behalf of health workers (Physicians for Human Rights 1988).

Physicians for Human Rights, an organization founded in 1986 by five Boston physicians to mobilize health professionals to advance health, dignity, and justice in defense of human rights sent a delegation to Santiago in October 1986. Drs. Carola Eisenberg and Robert Lawrence of Harvard Medical School, founding members of PHR, went to Gonzales and Rivas in prison and held a tightly-publicized press conference in Santiago. The PHR delegation drew international attention to the gross violations of medical neutrality by the Pinochet regime. The President and the Secretary General of the Collegio were released several weeks later.

My third illustration of medical conscience is the courage of the physicians in Turkey, who were imprisoned for "endangering the public order" when they testified to torture on prisoners (Physicians for Human Rights 1996). Dr. Cumhar Akpinar was arrested for providing forensic reports. The Central Council of the Turkish Medical Association and the Ankara Medical Chamber actively protested imprisoning a doctor for having "performed his duties in line with the ethical principles for the profession." Even though they were under police surveillance, more than 100 Turkish physicians attended his trial in solidarity with Dr. Akpinar (Committee on Human Rights Correspondence 1996). After a long legal process, he was found not guilty on 30 December 1999.

Doctor Alb Ayan, a Turkish psychiatrist who helped to found the Human Rights Foundation of Turkey, worked at its treatment and rehabilitation center in Izmir. He was harassed repeatedly by the Turkish authorities for documenting the stigmata of torture on the prisoners he examined. He has been a defendant in 41 cases during the past decade. The Committee on Human Rights of the U.S. National Academy of Sciences wrote to Turkish authorities in defense of Dr. Ayan. After lengthy trials, periods of imprisonment, and numerous costly court appearances, Dr. Ayan has been acquitted of all but two cases. For the academic year 2005-2006, Dr. Ayan has been appointed a "Scholar at Risk" at Harvard University.

The official response to the horrors at Abu Ghraib, Afghanistan, and Guantanamo has been to dismiss them as aberrations by a small number of rogue military police soldiers. The role of the DoD, the Administration, and the military command has been denied. Yet, a memorandum from Alberto Gonzales, presently the Attorney General, advised the White House that the "war on terrorism" makes some elements of the Geneva Conventions "obsolete". The Schlesinger Panel (2004), appointed to review DoD detention operations, recommended that: "All personnel who may be engaged in detention operations, from point of capture to final disposition, should participate in a professional ethics program that would equip them with a sharp moral compass for guidance in situations often riven with conflicting moral duties." Can we trust the very people whose policies led to the violation of ethics to prepare a new code? Who will guard the guardians? A top level commission, not beholden to this administration, should be appointed to review all of the evidence, assign responsibility for dereliction of duty, and propose a system of public accountability to prevent recurrence.

What of the complicity of behavior health personnel? The American Psychological Association appointed a Presidential Task Force to study the matter. To my dismay, it has concluded that psychologists can "support an interrogation and make use of confidential information in medical records...as long as it is not used to the detriment of the individual's safety and well-being" (Evans 2005). The caveat "as long as" defies belief" the interrogations in question have been designed to place intolerable stress on the detainee threatening his "safety and well-being"!

Contrast this position with that of psychiatrist Stephen N. Xenakis (2005), a retired Medical Corps Brigadier General, who directed major medical programs during the 1991 Gulf War. He has stated forcefully that health workers in the military "have a common duty...to provide care according to high standards of medical practice...and...to report any signs of physical or psychological abuse...Unlike soldiers, doctors have a duty to patients as well as to country. That is what separates U.S. military physicians from the German doctors who aided the Nazis in concentration camps and...the prison doctors who examined anti-apartheid leader Steve Biko."

This September, my wife enlisted a group of colleagues (Eisenberg 2005) to cosign a letter to the American Psychiatric Association urging it to condemn the use of highly coercive interrogation techniques by the United States, techniques that amount to torture and cruel, inhuman and degrading treatment; to enjoin the participation of psychiatrists in any of these activities; and to insist that the military provide specific operational ethical guidelines to protect the integrity of the psychiatric profession and the stability of military medical services. This September, The Board of Trustees of the APA adopted those principles: psychiatrists should not play any role in providing guidance, support, advice, monitory, or prisoner evaluation for interrogations, nor should they provide interrogators with any knowledge gained from observing detainees who are undergoing interrogation. To become official policy, the statement awaits action by the APA Assembly in November (Hausman 2005).

Health professionals who wish to affirm their opposition to torture can do so by signing on to The Call to Prevent Torture and Abuse of Detainees in U.S. Custody already endorsed by more than 1,000 physicians and other health workers. Log onto www.PHRUSA.org and click on the *"Torture"* link in the left column (on the home page).

If Physicians in the military have been silent for fear of court martial, that doesn't explain why civilian medical organizations have equivocated or remained silent. Have we been afraid to criticize government policy lest we appear "unpatriotic"? Have we created a professional culture in which one gets along by going along? A survey of students in six medical schools indicated that more than half report having seen and participated in unethical acts that put patients at risk (Feudtner et al 1994). Almost all students in the survey had heard physicians refer to patients in a derogatory way; two-thirds had witnessed unethical behavior by other team members; half felt themselves to be accomplices. Why had they gone along with what they knew to be wrong The reasons they gave included wanting to "fit in" and their fear of poor evaluations. What did being accomplices do to them? They reported feeling that their ethical principles had been eroded. Agreeing, faking a lab result or keeping silent when a house officer saves face by lying is not the same as acquiescing in torture; but it is no exaggeration to suggest that it is a precursor to the conspiracy of silence that covers up for medical malpractice.

From the time students enter medical school, they need to understand that, while their responsibility begins with maintaining high ethical standards in their own work, it includes confronting unethical

When Good Men and Women Do Nothing:

behavior wherever it occurs. Silence in the face of malfeasance is unacceptable (Dwyer 1994). We need to create an academic climate in which students challenge the missteps they see, despite personal risk (Eisenberg 1994). Fifty years on medical school faculties have taught me that the student who suppresses dismay at the mistreatment of a patient in a first-year clinic is no longer dismayed when he or she observes a similar event as a third year clerk and will be guilty of it as a house officer. (obligation to recognize) The house officer who tolerates unethical behavior will become the Assistant Professor who delays taking a stand until tenure is acquired. Sadly, the moral habits acquired on the way to tenure will guarantee having become so inured to ethical lapses that the new Professor will be bold only in defending space, salary, and parking privileges. Conscience atrophies without exercise.

If medical schools and teaching hospitals fail to instill in graduates a commitment to the human rights of their patients, the source is not far to find: lapses among the Faculty that pass unchallenged. We must construct an academic environment that fosters confrontation of problem behavior wherever it occurs. The medical curriculum should engage students and house officers explicitly from the first year in addressing the day-to-day dilemmas they face when peers or superiors mistreat patients or put them at risk. We need a clinical ethos in which lying — or remaining silent — to cover up a lapse in patient care becomes as reprehensible as the lapse itself (Bosk 1979).

When Elie Wiesel (1986) accepted the Nobel Peace Prize, he said: "I swore never to be silent whenever wherever human beings endure suffering and humiliation...Neutrality helps the oppressor, never the victim. Silence encourages the tormentor, never the tormented..." It is time to add a codicil to the Hippocratic Oath: "I swear never to be silent whenever wherever human beings endure suffering and humiliation."

Contemplating Pandemics: The Role of Historical Inquiry in Developing Migration Strategies in the 21st Century, 2006

Howard Markel, M.D., Ph.D., Professor of Pediatrics and Communicable, Diseases; Director, Center for the History of Medicine, University of Michigan

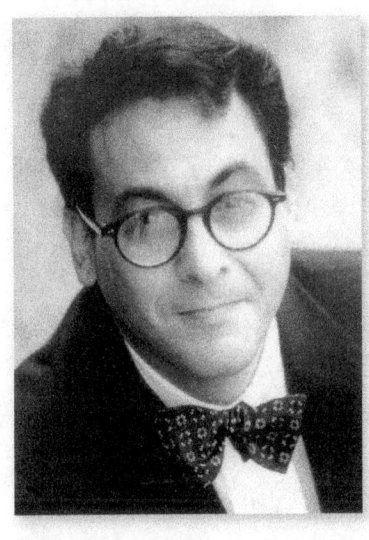

Well, thank you Phil, and thank you John, for those kind words. It is just a wonderful honor. And thank you to the Waggoner family and distinguished guests and colleagues who came here today. You know I--it has been a wonderful day thus far. I cannot remember spending so many consecutive hours with psychiatrists and not having to pay for it. So I am very delighted by that. Phil asked me to mention that there are ethical components to this. So I will say the word ethics. Ethics. Ethics and values. There was a Norman Fost who was a pediatrician--he is a pediatrician anesthetist, once said, "You know if you took all the medical ethicists in the world and laid them end to end, that would be a good thing." You could say that about medical historians as well.

This work that I will be talking about today--I have several colleagues in the back. Dr. Alexander Stern, Dr. J. Alex Navarro, and Alexandra Sloan who are working with me on this project. I would be remiss--I

Contemplating Pandemics:

am the front man, but they have been working on this project as well. This really just snow balled. It really began as Phil mentioned, I have been looking at issues like quarantines and epidemics for almost twenty years, but really the history of them with the hopes that they would have some implications for public policy, but after a few years, not really expecting that to happen.

About a year and a half ago over just before the July 4th weekend, a gentleman from the Department of Defense called me. This was a physician and who worked for the Defense Threat Reduction Agency and he said, "Well, we know your work and what we would like you to do is to look at some escape communities. There were several communities in 1918 that completely escaped the Great Pandemic of 1918. And the reason that we would want to look at this is that we are trying to figure out what we can do to protect our men and women in uniform to avoid a potential worst case scenario pandemic." And so I chuckled to myself and I said, "Well, Doctor, history doesn't really work that way and I am not sure that is the study you'd like to do." And he said, "No, that is precisely the study we want to do." And I hemmed and hawed a little bit more and I tried to get out of it. And then finally I said something to him that I say to lawyers when they call me to testify. I never do, but I always say, "Hey, you know I'm very expensive." And then with lawyers, that always ends the conversation. This time the man from the Defense Department said, "Professor, we are the Defense Department. We have trillions of dollars at our command." And so I paused and I said, "Well--hang on. Let me get Dr. Markel to the phone." And that began basically the work that I will be talking about today.

Although the possibility of a devastating influenza pandemic akin to the one experienced in 1918 gives most of us reason for pause, if not the outright shudders, the theoretical, practical, and intellectual questions raised by such a crisis are fascinating to say the least. What would we do if faced with the widespread human-to-human transmission of H5N1 or some other novel influenza virus variant? How would our medical

The Role of Historical Inquiry in Developing Migration...

system cope with the burgeoning numbers of cases needing immediate attention? How would public health agencies in the federal, state, and local levels respond? And how would the less developed nations of the world cope with such a crisis? What might be the economic, political, and social ramifications of such an event? These and so many other critical questions boggle the mind and yet we must, and hopefully will, develop a framework to help us come to some consensus about how to approach this and other microbial threats looming in the distance today.

And yet, most of us, regardless of the intellectual discipline we affiliate with, are rather uncomfortable making bold pronouncements and strategies because there is so little practical data or experience to work with. This, I think, is where historical inquiry can be of some value given that we simply do not have that much solid data on the means of mitigating or containing, worst case scenario, influenza pandemics, in our modern era. I will discuss why exploring the historical record of the 1918 pandemic may help to unleash a body of clues and suggestions. And just parenthetically, I am sure most of you know this, but in 1918 anywhere from fifty to one hundred million people died of influenza. The attack rate was twenty-five to fifty percent of all people who encountered it got the flu, and the mortality rate was about two percent. If you compare that to seasonal flu, where there is about five hundred thousand deaths worldwide and the death rate is zero point one percent at best, so we are talking about a worst-case scenario. And the 1918 pandemic is probably the worst pandemic in human history.

Most compelling to me as a historian of infectious diseases is that the 1918 flu pandemic provides with appropriate retrieval methods, perhaps the largest database ever assembled in the modern post-germ theory era on the use of non-pharmaceutical interventions to mitigate pandemic flu in urban centers. Now that fancy term, non-pharmaceutical interventions, I will get into in a moment. The key, however, is extracting this data in a rigorous and scholarly manner from the historic--from a wide swath of archives, libraries, microfilm reels, documents and so on that

Contemplating Pandemics:

are literally scattered across the United States. Perhaps more compelling to policy makers is the question in experiential data of how large numbers of people respond when a pandemic appears, but vaccines and antivirals are neither affective nor widely available. History suggests that when faced with such a crisis, many Americans and more formerly American communities will adopt in some form or another what they perceive to be affective social distancing measures and other NPI. And this is precisely what the nation did in 1918 resulting in a wide spectrum of outcomes and experiences.

So how can historians, mathematical modelers, epidemiologists, statisticians, and public health professionals make some sense of and exploit this historical data to inform decisions today on how best to employ or discard various NPI strategies? And can we or how can we evaluate their costs and benefits in a manner that includes a polyset of social, legal and ethical menses?

Before I get to that, I would like to give you some background on contemplating pandemics and several historians have been thinking very hard about epidemics and pandemics over the last several decades. One particular model that I liked was articulated by Charles Rosenberg who is a wonderful historian of American medicine and he constructed something that he calls the Four Act Model of an Epidemic. And he is really basing it not just on his reading of a wide variety of historical sources on epidemics, but a novel that is probably well known to everyone in this room, The Plague, by Albert Camus. Now I am very jealous of Albert Camus. He writes beautifully and I have been studying epidemics for a long time and this guy has got it down perfectly. It is actually probably the most perfect document if you want to read about epidemics. It is something that I always assign to medical students who are in search of information even though it is a novel, not a historical source.

But you will remember in the Act One, is what Rosenberg calls progressive revelation. If you remember the book, it has one of the most remarkable, albeit, disgusting openings in all of literature. When leaving his surgery on the morning of April 16, Dr. Bernard Rieux felt something soft under his foot. It was a dead rat lying in the middle of the landing. On the spur of the moment he kicked it to one side and without giving it a further thought, continued on his way downstairs. Only when he was stepping out onto the street, did it occur to him that a dead rat had no business to be on his landing. Well, that is exactly how the most epidemics or pandemics begin--with an odd occurrence that you do not give much thought to it. Something is afoot, no pun intended, but you really have not put things together. And that is a real problem because the time between putting that first event together with what might happen, is the time when the microbe can multiply and can infect other people.

This brings to mind the second act of an epidemic. Now you have more cases going on, but you still do not know what is going on and we call this managing randomness. This is a part of a painting called the Triumph of Death which is about the Black Plague of Europe by Pieter Bruegel, the elder. And how does the society make sense of these random events of people developing terrible symptoms and dying and new people developing those symptoms as well? What is in their own framework of understanding? What other beliefs of God or of science and what have you, and how these belief systems work, have a lot to do with how people put together or figure out what is going on?

The third act that Rosenberg talks about is something called negotiating public responses. And so once an epidemic is recognized, the public typically demands collective action of some kind. And the history of epidemics is littered with tales demonstrating the importance of bold and decisive leadership and the costs of ineffective or incompetent crisis management. And as many a student--historians of the tug of war between the public and those charged with protecting their health have noted that the operative word in public health is public. So in those efforts that fail to generate a strong consensus among the multitudes constituting a community which takes into account cultural values and attitudes, social and class hierarchies, economical and political

Contemplating Pandemics:

imperatives. If you don't do all of that, very little is accomplished in any attempt to reign in disease. In fact, sometimes you have people working at cross-purposes because they are offended by your actions.

The fourth act, subsidence and retrospection, is perhaps the most frustrating to those of us who study epidemic or work in the field. I have this quote here from T. S. Eliot's, *The Hollow Men*. "This is the way the world ends, not with obeying, but with a whimper." And that is precisely how most pandemics end. People forget. There is something I call profound amnesia. Let me illustrate. A few years ago when the SARS Epidemic was brewing, it was all SARS all the time. Now, for most people, it was either annoying or troubling. For me it was great business and so it was really quite remarkable how many people were calling me at that moment. And I was on the MacNeil/Lehrer Report and I was making this particular point. I said, "What is going to happen in the future?" Now historians by definition are uncomfortable predicting the future, but I hazard a guess and I said, "I think the SARS Epidemic will end in eight, ten, or twelve weeks, but what bothers me most, Mr. Lehrer, is that everyone will forget about it and that we won't take the steps we need to prevent the next one from happening." And I will illustrate this. If I call you twelve weeks from now and say, "Jim, I want to get back on the show to talk about SARS," he will say, "That is history." I did that twelve weeks later. The SARS Epidemic was over and I never got through to Mr. Lehrer, so it was a nice experiment.

But of course, while this four act model is very intriguing, not all epidemics and not all pandemics subscribe to the strict narrative structure as prescribed by a four act claim. And so some of the work that I have done over the past couple of decades, is a model that I call the Light Motif Model of Pandemics. Let me go through some of these themes. These are themes or ingredients in the mix. They do not always appear in the same proportions and sometimes some of them or a few of them are not in at all, but you can pretty much count from epidemic to epidemic that you will see most, if not all of these themes.

The Role of Historical Inquiry in Developing Migration...

The first one is that epidemics are almost always framed and shaped, sometimes advanced, sometimes hindered by how a given society understands a particular microbe to travel and infect others. So let us say, it was an epidemic of cholera--a pandemic of cholera in the early 19th century when the theory of the best medical science of the day thought that cholera pandemics were spread by measthmus(?), some type of polluted air that came from rotting organic material that somehow spread disease. Your approach to containing that epidemic would be very different than if you subscribed to the germ theory of--that explained that a particular microbe caused that disease. You might want to clean up the environment or the streets or what have you, but it would be a very different approach.

Another theme is the economic devastation typically associated with epidemics, could have a strong influence on the public's response to a contagious crisis. Now let us face it, epidemics or pandemics cost a lot of money. If you close a seaport or an airport, if you stop convention traffic, if you order business closures, you cost a lot of money. SARS cost the world economy over sixty billion dollars. The projections on if there was a worst-case scenario flu pandemic tomorrow or next year, the worst-case scenario projections in America--the United States of America alone, would be six hundred to seven hundred billion dollars. That is just the United States. So it costs a lot of money and so you--if you are going to close things down, if you are going to restrict movement and so on, you want to be sure that you are right for a lot of reasons beyond money, but that is one of them. And when people start losing money, they start complaining. And if they start complaining, they might not comply with the restrictions you might want to suggest.

The movements of people and goods and the speed of travel are central factors in the spread of a pandemic disease. This is a photograph of some immigrants coming into Ellis Island back in the good old or not so good old days when immigrants were coming. Twenty million came between 1880 and 1924. You had at least a seven to ten day lag time between the time those people left Europe and got to America or if they

Contemplating Pandemics:

were coming from Asia, you had about a 14 to 20 day lag time. So that if they had a contagious disease en route, it might already manifest itself before they got to, in this case, an American port and you could diagnose them and or quarantine and isolate them.

Today when you can get from anywhere to anywhere else in less than 24 hours and then you can go somewhere else on a hub and travel quite extensively, we do not have that leg up. So germs are traveling in a much faster rate whether they travel in the bodies of human beings or in insects or on cargo or what have you.

Our fascination with the suddenly appearing microbe that kills relatively few in spectacular fashion, too often trumps our approach to infectious scourges that patiently kill millions every year. This is an op-- [inaudible] that I did for the New York Times a few years ago. It was during the SARS crisis and you can see the bigger squares, they are not to scale, but the bigger squares, tuberculosis killed two million a year, eight million cases. Malaria kills about a hundred every hour. Hepatitis B and so on and that variant in that very corner is SARS. Because of that date, that was about May 1--April 30th of 2003. There were only 353 deaths in about five thousand cases. By the end of the SARS epidemic, there was about 800 deaths in eight thousand cases. But we love the sudden and scary and we do not pay enough attention to the infectious scourges that are carting off literally hundreds of people every hour. In the last hour alone, fifteen hundred people, half of them were young children, died of some infectious disease. Most of them are TB, AIDS, and malaria, but do not forget diarrheal diseases as well.

Wide spread media coverage of epidemics is hardly new and it is an essential part of any epidemic. The press has been with us for many, many, many, many, many decades and they have been covering epidemics quite extensively during that time. And how they write those epidemics up plays a critical role and there is good reporters. There is not so good reporters, but how that information is spread about can have a real impact on your public health management.

The concealment of contagious problems from the world at large has often proven quite deadly in epidemics past. Now, most famous in recent times was the SARS crisis. Now we knew there was--it came in retrospect we know there was cases of SARS in the Guangdong province of China for at least three months before the Hong Kong cases reported in early February of 2003. And yet for political or nationalistic reasons, they were concealed which gave the microbe a leg up in traveling and infecting other people, but this is hardly the first example of this. One of my favorite cases has to do with the cholera pandemic of 1892 which was a huge cholera pandemic and when it got to Hamburg, Germany, which was the largest port in the world--the largest seaport in the world, the German government simply concealed that they had cases and sent boat loads of people all around the world so that it spread further. They concealed the cases because they were afraid of the economic ramifications. You know, if we admit that we have a terrible cholera pandemic, no one will want to do business with us. It is kind of backwards reasoning because after a while, no one wanted to do business with the Hamburg port because they were afraid of getting cholera and that is similarly the case with China. China really had to clean up its act after SARS and be a lot more forth coming with surveillance data post-SARS than pre-SARS because they are part of the world economy as well and they wanted to maintain that role.

To me the saddest theme of epidemics, perhaps the saddest theme of epidemics throughout history has been the tendency to blame or scapegoat particular social groups. This is a cartoon from Judge Magazine in 1892, you will see it is a Dutch immigrant and a Russian Jewish immigrant walking arm and arm with a shrouded figure and it is called Asiatic cholera and Uncle Sam is looking over the wall there quite frightened. Lest you think this is just an artifact of the good old bad old days, here are a couple of cartoons that happened during SARS, so the Great Wall of China being quarantined and a particularly offensive cartoon, bad Chinese takeout. We are not immune to blaming people and so-called socially undesirable groups have often born the brunt of this and

Contemplating Pandemics:

that is particularly a problem, not just for the ethical or social reasons, but too you have consider that if a particular group feels scape goated and blamed, they may not cooperate with you. And when you are talking about containing a contagious disease, if people are not working with you or do not trust you for whatever reason, that actually hinders the public health rather than helps it.

The study that we did last year that will lead to what I will talk about in a moment was these escape communities that I mentioned and this is just--the work of this is--the full report of this is on a website which is listed right on the slide and the shorter version of the report appears in the December 2006 issue of Emerging Infections Diseases which you can get online right now but there is the reference if you would like.

Several of the places that we looked at like Fletcher, Vermont, which is a tiny hamlet then as well as now, it had a population of about 750 people, but probably simply too small to really suggest they did anything. You know, they did do some quarantine and isolation, but it was simply too small to make a lot of conclusions about it. By the way, Fletcher, Vermont, narrowly escaped a bad flu outbreak because they had local dances and one of the visitors to a dance was a soldier from Fort Devens outside of Boston, if you have read about the flu pandemic. That was one of the epicenters of the flu and it is just luck that this particular soldier did not have flu and did not infect the entire town of Fletcher, Vermont.

But a couple of other escape communities that we looked at Trudeau, TB Sanitarium and Saranac Lake, New York, and the Western Pennsylvania Institution for the Blind, had a remarkable period of escape from the flu and there is a lot of reasons. One, they shut themselves off, something that we call protective sequestration. I will talk about that in a moment. They literally close their doors from the outside world. It was a bit harder in Pittsburgh, which was a bad flu town. They actually closed their doors from the city proper. Saranac Lake was a bit more remote. But these places were already de facto quarantine islands, if you will. If you think about how people treated those with tuberculosis, they put them in sanatoriums far away from them and how people treated those with physical disabilities, being blind, handicapped, and so on. They were often in homes for the blind, for the crippled, for the ruptured, for the insane, and so on. So these were already separated places from society at large.

What work was more interesting actually was the United States Naval Training Station at Verba Buena Island in San Francisco and in Gunnison, Colorado, a mining town. The Naval Training Station literally shut itself off. It is right in the San Francisco Harbor. You can see the pilings in that picture are what becomes the Bay Bridge. That is a photography from the 1930s, but it is literally in you know, San Francisco, but in the harbor. But the Commandant shut the doors, so to speak, of Verba Buena Island three days--two to three days before a flu hit San Francisco, so there is no traffic from San Francisco or to San Francisco during an almost two month period of time. And all these sailors and their Naval officers who are on this island were basically flu free until they opened up the gates and then some cases started trickling in. Similarly, in Gunnison, Colorado, which was a mining town in the Rockies, the Public Health authorities closed the town, barricaded the roads with police officers manning the barricades, prevented the train from actually coming into the town proper without being inspected. People who did come into the town were quarantined for a particular period of time and so on. And indeed, for almost a four-month period of time, Gunnison was influenza free. This is a striking comparison to many of the towns that were surrounding it that had terrible flu outbreaks.

But the problem with protective sequestration is that it is a rather difficult thing to enact and so the best prescription that I could give the Department of Defense is that if you are a remote mining town or if you are in violent run by a Naval Commandant, you should shut yourself off from all interaction with the world. That is not a prescription that you can really enact in many places in the United States today.

Now this led to the study that we are doing now for the Department of Health and Human Services as well the Centers for Disease Control

Contemplating Pandemics:

and Prevention. And in a way it was a study I had hoped we would do a few months before when we were assigned the task for the Department of Defense. The reality is that there is hundreds of cities in the United States that had varying flu experiences. So if you read the grand sweeping narratives, the best selling books about influenza, it is all about the carnage that was brought on by this microbe and that hundreds of thousands of deaths in the United States alone. There are about six hundred fifty thousand deaths due to flu in America that year.

And yet, but we find when we take our microscope, our historical microscope and start looking at the individual experiences of these cities is that not every city had the same experience and some had better experiences. So the question is what did they do right or what did other cities do wrong? And what non-pharmaceutical interventions, quarantine, isolation, school closure, what worked and at what point should you pull those triggers and when should you release those triggers? Now here is the rub.

History is not a predictive science. It should not be looked at as an oracle of what is to be with all due respect to George Santayana, who said, "You know those who ignore the past are condemned to repeat it." I love that because it is good job security for me, but it really does not work that way. History does not repeat itself in exact circles. There are cycles and a relicenses and of course history, I firmly believe, can inform the present and the future, but it does not provide a blueprint for what is to come. Moreover, there are lots of ways to extract historical data and many of them are wrong. Okay, this is a very complex data source. How do you look at this data?

There are certain terms that are used even in the very narrow historical framework of a hundred years that certain terms like vaccine mean very different things in 1918 compared to today. Terms like quarantine can mean different things. Where do you get the primary sources? So there is lots of secondary sources on deaths in various cities and of course just like a game of telephone operator, which I am sure everyone played as a child, as you get secondary tertiary, quaternary sources, you start getting the story changed a little bit. So how do you find the best data available? And that is really what our team at the Center for the History of Medicine has been doing. We have been scouring the National Archives, the Library of Congress, the University of Michigan libraries, and a bunch of libraries and archives around the country to find the best possible data that we can to figure out these questions.

You also need to be intimately familiar with the social, cultural, and intellectual history of the region and period under study and attempt to explain the differences than compared to today. In 1918, the United States is a very different country than in 2006, so we can talk about that during the question and answer period, but most people do not have automobiles yet, trains are the major means of long distance travel. There is rapid communication, but in the form of telegrams and for some people telephones. Newspapers are very active then, so there is good media communication. People live in a more of a cash economy so they are used to going to the bank everyday. There are no refrigerators yet, so people grocery shop on a daily basis or they need to buy cakes of ice to put things that are perishable. So there are all of these issues that need to be thought of and discussed when you think about comparing then versus now.

So the study that we are doing now for the CDC and that we are advising the White House, the Department of HHS, and the CDC which are struggling to come up with some set of guidelines of what we would do in a worst case scenario. So this is not a 1957 or 1968 flu pandemic scenario. Those were flu pandemics, but really not many more people died during those pandemics than would die during seasonal flu, about a half a million. We are talking about the worst-case scenario of a hundred million deaths worldwide, two percent mortality rate, and a twenty-five to fifty percent attack rate. We are also talking about the other things as well, but this is the worst-case scenario.

And so the thought is--let us look at 45 Americans cities and we wanted to look at as many cities as we can to increase the power of our

Contemplating Pandemics:

statistical analysis and try to look at these things of what they did. These are the 45 cities by the way that we are looking at. But we are looking at these NPIs. Now what are they? NPI is a very fancy almost Orwellian term, but they include making flu reportable disease, isolating sick individuals, quarantining households with sick individuals, school closure, protective sequestration of children or adults, cancellation of worship services, and closure of public gatherings such as saloons, theatres, and so on, staggered business hours so you can decrease congestion on trams and public transportation, mandatory or recommended use of mask in public, closing or discouraging the use of public transportation systems, restrictions on funerals, parties, and weddings, restrictions on door to door sales, community wide curfew measures and business closures, social distancing strategies for those who encounter others, public health risk communication measures and declarations of public emergencies.

Now the rationale of course, of all of these was to help mitigate community transmission of flu. We do not know yet, we are getting close to it, of precisely how much mitigation, if any, was achieved. In fact, I wrote this before I spoke to our statistician today. We are actually getting very close to finding that some cities had quite a bit of mitigation. And what is intriguing about this is that no systematic study--lots of people are talking, "Well, back in 1918 this happened or what have you," but no systematic study of the NPIs taken, the case incidence and death rates during 1918, and what occurred in these populated centers really exists. This is a glaring lacuna both in the historical literature as well as in the public health literature.

Now we are working from the hypothesis that coordinated layered strategies of NPIs taken early during the 1918 pandemic may have helped some cities experience lower death and case incidence rates as compared to those with less organized or less comprehensive strategies. Now we fully appreciate that NPIs are not expected to prevent a pandemic or to have any impact beyond the time of their implementation. Instead, the primary purpose of these strategies is one, to reduce the attack rate at peak incidence, two, reduce the death rate at peak incidence, and to shift the epi curve to the right, thus delaying the impact of the pandemic.

Now think about this. This is I think remarkably exciting because if you could delay the rise of cases and the rise of deaths and flatten the epi curve and lengthen it over a period of four to six months, that would be enough time to create vaccine in the 21st century as well as it would not lead to a glut of hospital beds or lack of or rather a glut on the hospitals or other critical infrastructure. So if you have a rapid peak, your hospitals are filled to overflowing and not only can you not take care of the flu patients, you cannot take care of the other patients who we take care of on a daily basis who have a variety of other diseases. The conventional wisdom is that these NPI interventions have little if any effect on the United States during the 1918 pandemic because despite their use, virtually all United States communities were severely affected by this. But what the historical record is showing quite clearly is that some cities were more severely affected than others and indeed in terms of influenza mortality and morbidity rates, there is wide variants among these 45 cities. But the problem is that during the pandemic, the critical data that we would love to have that we would probably have if we were making a prospective study is not always there.

Take for example, case incidence data. So case incidence data varies from one city to the next and it is not always kept in the same way. So it is not nearly as reliable as we would like. With that data, it is a lot better, but there is a lot of secondary sources from the 1920s that sort of changed the data or made mistakes in terms of tabulation and so that you can get very different results if you do a statistical analysis in terms of the ranking of each city and which city was more successful more than others Fortunately our intrepid crew of researchers have found what I call the bedrock of death data for the flu pandemic. The National Census Data kept very good death data for the several years before the 1918 pandemic and during the 1918 pandemic for both pneumonia and influenza and so that we can actually construct an excess mortality rate and look at the death rates and suggest that it would be about seven to ten days after the case, roughly, if you think that is how--the average time people who had flu and died of it.

The outcomes of our study will be, as I said, the shape and slope of the epi curve, the death rate at the peak of mortality, and the time factor between initiating NPI and the height of the peak. Another source that we have been using are newspapers and this is very arduous work because you have to go through literally hundreds if not thousands of microfilm reels to extract each article. But it is really a remarkable source. Now far be it for me to ever say everything in the newspaper is true, especially if it is under my byline, I would be very nervous about that. But using newspapers to find out the days when the strategies--these triggers were pulled on and off is probably the most reliable source that we have. In fact, far more reliable than municipal reports and things like that. So we have been looking at every--about--there are 45 cities we have been getting two or more newspapers per city so that we can also evaluate in terms of circulation, social demographics, as well as political slant of that newspaper may have, but also to get these nuts and bolts kind of numerical quantitative data that we can measure some of these things.

The questions that we are asking is first, can an orchestrated strategy of layered NPI applied early and kept in place for appropriate periods of time lower the R0, the reproductive rate of an epidemic, flatten and lengthen the epi curve or even delay the appearance of an epidemic? Second, is which NPIs appear more effective than others? What factors promoted or detracted from the effectiveness of NPIs? For example, mandatory NPIs are not always as effective as voluntary NPIs. Did the timing and layering or a combination of these NPI play a role and is there a relationship between when the NPI were ordered, the number and the type of NPI used, the duration of these NPI, and the compliance among those so ordered? Were these NPI enacted smoothly, haphazardly, belatedly, or with inadequately enforced compliance or affective or ineffective leadership? And was there a communal push back or in successive waves? There were four waves to the 1918 pandemic, something that we call epidemic fatigue. So let us say the second wave of the pandemic was the most deadly in terms of morbidity and also in terms of cases as well.

The third pandemic which followed right on its heels, people were a little bit tired of being ordered to not go to saloons or movie theaters and so on. So it is very difficult to get people to adhere to restrictions when they last more than a week or two, let alone twelve weeks and then you repeat them only a few weeks after that. And in today's hyperactive world, I think people are even less patient than they were in 1918 so that may be a day or two is when the natives might start getting restless.

And finally, what broad historical lessons can we learn as we develop pandemic strategies today? Now there is a wonderful book by an epidemic(?) historian Alfred Crosby called *America's Forgotten Pandemic - the Influenza of 1918*. I still think that is the single best one volume account of the 1918 pandemic and he noted that in human terms, the pandemic was not one overarching story, but instead thousands of separate stories with different origins and outcomes from the flu victims, their families, and their communities.

Now while we do not have any auricular commandments from this work, what I can tell you is that each city not only had a different experience, that there are different things that you can do that might allow you to prevent--or not prevent, but contain or mitigate an epidemic. Now I am not going to go through all these cities very closely. I can do this in the question and answer period, but I think I will skip through them a bit, but let us take a look for example, at Pittsburgh. And what you see, Pittsburgh did not have a very good experience with the flu pandemic. It was a large city. It was an industrial city. It was racked by political class and racial tensions and what this shows is the death curve, the death epi curve during the second wave of the pandemic as well as the various NPIs that were used, and how long they were used for. Those are the bars on the bottom and what you see, for example, is that they applied many

Contemplating Pandemics:

of these, particularly school closure, very late in the pandemic after flu already started to rise. School closure by the way, is one of the things that the CDC is most interested in as a flu mitigation strategy for the 21st century. It is a very problematic mitigation strategy because so many of us rely on the fact that our children are going to school. There are many dual working parents or single parent homes, so that it creates a problem in terms of daycare. There are millions, ten to twenty million children everyday who get their basic nutrition in school lunch programs so that needs to be accounted for as well. And yet on the other hand, it is very intriguing to think about closing schools because anyone who has spent any time in a daycare facility or a kindergarten room or a first grade room knows that young children do not have the best respiratory etiquette. They sneeze on each other. They cough on each other. They blow their noses on each other and so on and when you think about high school kids, they have a different form of bad respiratory etiquette so that closure of schools might be something to think about.

I want to go quickly but, Denver for example, which had an early public closure of school. You can see a bimodal curve. Now it did not do all that well. It had one of the worst records in the country in terms of morbidity and mortality, but this bimodal curve is very interesting because it suggests that if you pull the trigger early enough, you might get the diminution of cases in this. And then when they released the trigger you can see when they released the trigger you start having cases rising up again so the city actually serves at its own control about what might have happened with these NPI strategy.

Newark had a disastrous experience. As you can see it had a very sharp curve and one of the reasons has less to do with what we can find in the quantitative data and it really explains--or illustrates the importance of qualitative historical analysis is that if you start looking at the way Newark governed itself, there are quite a lot of infighting between the mayor and public health department, and the State of New Jersey's Public Health Department, so they could never agree when to pull the triggers, when to release the triggers. It was based in just chaos and so it really brings up an issue is that when you have your leaders fighting and against one another, it is very difficult to orchestrate a good strategy of disease containment. Chicago is a very similar story as well.

But Milwaukee on the other hand, which is one of the healthiest cities in the country at that time, had a very low incidence and again has the same bimodal kind of a curve that goes exactly with these public closure order and school closure orders. So it is very intriguing as we are coming up with guidelines today. The best city in the country, bar none was St. Louis. Now, St. Louis really benefited from a very sharp public health officer named Starcloth who ordered school closure and public closure orders almost immediately when the first case of flu struck and kept them in place for along period of time so they had a very well co-ordinated and early proactive local response. And if you look at their curve, it is a bimodal curve as well, but it is very low. It is below forty cases per hundred thousand so that is very intriguing.

Well, based on the data that we have collected so far and we will be reporting this out in the next several weeks and hopefully you will be hearing about it. We have presented some of this data already to the Institute of Medicine and we will be presenting it at a CDC stakeholder's conference and then we will be preparing it for publication. Is that--the first issue is that long standing investment in public health infrastructure, experience with epidemic response and the building of local trust by health officers appears to have facilitated NPI implementation in every city that we looked at. So that compatible and smooth relationships between key authorities such as the mayor and the health commissioner, appears to have facilitated the coordination and implementation of NPI, but that does not demonstrate the NPI themselves were affective or appropriate, nor did these amicable relationships always guarantee ultimate success. Sometimes the microbe gets an upper hand as well.

Conversely, the implementation of NPI can be derailed by political and administrative tensions and the inconsistent behavior of key

Contemplating Pandemics:

authorities such as the mayor or the health commissioner. Other quantitative observations that while many scholars have focused on the cumulative death rates or the overall experience of individual cities with the flu pandemic, we believe this approach is less useful when assessing the potential efficacy of NPIs since it appears that their most extensive application occurred in the weeks between October and December of 1918, what is called the second wave of the pandemic. Cities with the bimodal curves, like St. Louis, Milwaukee, Denver, that appear well tied to NPIs may have had similar cumulative death rates as cities that did not implement the da--the same menu of NPI or even at all, but this does not suggest however, that the NPI had no impact. Quite the contrary. It may mean that for NPI to have an impact, they must be applied early in a--and in a sustained way. And that to me is the sixty-four thousand dollar question, because it is a very difficult situation to find yourself in to pull that trigger if you are the health officer of the community. If it is too early, people complain because people do not like to be restricted, money can be lost and so on. If it is too late, people die. So how do you hit that sweet spot, so to speak, is a very, very difficult issue.

It is interesting to note that based on preliminary observations of St. Louis, Milwaukee, and even Denver, when compared to many of our other cities, that the NPIs may have lowered the initial peak and were followed by a second delayed peak after some of the interventions were rescinded. Unraveling the complexity of these qualitative and quantitative observations is the challenge of this remarkably large study that we are doing with the CDC as we continue to systematically examine the historical record. For example, time does not permit me to delve into the nuance difference in public health, administrative structures, or political infighting or collaboration, the social responses to these NPIs and other critical issues such as immigrant communities or other ethnic communities might have an impact on how these things played out. Rest assured, we are looking at this for our broader study. But when completed, we believe that the final report that we produce as well as a

The Role of Historical Inquiry in Developing Migration...

web-based influenza archive that we are going to produce will constitute the single largest database on NPIs ever trad--taken during a human pandemic. And it will be easily accessible for scholars to look at and to challenge our observations and our interpretations.

While I spent a great deal of time discussing the historical lessons of pandemics during this last hour as well as how they can impact on society at large, I am very eager to discuss your questions and queries about this work and what we might do to better protect the nation's health. I would also like to conclude by noting the remarkable change over time that makes a future influenza pandemic so strikingly different from those of the past. Specifically, this is essentially the first pandemic in human history that we have had some semblance of advanced warning and hence, the opportunity to prepare. That is truly a great change over time and when you combine that with the advances in virology, surveillance, rapid communications, epidemic modeling in other fields, there really is the exciting hope that we can apply these methods to a pandemic's rapid mitigation if not containment or outright prevention. All of the light motifs that I mentioned were still at risk for them coming up--for them rearing their ugly heads and a host of other bad human behaviors or panicked human behaviors. But I have always been a great proponent rather not of panic but of informed concern. When you panic in the midst of a crisis, rarely do good things or good strategies come to play. But when you plan for a crisis in--before it occurs, it does not mean you are always going to be right in what you predict, but you are a little bit better prepared to handle those issues as they come up. Please be assured that as a pandemic does--if a pandemic does occur, there will be no blueprint that can be religiously followed and it will have to be changed by day by day just as all of us would do at a patient's bedside. I mean I look it as public health as really the doctor patient relationship at large. So if you are at a bedside seeing a patient and the data is one--presents one picture and then the next day things change, you change your treatment plan. And again with a public health situation, we may have to change

Contemplating Pandemics:

our treatment plan day by day, but with open and honest communication I really do believe that can happen.

And so I guess I will close and I am historically optimistic and hope the lessons from the past and the present can facilitate productive, ethically, and socially appropriate strategies that will mitigate the microbial threats that sadly but inevitably loom on our horizon. Thank you very much.

End of file

Ethics, Genetics and the Future of Sport, 2007
Thomas Murray, Ph.D., President, The Hastings Center,
Garrison, New York

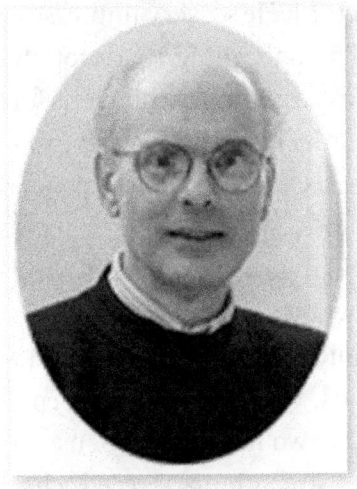

When I first was recruited to Case Western Reserve School of Medicine to create a bioethics center what I discovered immediately that the best allies you could possibly have were experienced clinicians who had the universal respect of everyone in the school. And when they voted with their feet and they came and they said this was important and they took part in our teaching and they led by example. That made my job possible and easy and pleasurable and my sense is that Doctor Waggoner was a person of that sort. So I'm just delighted to be here in his name. And of course my son-in-law, Matt Rennie, who is now an assistant sports editor at the Washington Post just thinks it really cool that his father-in-law is finally getting to appreciate the glories of Ann Arbor and UM. So that's a great pleasure as well. And he's done well by us. There are two beautiful grandchildren in Takoma Park, Maryland, in part with Matt having played a role in that.

So I'll tell you just a little bit about how we got into this issue of performance enhancement in sport. I was at the Hastings Center. I've had two stays at the Hastings Center. I went there in 1979. I was there through 1984. Very early in that first day we got a grant from the National Science Foundation to look at non-therapeutic drug use. There's the usual sort of familiar form which is drug abuse. But then there was this other interesting possibility that someone would use drugs not for pleasure but to try to actually be more effective for performance enhancement. I took on the role of sort of tracking that down and thinking about that and pulling together a research group to see what we could learn.

So in traditional Hastings Center style I went to try to get the facts straight. Friends of mine had gone into journalism from college and so some of them are doing sports and they introduced me to a variety of athletes. I met Julius Irving in that context, Doctor J. He's a very impressive human being, physically very handsome. The only thing that's totally out of proportion is his hands. They are half as large as they should be for a person of his size. So when I shook hands with Doctor J. I just felt like I was being enveloped. And I met other athletes, Olympians. I met people involved in sports, sports officials, sports athletes themselves, coaches and the like. And we learned a great deal about how, why athletes were using performance enhancing drugs and how they understood that use and what it meant to them. The drugs of choice at that time, we're talking now about 1979-80 were anabolic steroids, various synthetic forms of testosterone and stimulants. Those were the two main drugs of use in sport at that time. And we assembled the research group, learned what we could. I wrote a couple of articles and I thought that was that.

Well, then the U.S. Olympic Committee sort of discovered what I had been up to and they started inviting me to their anti-doping committee's meetings and they made me a member. I did that for about 16 years. Of all the voluntary things I've done it was by far the most miserable. You would be flown off to distant airports. On weekends you'd spend the weekend in a hotel meeting room, sometimes with no windows and you would be talking about athletes peeing into jars and then you would leave and you never knew what happened. I mean, the USOC quite frankly wasn't all that serious about drug control for a very long time with just a very short exception when Baron Pittenger was the executive director. I'd come home and I'd be full of frustration and then my wife would just say, "Quit." She's very sensible. She'd say, "Quit. Don't do that anymore. You don't get any money. You just take your time. It takes you away from your family." And "Nothing good happens from it." And after 16 years she was basically right.

Things have changed a bit we think with the introduction of the world anti-doping agency and the various national agencies in the U.S. It's the U.S. Anti-Doping Agency or USADA. You actually have a person who has now joined the University of Michigan family. Doctor Don Vereen who can tell you something about the history of this. And Don's an old friend of my sitting right here. You should all meet Dr. Vereen. Now having done this work we never had any money to do any more research until about four years ago when I was able to get some grants and begin our work.

So let me now tell you the story about what I've learned in these. Now I'm going to frame the discussion this way. We're looking at the general question of how to use biomedicine, when and how to use biomedicine in pursuit of human goals. Sport is one realm of human endeavor. Despite what the football coach told you in high school it's not all that matters, but it can be important. And I think it is important in a lot of ways in sort of telling us about our own humanity. So I'm going to think about the meaning of sport as a human activity and I want to offer just a thesis that a useful way to think about excellence in sport, and here I don't just mean Olympians or professionals. I mean if you get out and you play tennis or you play golf or ping pong or softball or in my case I got bicycling, excellence matters for all of us. I mean it's sort of reaching wherever our natural talents take us and whatever we do to perfect those talents.

Now I use this old-fashioned word virtuous perfection. I'll tell you why. It may come as a shock to you to know that I'm quite confident that I could win the 100-meter dash in the 2008 Olympic Games. All I need is the right equipment, a baseball bat to break the legs of the people who are running with me. So that would not be a virtuous perfection of my natural talents. I don't even have that good of a swing in baseball so you can't go that way either. So by virtuous perfection I just mean the things that we do that are admirable. They could be admirable in many realms of life.

Now over the years I've collected all kinds of objections to the proposition that we should try to control the use of some kind of performance enhancing drugs in sports. So these are all objections to the idea of drug control. And I've found five that strike me as the most common and the most philosophically interesting. One is the claim of incoherency. Two is the line drawing problem. Three we'll call the resistance is futile objection, Star Trek fans will recognize that one. The appeal to individual liberty is the fourth. And the romantic promethean view will require a little more explanation than the others but call that the fifth.

Here's the incoherency claim. The idea here is, look, there's no way to tell the difference between the various things an athlete might do to enhance their performance. I mean suppose somebody has really, really fancy running shoes and somebody else doesn't. Well, the really fancy shoes are going to allow them to run faster. I understand there are golf clubs now that you can be not very good drivers but you can still hit the ball far and straight. That's an equipment change. What's wrong with that? The claim is that it's incoherent to try to make any distinctions among any of these ways of enhancing performance. And if that's true then there's no difference between eating well and taking gobs of anabolic steroids.

Well, this is a plausible objection. I often think in terms of analogies and cases so I tried to create a case. Now imagine that someone shows up for, we'll make it the New York Marathon. Shows up for the New York Marathon having appropriately registered, prepared to set off, number pinned to her back but she's had the creativity to wear these really cool shoes that have wheels on the bottom. She's brought roller blades. Then just imagine that the marathon never thought to ban roller blades and so she sets out and she covers the 26 plus miles faster than anyone else. Would you feel that she genuinely deserves to be crowned the champion of the New York Marathon? All of you who believe that please raise your hand. All of you who believe she doesn't deserve to be crowned the champion please raise your hand. You folks have just put to rest the incoherency objection because you see the difference between running shoes and roller blades for the New York Marathon. Maybe we can't fully articulate why that distinction matters yet, but we sure can tell the difference. That's enough with the incoherency claim.

Our critic steps back and says all right, all right. There might be differences but there's no way you can draw a line that isn't going to be arbitrary and that when you do something that's arbitrary it's inevitably bad. Fair enough. Let me suggest something here. Let's suppose that I tell Doctor Margolis "Doctor Margolis we are going to give you an award of ten million dollars. And Doctor Greden, we're going to give you a hundred lashes." It might actually be easier than being Chair of Psychiatry. But you said, "Why are you doing that?" And I said, "I don't know. I just feel like it." Well, that's arbitrary and that's wrong. When you treat people for no good reason differently in that way, punish and reward, that's a moral fault. So if drawing a line is arbitrary in that way it's a terrible problem.

Now let me ask another question. What's the distance between the pitcher's rubber and home plate in baseball? 60 feet, 6 inches, what a goofy number, not even a round number, 60 feet, 6 inches. That's arbitrary. Let's say that we take that objection seriously. We say you're right. That's an arbitrary distance. We're not going to enforce it. Do what you want. What happens to baseball? I've actually asked some pitchers this question and they say, "I'm going to get right up on top of the catcher and I'm going to just throw the ball. And the batter will be helpless." The only chance the batter would have to get his bat on the ball at all would be just to hold out in front of home plate. Baseball would be reduced to a game with a pitcher, a catcher, a bunter and seven infielders. Well, if you like baseball that doesn't look at all like the kind of sport that you enjoy. So is 60 feet, 6 inches arbitrary? It sure is. It could've been 60 feet or 61 feet, the game wouldn't be all that different. But if you made it 5 feet it would sure be different. Or if you eliminated the rule altogether it would be different.

So here we have a case where we've drawn a line and drawing the line at 60 feet, 6 inches is defensible, drawing some line is defensible. If you didn't have a line the sport would basically disappear. And drawing it in this particular place, 60 feet, 6 inches, is not unreasonable. It could've been 60 feet, 7 inches or 5 inches or 60 feet or 61 feet. You'd still have something that'd look like the baseball that those who love it love, but you couldn't draw it at 5 feet and you couldn't draw it at 120 feet. It would be a completely different game. So you have to satisfy two conditions. One is that drawing some line is defensible and secondly that putting it in this particular place is at least okay. There might be other places you could draw it but it still preserves the meaning in the activity. That's the key point. Yes, 60 feet, 6 inches is arbitrary in that sense, but that doesn't make it bad. In fact, if you didn't have it what you cared about the sport would disappear. Anabolic steroids prohibited, nutritional supplements permitted. There's a line in between the two. Does the line get a little difficult and fuzzy at times? Yes. If you eliminated the line would what we care about in sport disappear? I'm going to argue later that it would.

Now the resistance is futile objection. Notice in the first place here the claim is you can try to ban steroids, you can try to ban HDH, you can try to ban EPO and endurance sports. It's not going to work. Athletes are going to use it anyway. And quite frankly what happened in the past Tour De France at least a year before would seem to underscore that this objection is sometimes correct. Athletes will use it no matter what you do to try to stop them. But notice in the first place that it's not an ethical claim. To say that resistance is futile isn't to say that it's wrong to try to enforce rules. It's basically two different predictions. One is that if you try to control drugs in this sport you won't succeed. And secondly it'll be even worse if you try to enforce a ban. There'll be bad consequences of various kinds. Well, that's not an unreasonable argument. But it ignores a couple of things.

Let me give you another example. I live an hour north of New York City and it doesn't happen so often there, but in New York City it's been known that people drive automobiles that don't belong to them. You've heard of this phenomenon? Does it ever happen in Ann Arbor? Well, suppose I come to you and say well, the fact that you have car theft in Ann Arbor, why try to ban it? I mean, people are going to do it anyway. I mean, that doesn't convince you, does it? Well, control is never perfect. It's not perfect in banning criminal activity. It's not perfect in banning drug use in sports. The fact that it's imperfect is not in and of itself an argument to not attempt it because some good comes from the effort to control. You damp down the activity. You've made consequences for it. Successfully controlling something requires, among other things, the public conviction that the effort to control it is right. That's what happened with prohibition, there wasn't strong public support of prohibition. And you need it reasonable infective, not perfect but infective enforcement. We'll put this one on the side and say they've got a point, but that's not a compelling reason not to attempt it if you can get support and if you can enforce reasonably well.

Now the argument for liberty. This is the one we dealt with 25 years ago at the Hastings Center when I talked to the athletes. This is what we learned because at the time there were people making arguments, well look this is the use of anabolic steroids or other performance enhancing drugs in sport. It's just an expression of individual liberty. We should allow athletes to do it. They're just trying to succeed. They're trying to be the best they can. So that was the positive argument.

Then there was the negative argument. You all know what paternalism is? Roughly speaking paternalism is doing something to or for another person in what you believe is their interest but without their permission or consent. It has its place. We're going to take care of two of our grandchildren. If my three and a half year old granddaughter Tess wants to run out and play in the middle of the street my reaction is not going to be, "Yes, Tess, I respect your autonomy. If you wish to play in traffic that's your"--I'm going to say, "Get in the house." Paternalism has its place but it doesn't really have much of a place with say a 25-year-old elite athlete.

Ethics, Genetics and the Future of Sport, 2007

So when athletes were being told, this is the case in the early 1980's, that you shouldn't take anabolic steroids because number one you'll hurt yourself. And number two they are ineffective. Athletes weren't convinced. For one thing they were effective and they knew it. The athletes knew that. And for the other, I mean, the paternalism argument just didn't wash. I understand that there are people who in winter will go on top of a mountain, strap boards to their feet and careen down mountains at 60 miles per hour. Can you believe this? Downhill skiing. Now if I tell someone who does downhill skiing, "Don't use anabolic steroids. You might hurt yourself." They will look at me as crazy. Just somebody not to be taken seriously because we've encouraged them to take these very significant risks and it's not just downhill skiing. There are a number of sports that carry a significant risk. We not only permit it we encourage it. And then we say don't do this other thing because there's this slight probably you might hurt yourself. It doesn't wash. So paternalism, that's not going to be an effective argument against drug use in sport for adult athletes. It will work for young athletes, but it will not work for mature athletes.

In our project what we discovered was that when athletes who worked very hard, particularly the ones who got to elite or quasi elite level, didn't want to lose and didn't want to abandon their sport. And in the absence of effective drug control the only option we've left them is to level the playing field by using the same drugs being used by their competitors. And that's the story we heard. That is why drug use was endemic in at least a number of sports and continues to erupt as endemic in sports from time to time. Until you can assure athletes that they've got a reasonable chance to compete on a level playing field you will have lots of pressure on athletes to use drugs. So we talked about the coerce of power of drugs and sports. If the drugs are effective they make a difference. And if they're being widely used the pressure on an athlete to use them can be immense particularly when the difference between grand success and failure is measured in fractions of a second or inches. Somebody said that anabolic steroids and baseball don't let you hit the curve ball. That's probably true. However it makes that fly ball you hit instead of going to the edge of the warning track it lands in the second row of the bleachers. That's a big difference in baseball. And if that's the effect it's having then you need to take seriously whether you are going to permit it or try to control it.

Now to the last argument. This is philosophically the richest one. I've called it the romantic or promethean view. It has several elements. Number one it views human beings, all of us, as fundamentally self creators. We may decorate our bodies with clothing, with piercings, with tattoos. We try to perfect our minds. It could be as works of art. Some people see their body as a canvas or it could be in pursuit of particular other kinds of goals, performance related goals.

It's essential, I think, to understand the cultural and philosophical context and implications of this view. One thing it does is it valorizes. Basically it kind of holds up for praise unfettered will or willfulness. If we want this thing to be this kind of thing, that's what matters, and our capacity for self manipulation. Of all the things that we are as human beings, all of the beings whose lives are lived in these powerful and immensely important webs of relationships that we have, the things that this view pulls out are the human willfulness and the human capacity for self manipulation. You will find many representatives of this view out there and they will be arguing that not only should we permit drugs in sport we should actually celebrate it because it's another form of human self creation.

Now some sports do that. Body building. I understand people have even gone on to become governors of states after having careers as this, but I don't believe that myself. In body building they literally are seeking a particular form and drug use was not just prevalent it was a necessary element, I think. It may still be in body building. But body building's not an Olympic sport. It's a different kind of activity. Now I'd asked what's the relationship of this kind of unfettered pursuit in self manipulation to human flourishing, which is a fancy word just for saying what makes for good lives for people, for men, women and children? I leave that as a question.

Now one of the implications of this view is spelled out by a film critic, Noelle Caskey, who does not support this view herself but she describes it. She says, "Anorexia is the cultivation of the specific image as an image. It is a purely artificial creation and that is why it is so admired. Will alone produces it and maintains it against considerable odds." Now you see how this is exactly an example of the kind of willfulness and self manipulation I've just talked about. But here it's actually used as a description of a condition which can be a terrible disease and indeed a lethal disease. One should be cautious about how far to take this notion about the human prometheus.

Now what I worry about is a little more down to earth and that is the triumph of the performance principle. By that I just mean the pursuit of maximum performance by any means, whatever means at whatever cost. There's a sport called power lifting which is like weight lifting in that they're lifting weights. But it's not an Olympic sport. It's got a different set of governing bodies. In fact, it's got many, many different associations. Some of them are drug free or at least so advertise themselves. Some of them basically say we do no testing so come in and do whatever you can and just get those weights up there. And so power lifting provides a very interesting experiment in nature of what will happen if you remove any efforts to control performance enhancing drugs in sport. And I think the jury's out. I'm not sure what it's in the end going to tell us. But it's a real phenomenon. It's going on right now and we're continuing to pay attention to it. In my most recent project we have two world champion power lifters, a husband and wife team, who are now actually professors at the University of Texas, who have been studying the evolution of power lifting and particularly the role of drugs in power lifting. They have a great chapter in the book that will be coming out soon. My sense is that the power of the performance principle will unavoidable triumph if you refuse to set any limits. If you refuse to draw a line anywhere you are basically saying do whatever. It will result in greatly increased health risks to people who then pursue those limits.

Now here I try to make maybe a subtle distinction. I've already said that telling a downhill skier you shouldn't take anabolic steroids because it might hurt yourself was paternalism and tough to justify. Yet I want to be able to say that it makes sense to have rules to govern a sport that would reduce the likelihood that people will in fact be driven to these extremes. So yes I am doing the rules for more reasons than just to protect them, but it will have the impact of protecting them if we're successful in enforcing the rules and I would argue that's defensible.

Now I also think that if the performance principle triumphs we're going to lose what's meaningful about sport. And I'll say more about that. Now don't get me wrong. I'm not against all forms of biomedical enhancement. There are lots of things we can do to enhance human form and function and many of them, I think, would be quite desirable. So again I made up a hypothetical years ago. Let's imagine that a neurosurgeon who does the most sensitive and delicate operations is concerned about the normal tremor that all of us have. If you hold your hand out here and you watch it closely enough, see you've got a little bit of a tremor. There's nothing unhealthy about it, it's just part of normal human physiology. Imagine that a drug comes along that it's noticed that one of the side effects of this drug--and it's a pretty innocuous drug that's used for other things, but one of the side effects is it just knocks down that tremor so your hand becomes much steadier. A neurosurgeon gets the idea that if I took that drug maybe that would actually steady my hand during this procedure. So I'm going to try it. And then take this hypothetical further on, many neurosurgeons try it. They actually run a randomized controlled clinical trial to see what the results are and the results are unequivocal. The patients of neurosurgeons who have used the drug do better, faster recoveries, fewer complications, more successful surgeries than the patients of the physicians who don't. That's the set up, now the question. The person in the world you love the most needs exactly one of these procedures. For some of you that person will be yourself. For some of us it will be somebody else. It will be our child or spouse or parent or whomever. It doesn't matter whoever that person is. And here's your choice. You go into the Ann Arbor Neurosurgery practice and you've got two options. Surgeon number one says, "Well, I think it is unnatural to use performance enhancing drugs. I think it takes away from my agency in the course of this surgery. So I would never use them." And the second surgeon says, "I use them every time I operate. My patients do better." Which surgeon do you choose for your loved one? Who chooses number one, the one who goes au natural? They are otherwise equal. Number two has better results because he or she uses the drug. Who chooses number two? I choose number two. It's hands down. It's easy. That's a performance enhancing drug. Now if you read the report of the current president's commission council they would seem to be opposed to that because it detracts. It's biomedical intervention. It seems to me they don't get it on that point.

What matters is the point of the practice. If the point of sport is to display natural talents and their perfection then drugs don't belong. If the point of neurosurgery is to make patients better and this drug without harming the neurosurgeon helps patients, what's the problem? It seems that one would embrace the use of a performance enhancing drug in that context. It's not the means per se. It's not that it's a drug or biomedical intervention. But it's the relationship of that means to the goals of the practice, to whatever it is we value about this activity and to in the end to human flourishing.

Quickly about genetics, the challenge of genetic enhancement in sport which people have called gene doping. It's the same techniques that are being developed towards gene therapy, could be used to try to improve someone's athletic capacities. So if we value in sport natural talents and their virtuous perfection what do we disvalue? And I think what we disvalue among other things are any interventions that would distort the relationship between those talents, their virtuous perfection and natural excellence. Now what makes a talent natural? Here it gets complicated. Athletic talents are by in large what geneticists will call complex traits or complex phenotypes. It's unlikely that any one gene is going to have much of an effect on athletic ability, but there may be some exceptions. I suggested some years ago the metaphor of the genomism ecosystem rather than beans in a bean bag, the old bean bag model in classical genetics. Think of genes as operating an extremely complex ecosystem with many, many positive and negative feedback loops inside each cell, then in the tissues, then in the body, then with the external environment. It's a very complicated, fascinating picture. But it means that you can't count on simple interventions having the outcome that you want for them to have. Can I suggest if anyone's interested they can download the report. It's a free PDF on the center's website on behavioral genetics, which it's the best discussion I've ever read and it's received broad praise. I didn't write it. Colleagues of mine did about trying to understand complex traits, particularly behavioral genetic traits. And athletic traits are behavioral traits.

Now how should we think about differences in natural talents because I was just trading emails with the sports writer, John Feinstein, do you know who he is? He is author of *A Good Walk Spoiled* and a number of other fine books about sports. He's going to come with us to Capitol Hill. We're going to do a briefing in the Senate office, the Commerce Committee hearing room, on genetics and sport in about a week and a half. And Feinstein's going to come and do it. And he was saying that he really wanted to be a basketball player, but he was too short and couldn't. And I said, well when I was twelve, and this was true, I was this height. And I had great dreams of being a basketball player. But I had a couple of liabilities. One is I never grew. Two is I weighed 125 pounds or so, so a breath of air could blow me out of the way. And three was at the top of my leap you could stick two credit cards under my shoe. So there are inequalities in natural talent.

Do you know the Kurt Vonnegut story? I can't remember the story's name but it's in one of his short story collections. But the handicapper general's job is to make sure that no one has a natural advantage over anyone else. So physically gifted and graceful people have weights tied to them. Very smart people have implants that emit shattering noises into their brain at regular intervals so they can't think for very long without interruption. Do we want to handicap the general model of sport? I don't think so. Should we think about and add the differences in natural talent as inequalities to be redressed or as just expressions of human variation that we can celebrate? And my take is that the Olympic movement opts for the latter. And I think the alternative is this romantical promethean triumph of the performance principle.

There's a new thing that's come that showed up. And that is the idea that one would not genetically manipulate, not try to change the genes in your cells, but try to test for particular versions of the genes. And so there's a gene called ACTN3 and there are a number of versions of it but one particular version, one particular allele looks like it's a stop mutation. So if you have this particular version you can't make the full protein product and so you don't get the protein. Now your cells function fine. It turns out that the protein's made in muscle cells. And there's another version called ACTN2 and people who have a double stop, two versions of the defective one in ACTN3 usually have healthy ACTN2 and there's no disease issue here. They're fine. There are no symptoms. However, some scientists have developed some early evidence that people who have two of the mutated forms, so they're not making any of the protein, they have faster twitch muscle fiber and may therefore be better adapted for sports like power sports and sprinting sports. Whereas people who have two healthy versions of it have slow twitch--are more likely to develop slow twitch muscles and so may be more suited for endurance sports. So for 110 dollars Australian you can get a kit, take a swab inside the cheek, put it in the vile, send it back to the lab. And they'll tell you whether you're a double no, whether you're one and one, heterozygote or whether you've got two full versions of the protein. And the claim is well you can use that to help decide what sports that individual ought to be in.

Ethics, Genetics and the Future of Sport, 2007

Well, who are they going to use this test for do you think? I mean, they're not going to do it for many 61-year-old bioethicists I think. It's kind of set for me. I mean, I kind of know what I'm going to be doing athletically or not. I'm a bicyclist. That's what I do. Who do you think they're going to use this on? Yeah. There is some activity among sort of barely adult athletes who are maybe wondering if they're elite athletes or not. But, yes, I think a lot of these are going to be children. Now if you go to the website of the company in Australia offering the test they will tell you it's not for children under 18. But they never see you. They just get the cheek swab you send in and they send you back the results. So are people using this test to ascertain whether their kid is going to be a marathoner or a hundred meter dash runner? Some people are.

How valuable is this information? My guess is knowing what we know about the complexity between genes and complex phenotypes that the information's going to be about as useless as you can get. It's not going to be worth 110 dollars Australian. Nonetheless people believing in the power of genes will still perhaps still young people towards or away from sports that they might love and might actually be well suited for. So that's the worry.

In the end we have a clash of meetings. How should we understand sport? How should we understand the meaning of the Olympic Games? And what the WADA, World Anti-Doping Agency, code calls somewhat vaguely the spirit of sport. They're hinting at something that I believe is important but needs to be spelled out more clearly. Should we see sport as exhibitions of maximum human performance and human self manipulation? Well, that's one view. It's not a crazy view and there are plenty of people out there who hold that. And if that view prevails then we probably will cease worrying about drugs and sports. Or should we see it as a celebration of human differences, as variations in natural talents admirably perfected? As people point out Michael Jordan never could play baseball. He couldn't hit the curve ball. So wonderful athletic talent in one realm does not necessarily translate to another. Is that how we should see the future of sport? And that's a question that we will be wrestling with and our children will be wrestling with and I think generations on to that will have to wrestle with because there will be many, many more ways of intervening pharmacologically, surgically, with various kinds of biomedical devices and prosthesis. All of which sport will be confronted with and will have to make decisions about should this be part of the sport or should it be given its own special niche in sport or should it be banned from sport? And that's a question we'll all have. These are my coordinates and this is where I work. And if any of you are in the area give us a warning and we accommodate visitors every time we can. It's an interesting group of people I work with, herding cats but they're smart cats. Thank you very much.

Beyond Band-Aids: How to Cure America's Sick, 2008
Ezekiel Emanuel, M. D., Chair,
Department of Bioethics, The Clinical Center of the National Institutes of Health

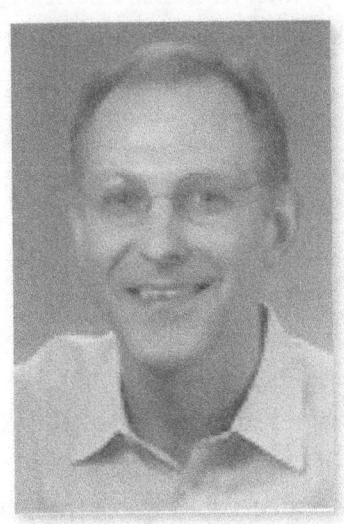

W<!---->ell, it's wonderful to be here. And this is actually only the second time I've been to the University of Michigan despite having grown up in the Midwest, in Chicago. And I will say I nevertheless feel a very close attachment to the institution. For one thing one of the most important mentors in my life at the Dana Farber Cancer Institute, Dan Hayes, is a faculty member here and a man from whom I learned a lot. The former dean here is a very close friend, Alan Lichter, who I constantly get sage advice from. And the medical school has been wise enough to accept three of the fellows from my department here. And they have thoroughly enjoyed the place so it has left me with a very soft spot for the institution and I appreciate your turning out.

One of the things that Doctor Margolis did not mention is that I do a lot of surveys in my research and despite not getting informed consent from you I am going to do a little bit of a survey here at the start of my lecture. The first question is considering all aspects how well do you think the American health care system functions? Who thinks it functions very well? No one? Maybe one. Moderately well? A fair number of people here. Fairly well? Maybe the majority at fairly well. Not well at all? All right. Second question, considering all aspects how happy are you personally with the health care services you personally receive? Very happy? A lot of people there. Moderately happy? A few more. Fairly happy? Not too many. Not happy at all? None. This difference between the way you view the health care system and the way you view your own personal health care services is a very important data point. And it's actually an important barrier to health care reform which we're going to come back to at the end of the talk.

Now I think that this cartoon summarizes it pretty well. Between congratulations on your left and get well it says good luck with the American health care system. The American health care system has really combined two parts. One part is how we pay for care, how we actually pay doctors. And the other part is how we deliver care, seeing patients, admitting them to the hospital. And I want to submit to you that both parts, both the financing part and the delivery side, are broken. The financing part is inefficient, inequitable and increasingly fiscally unsustainable. And in a few seconds I'll review the data on that. The delivery system, again how we deliver care to our patients, is fragmented. It's not designed to care for chronic illness even though chronic illness accounts for 70 percent of the dollars we spend. It delivers haphazard and I would submit poor quality. And we have a very high use in this country of unproven and marginal therapies. And again, we'll discuss some of the evidence for each of these.

True health care reform must fix both the financing and the delivery side. I think this is a very good litmus test for any health care reform proposal you happen to see. When a politician proposes a health care reform and you listen to it you ask yourself does it solve the financing problem, does it solve the delivery system problem? If it doesn't do both you can be sure it is not a going concern. It is not sustainable. The unfortunate fact is that in this political year and the debate about health care reform in America today we are focused on the financing side and trying to get to universal coverage. We say almost nothing about delivery system reform and that is a serious problem which we'll return to.

How to Cure America's Sick, 2008 Ezekiel Emanuel, M. D., Chair,

Now if I locked all of you in a room, gave you a sheet of paper and a pen and said what would you want a good health care system to achieve? You would fill up a page with lots of ideals that it should achieve. Now we can't talk about 30 or 40 different things. I can talk about seven and that's probably itself too many. The first three coverage, cost control and quality I don't think there's any disagreement on. The fourth one, choice. We live in a country where you can go to the supermarket and choose from 50 different jams, probably 75 or 100 cereals. It's going to be very difficult not to have choice built in to the health care system. We will not tolerate that. We also need a system that has fair fiscal responsibility where the rich pay their part and we subsidize the poor rather than having the poor subsidize the rich as we do today in our current system. If we want doctors to support a reform system we need malpractice reform. And last, we want a health care system that helps the economy rather than dragging it down and creating problems for employment and businesses.

Well, how does the current system match up to these goals? And I'm not going to go through each one of them. You already know because everyone pummels you with it that 47 million Americans are uninsured. Probably what you don't know is that between two-thirds and three-quarters of those uninsured are either full-time workers or members of families with a full-time worker in it. That is completely, completely un-American. The rules of the game in this country are if you work hard, you play honestly, you're supposed to get the benefits of our society. Not getting health care insurance even though you pay taxes and therefore support health insurance for other people is not part of the American social contract. Worse even is the fact that 9 million children who couldn't possibly afford to provide themselves with health care insurance don't have coverage. We should be ashamed of that.

Cost control. In 2006 the last year for which we have reliable data we spent 2.1 trillion dollars on health care. No. I did not by mistake add three extra zeros there. That is what trillion looks like. That's one out of every six dollars in your wallet going to nothing else but health care.

Beyond Band-Aids:

Now I'm at the University of Michigan and I know you guys are really smart but I would venture to wager you don't really understand how big a trillion is. So I am just going to help you here. How many seconds ago is a million seconds? Last week. How many seconds ago is a billion seconds? When Richard Nixon resigned the White House. How many seconds ago was a trillion seconds? 30 thousand B.C., 15 thousand years before a human being stepped foot on the North American continent. And we are spending two of those each year on nothing but health care. I was pretty sure you didn't know how big a trillion was. It's so big we're spending two trillion dollars a year. It's bigger than the GDP of China. Everything they spend in China for 1.2 billion people is less than what we spend on health care. It's bigger than the GDPs of France and Spain put together. But it's not just how much we're spending today. It's what I call the tsunami of the future. This is health care spending as a percent of GDP long into the future. If we don't do anything by 2082 there is only health care. There's either patients and the health care people taking care of them, nothing else exists in the economy. That clearly can't go on, but that's what the curve looks like if we don't do anything.

Now if you think about controlling costs there are two aspects to it. One is the waste in the current system. And I want to focus just a bit on the administrative waste which is mainly related to administrative waste with insurance from underwriting, sales, marketing, broker's commissions, billings. And then there is the long-term upward slope which is 50 percent of that slope is related to technology, the development of new technologies and the diffusion of existing technologies to patients with less and less indication for it and therefore less and less impact. Well, let's just talk about administrative costs for the moment. This is a quote from two economists from Stanford, "The need for more than 850 insurance companies to see and contract with millions of employers, underwriting each one, adds greatly to administrative cost." Typically administrative costs are on the order of 11 percent of premium. And this does not include the cost to employers to purchase and manage that health care spending. To understand how this could be different consider that Kaiser Permanente signs only one annual contract for the coverage of more than 400 thousand employees independent with CalPERS. That's a California Public Employees Retirement Plan. And the administrative costs are on the order of 0.5 percent of premium. That 10.5 percent difference between 11 percent and 0.5 percent is pure administrative cost with no health benefit. That is a result of a defective, broken health care insurance market. It's because you have to sell to each employer individually rather than to the whole country.

Let's talk about quality for a second. We have a terribly fragmented, nineteenth century, horse and buggy delivery system. Last year there were one billion office visits in the outpatient setting to doctors. A third of them were to solo practitioners operating alone. Another third were to doctors in groups of four or less. It's really hard to provide high quality care in those kind of small groups, hard to provide the infrastructure of computers, hard to coordinate care. The typical Medicare beneficiary sees seven different doctors in a year including five specialists. And if you have two chronic conditions in Medicare you see 15 doctors. Is that likely to get you good medicine? The WRAN study, many of you may be familiar with this published in the New England Journal about four years ago, looked at Medicare patients discharged from hospitals. And they assessed the quality of care they got on nine very simple measures. We're not talking about complicated chemotherapy, complicated surgical procedures. We're talking: was blood pressure measured and if it was high were patients put on the right medication to get it under control? Was cholesterol measured and if it was high were they put on the right medications to get it under control? Did they get a NUMA vaccine before discharge? Well, the chance of Medicare patients getting those nine proven procedures about 55 percent, flipping a coin essentially. And if you're a child on other measures the WRAN study found only 46 percent of the time you get proven measures, simple things again. We are not providing high quality care.

And then there is a lot of unproven costly therapies. So you may know that over 210 thousand American men will get diagnosed with prostate cancer this year. And you have a choice of three different therapies. There's watchful waiting. There's surgery, a prostatectomy. There's radiation therapy. And inside radiation therapy there are four flavors of treatment. You can get 3D conformal radiation guided by CT scans. You can get breaking therapy which is little radiation seeds implanted into the prostate. And then there's IMRT, Intensely Modulated Radiation Therapy. And then there's Proton B, not giving electrons but giving protons. These machines cost upwards of a hundred million dollars, have to be housed in football field sized buildings. And you can see the price difference here. Those are the Medicare reimbursement prices except for Proton B which is what Lul Melinda charges out in California. Eight full price differences. Now you might want to ask what's the difference for eight full price difference? I can't tell you. No one can tell you. There's never been a head to head comparison of these four treatments. I will tell you one thing. No one in this country believes that there is a survival difference and that includes the three thousand radiation oncologists in this country. Because last year at this time I went to their annual meeting, gave the plan of recession, showed this slide and I asked, "One person just get up and tell me I'm wrong." Not one of them did. At best based on single institution studies there is probably a 10 percent absolute difference in side effects. Now is that difference in impotence and proctitis worth 70 thousand dollars? I ask you.

Well, you also heard that I'm a breast cancer oncologist. I just picked on the radiation oncologists. Now I'll pick on the urological oncologists. A recent study in the Journal of Clinical Oncology showed that among men 66 years and older with low or moderate grade prostate cancer not receiving radiation or prostate surgery a third of them received castration, either chemical castration or actual surgical castration. This despite the fact that there's no evidence it improves longevity and we know it makes the quality of life a lot worse because they end up impotent. It's not recommended on any of the major guidelines either the AUA guidelines or the NCCN guidelines and yet a third of the time urologists are doing this. And the worst piece of information, in my humble opinion, academic urologists are not much better than private practitioners.

Drag on the economy. The average cost of employment based coverage for a family is 12 thousand dollars a year. To translate that for you when the University of Michigan gives you health insurance for you and your family that's like hiring another worker at minimum wage for the whole year. To give you health insurance it's hiring two workers. That is a serious drag. The way we've structured our health care system we link health insurance to employment and this has created a whole series of problems. First, over the last decade almost every strike has been linked to health benefits. The only strike that's not linked to health benefits was the Hollywood Writer's strike and no one knows what the h** that was about. Linking employment and health care insurance creates this problem of portability especially if you've had an illness. It encourages companies to outsource and off shore jobs as you well know in Michigan. And it actually leads to suppression of wages. Money that goes to buy the insurance doesn't go actually to wage increases.

So the real question is what should be done. What should we do? Well, you did hear that I work for the U.S. Government and the NIH and I'm required to say these are not the official views of the U.S. government or the NIH, the Department of Health and Human Services. But I will use this slide for a little civics test. You all know the guy in the middle. The guy on the left, Secretary Michael Leavitt. About one to two percent of audiences even at very educated places know that. Interestingly he controls more money in the federal government than anyone else, about a trillion dollars a year and we don't know who he is. The guy on the right? Zirhouni, right. You know him more interestingly and he only controls 28 billion dollars and only for one more day because he's resigned effective Friday. Not that late in the afternoon ladies and gentlemen.

Well, if you go around and ask what should be done in Washington you can come across literally hundreds of health care reform proposals and I am not joking, hundreds of them. As a matter of fact some of you may have

Beyond Band-Aids:

heard of the Center for American Progress which is a left leaning think tank in Washington run by John Podesta who's a former chief of staff of Bill Clinton, a very smart guy. And they have actually in the last 18 months issued three health care reform proposals. That's not because one has been adopted. It's because you want to get attention you release another health care proposal. But you don't need to think about hundreds of health care reform proposals or even ten. All health care reform proposals can really be boiled down to one of four flavors. The Guaranteed Health Care Access Plan which is our plan which is similar to the Wyden Bennett bill, incrementalism, individual and/or employer mandates, what they're doing in Massachusetts, or single-payer. So what I propose to do is to explain our plan and then like Fox news give a fair and balanced rendition of everyone else's.

So the Guaranteed Health Care Access Plan has ten planks to it. First, every American receives a certificate or voucher to receive a standard benefits package through an insurance company or a health plan. There's an insurance exchange set up and you get to choose which company you want to go with. The standards benefits plan is modeled on the program. It's essentially the health insurance that federal workers as well as congressmen and senators get. It's better than what about 85 percent of Americans currently have. The health plans have to guarantee issue and they cannot exclude anyone or coverage for any preexisting condition. In exchange for that everyone's included so there's no selection on that basis. And they get a risk adjusted premium which means they get paid more to cover people with emphysema or COPD or cancer or diabetes and less to cover the healthy 20-year-old University of Michigan students.

Second, Americans who get their certificate have free choice of any qualified plan which has to enroll them at no premium and no deductible. Typical people would have a selection of five to eight plans. In rural areas it might be only one. Americans who don't enroll are randomly assigned to a health plan by their regional health board. There are no cracks in this system. You cannot be excluded. You don't have to pay anything. No requirement for a mandate.

Certificates are funded by a dedicated value added tax. What do I mean by dedicated? All the money from the value added tax goes to health care, no general revenue. And the value added tax can't be siphoned off for other things whether it's social security, education, the environment, defense.

Fourth, people have freedom to purchase more services than the standard benefits package with their own after tax dollars. You want a wider selection of doctors, you want more brand name drugs, you want complimentary and alternative medicine, you want a better mental health package, you want concierge medicine and have a doctor come to your house you can buy all those services with your own money.

Fifth, the private sector organizes and delivers care and is accountable for it.

Sixth, the tax exemption for employment-based insurance is eliminated. So right now when the University of Michigan provides you health insurance you pay no income tax and no payroll tax on it. This is a huge incentive and a huge reason we have employment-based coverage. We get rid of that. Right now that tax deduction, single largest tax deduction in the American tax code, worth more than 210 billion dollars.

Seven, we phase out Medicare, Medicaid, SCHIP and all government programs. What does that mean? No person on those programs is thrown off but no new enrollees go on. So if you're 65 or you turn 65 in our plan the Guaranteed Health Care Access Plan you don't go on traditional Medicaid/Medicare you just stay in our plan.

Administration and oversight are by a national health board and 12 regional boards modeled on the Federal Reserve System. So people are appointed to the boards for long staggered terms nominated by the president, confirmed by the Senate, can't be removed for political reasons or making unpopular choices. They have their own funding stream because of the value added tax. They're responsible for setting the standard benefits package and adjusting it based upon the available money as well we changes in technology. They oversee the insurance exchanges that compete for people. They regulate the health plans and collect data from them. And they report to Congress.

Nine, we create an institute for technology and outcomes assessment to do two things. First, to evaluate new interventions, see why they're clinically effective, cost effective and compared to other things. And it collects patient outcome data from the various health plans and evaluates them and distributes that information to the public.

Finally, each regional health plan has a Center for Dispute Resolution and Patient Safety to do two things again. One is to adjudicate claims of patient injury. So they evaluate the claims and see whether in fact an injury has occurred and whether they should compensate them. And secondly, more importantly, they have responsibility, authority and financial resources to promote proven patient safety measures that are not widely implemented now because there's no champion and no resources for them. This prevents, we hope, a lot of malpractice.

Well, how does the Guaranteed Health Care Access Plan stack up against the seven goals I mentioned at the start of the talk? Guaranteed coverage, all, one hundred percent of Americans are covered regardless of income, age, job, health status or any other condition you can think of. There is no crack in the system. There's no employment-based coverage, Medicare, Medicaid and maybe a crack between someone falls through if they don't qualify for those. Everyone qualifies. There's no premium barrier. There's no deductibility barrier. And if you don't sign up, you're assigned. You cannot be left out of this system.

Controlling costs, we eliminate or reduce costs from insurance underwriting sales and marketing. Incoming subsidies, right now in Medicaid to decide whether someone's eligible the state has to decide what their income is. And investigate whether they fulfill other eligibility requirements. That is very expensive. That's completely eliminated in our system. No subsidies so you don't need even to look at what someone earns. And business no longer has to buy health insurance, saving money. You will see human resource departments at businesses shrink dramatically.

What about quality health care? Health plans that will receive the certificate and provide the coverage will provide an infrastructure, information and incentives for integrated care and coordinated care. If they have to report outcomes to the national health board and the regional boards that'll be a huge incentive for computerization and infrastructure changes to bring doctors and hospitals and home health care agencies and pharmacies together to provide better care at the right location. Providing a standard benefits for a fixed premium, we'll provide them a big incentive to cover only interventions that pass technology assessment and to figure out how to get rid of duplicative testing. Finally, because individual consumers, you, rather than your company or the government will chose the health plan there will be a big incentive to provide good customer service and high quality, persuading people that you are a high quality provider.

Freedom of choice, Americans will have the complete freedom of choice, which plan they want to go with, which doctor they want to follow, which hospital they want to go to and whether they want to buy additional services with their own money. We have financial responsibility. Everyone pays a VAT. You can't evade it if you buy something. And the more you consume the more you pay. The average American family where the median income in our country is now 50 thousand dollars will pay 45 hundred or less under our plan and get a benefit of 12 thousand dollars. That's a hallmark of progressivity.

Now practice reform I already mentioned, the two aspects of the Center for Dispute Resolution. And helping the economy, under our plan business no longer pays for health care. This eliminates the incentive for outsourcing and promotes the hiring of more workers because you no longer have to consider their fringe benefit so carefully. It will reduce labor management conflict and it will provide you as a worker complete portability. Further it will reduce a lot of taxes. Yes, we add on a value added tax but you have to understand how we pay for health care today. A third of the budgets across this country of states are devoted to health care through ensuring state workers, Medicaid, SCHIP. Under our plan

Beyond Band-Aids:

that goes away so state taxes can be dropped by a third. Now it may be true that governors won't give you every penny back. They might want to invest some of that in say the University of Michigan or K through 12 education, but you will see a huge drop in taxes. In addition, Medicare payroll taxes will be dropping over time as fewer and fewer people are on Medicare. And right now the federal government contributes about 150 billion dollars a year of general revenue into supporting Medicare and Medicaid and that will decline as well.

Well, you might be sitting there and wondering well, it sounds a little too good to be true. What's the price tag? That's a very legitimate question. Any health care reform has to pass the fundamental test of economic feasibility. On this slide I've shown you what we're paying for health care today excluding the Medicare population. So everyone under 65 what are we paying? I assume we can fold in the Medicare population dollar for dollar. Well, employment-based coverage, what employers pay and what workers contribute in premium in 2006, the last year for which we have reliable data, was 723 billion dollars. Medicaid and SCHIP were an additional 269 billion dollars when we exclude nursing home coverage. So that doesn't count the nursing. And then other safety net programs whether it's payment for pregnant women and children or other programs comes to at least 10 and some people think as much as 50 billion dollars. You add all that up and using government figures it's about one trillion dollars.

So one question is can the Guaranteed Access Health Care Plan provide coverage to all Americans for that one trillion dollars? Well, on the next slide I show you the answer is, of course, yes. Otherwise I wouldn't have put this one up, right? I'm not that stupid. So what you have here is the population under 65 of individuals who aren't in households and families in households, 258 million Americans not covered by Medicare. Here under annual premium you have the 2006 premiums for the high end, PPO Blue Cross and Blue Shield plan provided by the Federal Employee Health Benefits Plan. It's actually the Illinois version. It's the one I have. You can see individuals they have to pay five thousand plus dollars and for families it's eleven thousand, two hundred, two years ago. You multiply these numbers together and you get 944 billion dollars to cover 258 million Americans. Now I presume in the audience and I'm just going to take a guess there are one or two public health students who say, aha, but that is a distorted number because being a federal employee is a very good test of your health. And if we include the Medicaid population and the uninsured they actually are likely to use more services. One of the reasons they're on Medicaid is they can't work because of their illness. And that's absolutely right. So we know that Medicaid especially, not so much the uninsured, will use a lot more services. I could show you the calculations. It's around about 50 billion dollars a year of additional services they're likely to use. So add that and you come up with 994 billion dollars, round it off after all I'm a government employee, a trillion dollars. The same that we're spending today and not covering 47 million people and not giving most Americans as good a health package as the Federal Employee Health Benefits Plan. How is that possible? Well, for one thing we got rid of those 70 billion dollars, that 11 percent of premium. We get rid of most of that, so worth about 70 billion dollars. And that's almost enough to cover all Americans in the plan and give them a very good health plan. We rationalize the insurance market.

But economic feasibility is more than just covering everyone at current dollars. It's also long term cost control. What does the Guaranteed Health Care Access Plan do for long term cost control? Well, it has multiple cost control mechanisms. Because we don't believe that only one cost control method is going to be effective. We need all the horses pulling in the same direction.

First, there is what I like to call the reistat based upon the dedicated value added tax. Any increase in benefits, if Americans want more benefits they're going to have to pay for it through and increase in the VAT rate. This should provide a hard backstop limiting how much we spend and increased year to year. I assume given how much Americans love to

Beyond Band-Aids:

pay taxes it'll be a little difficult for congress to raise that VAT rate too much too fast. This will provide some breaks on the system and some incentive for efficiencies.

Second, by requiring people to provide additional services with after tax dollars they're going to look very carefully for quality and again, this will keep increases down. Competition among health plans [inaudible] a heavy emphasis on cost effective care, care that actually improves health at a reasonable rate. If you are skeptical of this role of competition let me just draw your attention to Medicare Part D. The new premiums are out and they're about 26 percent lower than anticipated at the start of the program because the big eight plans that cover 85 percent of the population, are competing pretty heavily to enroll people and have gotten remarkable efficiencies.

But the most important cost control is systemic technology and outcomes assessment. It will do two things for cost control. First, it will give us information about what's effective and what isn't effective that can be implemented and covered by the health plans. But more importantly it will send a signal upstream to those people who are developing technologies and drugs about what will be acceptable under the system. After all the big pharmaceutical companies are working on innovations and drugs today that'll be on market 10 years from now. They have to make determinations. How much will be paid for? What will the competition be? What is that playing field going to be like? The technology and outcome assessment sends them a signal. We develop a cancer chemotherapeutic drug for 55 thousand dollars that improves life expectancy one month, two months, it's unlikely to be covered or paid for. That will change what they invest their money in.

Well, that's the Guaranteed Health Care Access Plan. Now in an objective way let's consider the three other proposals. One is incremental reform and there are a variety of flavors of this. We could expand SCHIP to all children. We could have electronic medical records in all physician offices and hospitals and pharmacies. We could have medical savings accounts with catastrophic insurance over five thousand. McCain's health plan is based on three planks.

First, he proposes to eliminate the tax exclusion for employer-based insurance. I mentioned that to you already and he agrees that we should get rid of that and so you would have to pay taxes on the University of Michigan's contribution to health care for you. Instead he would offer people a tax credit, five thousand dollars to a family and twenty-five hundred dollars to individuals for however they got insurance, whether their employer provided or whether they had to go into the individual market and get it. And then he would allow interstate purchase of insurance in a more unregulated market. So you in Michigan could buy coverage from say Nevada or Arizona or an insurance company in Oregon or wherever.

Then he's got this whole sort of motherhood and apple pie list of things, everybody agrees to these: electronic medical records, pricing transparency when you go in, you know what your cat scan is going to cost, you know what your cabbage will cost and it can't be hidden, re-importation of drugs so we give Canadians a reason to come across the border for us, a little disease management, and then state insurance pools for people with pre-existing conditions. Senator McCain's proposal is incrementalism quintessential. It is a classic case of incrementalism.

Now the main appeal of incremental reform is not the quality or the adequacy of the reform, but it's supposed political feasibility. It is the triumph of politics over policy. No one says it's going to really fix the system because it doesn't fix any one of the goals. It certainly doesn't get the universal coverage. It doesn't have cost control. And it doesn't lead to an improved quality of the delivery system. It is not meant to achieve any one of those seven goals. Its single virtue is supposedly it can actually be enacted, given how easy it was to enact SCHIP reform or SCHIP expansion in this country I have real doubts about that political feasibility to begin with.

The Lewin group, a non-partisan health policy consulting group in Washington, did an evaluation of the McCain and Obama plans and they said that McCain's health plan would reduce the uninsured by 21 million, roughly 45 percent of the uninsured would get coverage and that's mostly by the tax credit. It reduces employer coverage by nearly 10 million so a lot of young people are likely to leave employment-based coverage because they can get a better deal with that tax credit outside. And its cost, two trillion dollars over 10 years so roughly two hundred billion dollars a year. So keep in mind 21 million people covered at a cost of two hundred billion dollars a year because I'm going to come back to that number in a second.

In addition, when individuals buy coverage in the individual market as opposed to their insurers they typically get less generous health benefits, a smaller package with higher deductibles and more co pays. And if you don't like red tape and paperwork this is a terrible plan because if you go into the individual market the insurers have to underwrite you and evaluate your risk. That is very administratively intensive and a lot of administrative cost. And finally, there is significantly worse protection for people with pre-existing conditions under Senator McCain's plan.

What about the other alternatives? Mandates. This is what they're doing in Massachusetts. It rests on three pillars. First, there is this mandate. You require individuals and their employers to buy health insurance even if only catastrophic coverage with a high deductible health plan. Second, you set up insurance exchanges. And again, this is where all the insurance companies have to offer the same package. And people can choose typically in the mandate proposal it's for the uninsured, the self-insured small businesses. It provides them lower rates and more selection. And last, if you can require people to get coverage you have to subsidize them. And the typical plan is to subsidize lower income people, usually up to 300 percent of poverty or 60 thousand dollars a year and/or subsidize small businesses for providing coverage to their workers.

The Obama plan is a version of mandates. The mandate in his plan is cover all children. All children have to get insurance through their families. And large employers have to do what's called pay or play. That is they have to provide coverage to their workers or they have to pay a penalty. And some of you may have seen recently an article in the *New York Times* where one of Obama's advisors would say, well, we didn't figure out what constitutes large employer. We didn't figure out what the penalty was. We just decided not to do that. They also would have an insurance exchange, a national exchange where all health plans, all insurance companies would have to offer the same benefit package and allow people to buy coverage. They'd have a competing national health plan run by the government open to everyone who couldn't get coverage through their employer or a public program. Again they would have a standard benefits package based on the federal employee benefit program like we do with guaranteed issue and no pre-existing condition exclusions. And finally, it has subsidies, 50 percent tax credit to small businesses to provide health insurance for people. And income links up to these for people to buy into the national health plan if they can't get coverage any other way. Then it's got, as I said, motherhood and apple pie. The same set of provisions that McCain has, electronic medical records, pricing transparency, re-importation of drugs, yadda, yadda.

Well, you might think of mandates as a fill in the cracks reform. It relies on the current system and tries to make as few changes as possible to the current system to get you as close as possible to universal coverage. Now given that I told you I was going to be fair and balanced you might think those are my words. They're not. They're actually the words of Jonathan Gruber, the MIT economist who developed the Massachusetts Plan. He and I were debating for John Edwards when Edwards was considering what his health plan ought to be and this is the way Gruber characterized his own plan, a fill in the cracks plan.

Coverage? Never gets beyond 97 percent and maybe not even that close. Why? Because while it provides subsidies to people up to 300 percent of poverty. There are people between 300 percent and 400 percent of poverty or 60 to 80 thousand dollars in annual income. Those people are not poor in American society. They are not poor and yet we're going to ask them to buy a 12 thousand dollar health insurance plan? A lot of them aren't going to be able to afford it and they're going to be excluded from the mandate.

Controlling cost? There's really no cost control in this plan at all. And the experience of Massachusetts confirmed these worries. Before they started they marked 620 thousand uninsured in Massachusetts, 11 percent of the population. According to an article recently more than 200 thousand previously uninsured residents have enrolled in the health plan but state officials estimate that at least that number and perhaps twice as many have not. The current estimate is at about 93, 94, 95 percent coverage, somewhere in that range.

But the real problem is cost control, making it unaffordable in the long term. Rising costs of health care will mean that employers will pay a penalty rather than provide insurance and allow their workers to get coverage through the state plan. States therefore are going to have to provide great subsidies. Now just imagine what's going happen in the next couple of years. We're going to go to eight, nine, ten percent unemployment so you're going to have a lot more people who need to get Medicaid because they're unemployed and have no employer. The recession is going to put a lot of pressure on employers and they're going to have to choose between keeping workers or getting rid of health insurance. This is going to create a dilemma for the state government. Either they increase taxes to pay the increased subsidies or they declare more people exempt from the mandate. Now if you're a governor sitting in a recession with 10 percent unemployment in your state what do you think you're going to do? Raise taxes or declare more people exempt? You don't have to ask me. Massachusetts insurers plan to raise 10 to 12 percent next year in 2008, twice this year's national average. If we continue with double digit inflation I don't think health care reform is sustainable. That's the guy running the Massachusetts health care insurance exchange, just listen to him. He tells you if we can't get cost control we cannot continue with this health care reform. And yet the plan doesn't have cost control.

Then there are the other problems, no real reform to improve quality of care. Freedom of choice might be better for the uninsured and the insurance exchange but not for people covered by their employer. Fair fiscal responsibility? Depends how you fund it. If you fund this health care reform by a payroll tax that is a very regressive tax. And helping the economy? Let me just say the following, if your economic plan is jobs mandating employers cover people is not consistent with that plan. It's an oxymoron. So you got to think about that. As I mentioned Obama's health plan is thought of as mandates -like because it doesn't have a mandate for adults.

The Lewin Group did an estimate. It suggested that it would improve coverage by 27 million Americans so 57 percent of the uninsured would get coverage, not close to the hundred percent. It would increase employer coverage by about 5 million and the cost would come in at 1.2 trillion over 10 years, round about 120 billion a year. So it in fact, covers more people than McCain at a lower price, but it doesn't cover a hundred percent at no price increase the way our plan does.

Finally, there's Medicare for all or Physicians Working Group for Single-Payer National Health Insurance, the single-payer option. It, too, rests on three major principles. The first is there's a single national health plan, a single public plan covering all Americans. We get rid of the insurance companies. We have one national plan. It would reduce administrative costs because instead of that 11 percent of costs that I mentioned about insurers you would have the 3 or 4 supposed percent that Medicare pays. You'd eliminate all those administrative costs of insurers. And, finally, the main cost control mechanism is negotiated fees and payments to doctors, controlling their prices, to hospitals, controlling their prices and you'd negotiate the price with drug companies, device manufacturers, medical equipment providers, etc. to keep costs under control. Well, I think the best way of thinking about single-payer plans is as a radical reform of the financing of health care tied to our current nineteenth century horse and buggy crafts model delivery system.

Beyond Band-Aids:

Coverage? It's certainly true that single-payer provides a hundred percent coverage with no gaps. Everyone's in the system. A hundred percent freedom of choice and it will certainly remove employers although I'm not sure help the economy. The key problems are no improvement in the quality of care, as a matter of fact institutionalization of our current system. No real cost control mechanism or really a failed cost control mechanism and worse the politicization of decision making.

As I mentioned if you want to get high quality care in America we have to have a new coordinated health care system. We need an infrastructure that brings doctors together with hospitals, home health care agencies, hospices, and the rest. We need information systems, electronic medical records so that they all have the same information in caring for patients. And it's real time with reminders, with safety measures built in. And we know that those things don't happen spontaneously because in the current system we don't have that infrastructure and we don't have those information systems by in large. So we need incentives to make that happen, right? Most doctors are willing to be team members as long as they're the captain. And to persuade them to coordinate and work with other doctors and hospitals and others requires incentives. I don't care what you call it but that organization that structure is going to give you the information systems, the infrastructure and the incentives. It's going to look an awful lot like an insurance company. You can call it some other name, but it is going to be an insurance company. And yet single-payer advocates are completely against that kind of intermediate organization.

Worse yet in my opinion, single-payer plans at least as currently advocated, institutionalize fee for service delivery system which we know does not encourage integration and coordination of care. It encourages the very fragmentation we have. The fragmentation didn't happen spontaneously. It happened because 80 percent of the health care system is paid fee for service. And this reform institutionalizes it. The main mechanism of cost control is setting prices for physicians and the rest of it. We know this is a failed cost control regime. We've seen that in Medicare.

How to Cure America's Sick, 2008 Ezekiel Emanuel, M. D., Chair,

And then there is the problem of decision making. If you ask single-payer advocates, well just imagine who's going to run the system, how are you going to have this administered. They think this guy is going to be the guy who runs it. But as we've learned you can't rely on a person. Because you might end up with this guy running the system and that wouldn't be good either. Hal Luft, a health economist formally of University of California San Francisco and now the Palo Alto Medical Clinic wrote in *JAMA* a couple of years ago. "Medicare which provides near universal coverage to U.S. residents 65 years and older is the prototypical single-payer model and routinely exhibits the problem of that model. Although permitted to arbitrarily set fees Medicare has found it difficult to do so effectively. Across the board fee changes elicit broad-based political reaction, narrowly focus changes to a sub rows of special interest lobbying. Patient advocacy groups often supported by industry and specialty societies encourage coverage for their specific service. Rather than market discipline Medicare is subject to political manipulation and bureaucratic rigidity. Single-payer advocates envisioning an equitable and efficient health care systems idealistically disregard the example of Medicare and the ethos of the U.S. political system. They are so focused on the evils of the insurance company and the evils of the drug company very little thought is given to how to actually run a system with minimal political interference that would strive for efficiency and high quality."

I want to end this talk in thinking about the politics of health care reform because we could have a million proposals but if we haven't thought through the politics we will not get it. There are many, many barriers to change. And let me mention just a few. The first is the rule of satisfaction, what you so wonderfully demonstrated at the start of this lecture. Most Americans want health care reform but they also say don't touch what I have. Well, it's very difficult to have health care reform and not touch your personal policy or your personal relationship. To the extent that 85 percent of Americans are covered and more importantly 93 percent of voters have insurance. This rule of satisfaction is a real barrier.

Beyond Band-Aids:

The second barrier is what I like to call is the James Madison rule of government. James Madison wrote the constitution and he had one objective in mind, prevent tyranny. And he made it very difficult to make big changes. So if someone got into the White House who wanted to be a tyrant it would be virtually impossible. That's why we have a system where you have to pass a bill in one committee of the house and pass a bill in a committee of the Senate, have the House vote on it, have the Senate vote on it. And of course they're not the same bill so you have to have a conference committee, then you have to go back and vote and send the bill to many, many places to torpedo legislation. We have gridlock in Washington. James Madison would've been proud. That's what he wanted. Then there's my favorite, Machiavelli's Rule of Reform. He wrote to the Prince, "There is nothing more difficult to carry out, nor more doubtful of success, nor more dangerous to handle than to initiate a new order of things for the reformer has enemies and all those who profit by the old order and only lukewarm defenders and all those who would profit by the new order." After all if you're in the old order you know what you're going to lose, that nice salary, that ability to charge a lot of money. But if you're going to benefit from the new order it's a little hypothetical, abstract, maybe it won't work out exactly that way, not sure.

Finally, there's what Stuart Altman a health policy expert at Brandeis says the rule of second best. Now I assume in this audience there are die hard single-payer advocates. Maybe some of you are for mandates. Maybe I've even convinced one or two of you to Guaranteed Health Care Access Plan. I hope there are no incrementalists. But we all have a second best, do nothing. For me, I'm not passing yours. This is a real problem in America and we saw it play out in California with Governor Schwartzenegger's proposal. But I am not pessimistic.

Now a great political scientist, great I say in this audience but I actually say it in all audiences, because he used to be a professor here at the University of Michigan in the political science department, John Kingdon, wrote that to get major change in America you need four things. Actually he wrote three things and I was uppity enough to think I could add a fourth. If you want major change in America four things have to come together at one point in time. First, you need widespread recognition of the problem. Second, you need a proposal that is agreed upon by the major actors. Third, and this is my emendation, you need a major actor or set of actors that are going to champion that proposal through thick and thin and over years. And last, you need a transforming political event to create what he called an open policy window to enact the agreed upon change.

Well, problem. I think we have widespread awareness of the health care problem. Actually when I talk to senators and congressmen, when I talk to their aides, if you even go to the McCain website and read his material on the health care you realize people really understand the problem. They understand the fact that we're getting more volume rather than quality, the fact that we're mispaying in the system, the fact that it's really broken. I don't think the problem is poorly understood. Of course we can educate Americans more about the problem, but I don't think that's the issue.

Policy? At the moment we don't have consensus on a policy. We have Senator McCain's proposal. We have Obama's proposal. We have our proposal. We have single-payer. Importantly many key stakeholders haven't gotten off the fence. You are in Michigan. The big three are complaining about the health care system. They complain bitterly about it. But tell me what they're for. You don't know. They have not come off the fence and told you what they're for. There's a difference between whining and making a positive proposal. Even the head of Wal-Mart whines about the system but that is not the same as saying we want the following five elements in a health care reform plan. So business is one group that hasn't gotten off the fence. Governors are another group. I have no idea why governors are so passive in the current system. They are handcuffed by the 32 percent of their budget going to health care, preventing them from doing something about education or the environment or whatever else they want to do. But they have not said we need leadership from Washington in unison and we want the following parts to the plan. And finally, there are patient advocates. So the champions we need I think are those three groups.

And finally, we need a transforming political event. That transforming political even by definition is unpredictable, not only unpredictable to you and I who are not politicians but unpredictable to politicians. There's actually been some really interesting studies about how well politicians understand when a moment of change is going to happen and which bill will be passed. They're worse than you and I at predicting that actually. But I think the financial crisis we're in may be that transforming political event. And let me give you six separate reasons for that.

Reason one, when you bail out the banks and Freddie and Fannie and AIG with hundreds of billions of dollars who's going to talk about socialized medicine anymore? When you socialize Wall Street no one can credibly talk about socialized medicine as an epithet of negativity. You just will not hear it. So we might actually get an intelligent discussion about health care reform without slinging this nonsense of phrases.

Second, when you spend seven hundred billion dollars maybe, maybe not to fix the economy suddenly spending two hundred billion dollars doesn't look so expensive. It's chump change. Everything is a matter of perspective.

Third, in this very uncertain fiscal time a lot of American families are going to worry about being unemployed, having their employer cut off their insurance. They're going to look for a safe harbor and having a guarantee of insurance may be a very important safe harbor that they want from the government.

Fourth, that fiscal insecurity might also make Americans willing to compromise instead of the gold-plated Cadillac coverage they might be willing to accept a more basic coverage but as long as it's guaranteed through thick and thin.

Fifth, there are employers. They may not be able to afford health care insurance. They may want to get it off their books. They may want to compete without it. And the recession that's coming may induce them to be more active on this.

Finally, sixth, you remember I said remember the figures for McCain and Obama. McCain covered 21 million people at a cost of 2 trillion dollars over 10 years. Obama covered 27 million people at a cost of 1.2 trillion dollars over 10 years. And I showed you that we could do it for zero. Well, let me tell you the Lewen Group hasn't assessed our plan, but it's assessed the Wyden Bennett bill. And that bill which covers all Americans gets rid of employers, very similar to our bill, Lewen estimated that they get a hundred percent coverage, costs zero. As a matter of fact it saves 1.4 trillion dollars over 10 years. So what you have is the very important phenomenon that more comprehensive health care reform is actually cheaper in the long term. Given the debt pressure of the fiscal crisis and the need to spend seven hundred billion dollars to bail out Wall Street this may induce congress to actually do more. Now I have to admit until two months ago I was talking about health care reform in 2013, not in 2009. But I think this fiscal crisis may have changed the landscape. I can tell you all the negative reasons I just offer that as an idea at the end here.

So for those of you who are politically engaged and want to learn more about Health Care Guaranteed you can look at that website. It's not run by me; it's run by two guys out of Seattle who are active in this. If you want to look at details like technology and outcome assessment or the taxes or independent administration or how you have competition you can go to freshthinking.org. I'm really meaning if you want a good paper that will put you to sleep like that, freshthinking.org.

Finally, one of the things that happens when you become an author is you become completely shameless. So we have published a book that summarizes and expands on the things I've mentioned today and it is available as Phil mentioned. Thank you very much and I look forward to your questions.

Redressing the Unconscionable Health Gap: A Proposal for a Global Plan of Justice, 2009

Lawrence Gostin, J.D., L.L. D., Associate Dean and Professor of Global Health Law, Georgetown University Law Center

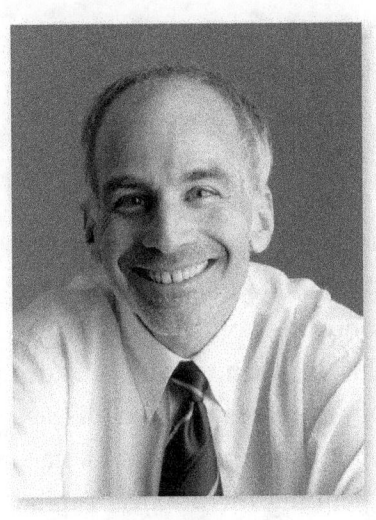

Good afternoon. Thank you all for coming. I know it's late in the day. I wanted to add my thanks to Dr. Philip Margolis for being such a gracious host and really being the inspiration behind this series. It's wonderful. And I welcome the Waggoner family who are delights and I've really been privileged to meet you. Ray Waggoner was somebody that I feel honored to represent here because he believed in at least two things that I believe in passionately which are mental health, humanity and ethics. And that really is very important to me. I gave a talk at Grand Rounds this morning on mental health and human rights. Mental health was my first love other than my wife. And I've moved from mental health to AIDS and then public health and now global health. It's very hard to get my hands around the global health area.

I'm going to be talking about a topic of global health governance and what the grand challenges are. I'm not going to per se talk about my global plan for justice but actually even a bolder proposal, the framework invention on global health. The global plan for justice idea is going

Redressing the Unconscionable Health Gap:

to come out in the *Lancet* in the next month. The longer version will be coming out in the *Harvard Journal of Law and Policy*. I want to apologize for two things. One, I'm a lawyer so I just talk - no PowerPoints. And normally I wander around the audience, but I was really tethered to the microphone so I'm just going to be a good boy and sit at the podium nicely. And secondly, I don't normally do this and I haven't in any of the other lectures, but I'm going to read my lecture because I have so much to cover that I want to be able to cover it in a way that's efficient.

This lecture searches for solutions to the most perplexing problems in global health. Problems so important that they affect the fate of millions of people with economic, political and security ramifications for the world's population. No state acting alone can insulate itself from major health hazards. The determinants of health: pathogens, air, food, water and even lifestyle choices do not originate solely within national borders. Health threats inexorably spread to neighboring countries, regions and even continents. It is for this reason that safeguarding the world's population requires cooperation and global governance. If I am correct that ameliorating the most common causes of disease, disability and premature death require global solutions then the future is demoralizing. The states that bare the disproportionate burden of disease have the least capacity to do anything about it. And the states that have the wherewithal are deeply resistant to expending the political capital and economic resources necessary to truly make a difference to improve health outside their borders. When rich countries do act it is more often out of a narrow self interest or humanitarian instinct, as in Haiti, then a full sense of ethical or legal obligation. The result is a spiraling deterioration of health in the world's poorest regions with manifest global consequences for cross border disease transmission and systemic effects on trade, international relations and security.

This lecture first inquires why governments should care about serious health threats outside their borders. And I explore the alternative rationales of direct self interest and lightened self interest and national

A Proposal for a Global Plan of Justice, 2009

security. Second, I examine the compelling issue of global health equity and ask whether it is fair that people in poor countries suffer such a disproportionate burden of illness and death. Here I will briefly explore a theory that I call a theory of human functioning to support a more robust understanding of the transcending value of health. Third, I describe how the international community focuses on a few high profile, heart rendering issues while largely ignoring the deeper, systemic problems in global health. By focusing on what I call basic survival needs the international community could fundamentally improve prospects for the world's population. And finally, I explore the value of international law itself and propose an innovative mechanism for global health reform, a framework invention on global health.

My proposal in a nutshell is to establish fair terms of international cooperation with agreed upon mutually binding obligations to create enduring health system capacities, meet basic survival needs and reduce the unconscionable inequalities that exist in global health. I'm quite torn about this proposal because on the one hand most of the people I've talked to, and I've talked Bob Zoellick, head of the World Bank, Margaret Chen at WHO and others, support it as an underlying theory. On the other hand the political realities are dim and make me very dispirited at times. Next month I'm going to Oslo because I had one piece of good news, the Norwegian Parliament has adopted the framework. And I'm going to be championing it in the international arena. So all I can say is go Norway.

It's axiomatic that infectious diseases do not respect national borders, but this simple truth does not convey the degree to which pathogens migrate great distances and pose health hazards everywhere. Human beings congregate in travel, live in close proximity to animals, pollute the environment and rely on overtaxed health systems. The constant cycle of congregation, consumption and movement allows infectious diseases to mutate and spread across populations and boundaries. These human activities and many more have profound health consequences for people throughout the world and no country can insulate itself from its effects.

Redressing the Unconscionable Health Gap:

The world's community is interdependent and reliant on one another for health security.

Powerful reasons therefore exist for governments to pay close attention to global health, not only for the sake of people in faraway places but to prevent potentially catastrophic social, economic and political consequences for their own citizens. But beyond narrow self interests are the broader and lightened interests in redressing extremely high rates of disease and premature death in the world's poorest regions. There is a strong case that a forward looking foreign policy would seek to reduce the enduring intractable diseases in developing countries and it's my profound hope that president Obama's Global Health Initiative, which I hope he will talk about tonight, may redress some of these.

Epidemic disease dampens tourism, trade and commerce as the 2003 sores outbreaks demonstrated. Animal diseases such as foot and mouth, BCS and pandemic influence, whether H1N1 or avian influenza, also had severe economic repercussions. In the avian case it included mass culling of flocks and herds, trade bans on beef, lamb or poultry. And it's predicted that massive economic destruction would ensue from a pandemic of human influenza, one that was more pathogenic than the current H1N1 with a projected loss of up to six percent in global GDP.

In regions with extremely poor health economic decline is almost inevitable. AIDS in sub-Saharan Africa accounts for 72 percent of global AIDS deaths. Average life expectancy in the region is now 47 years, when it would have been 62 without AIDS. And for some of the worse affective countries such as Botswana life expectancy has declined from 76 to 34 years of age. Most of the excess mortalities among young adults age 15 to 49, leaving the countries without entrepreneurs, skilled work force, parents, teachers, political leaders. The World Bank estimates that AIDS has reduced GDP by nearly 20 percent in the hardest hit countries. And AIDS, of course, is only one disease in countries experiencing multiple epidemics of starvation and massive poverty and regional conflicts that devastate the population. Countries with extremely poor health become

A Proposal for a Global Plan of Justice, 2009

unreliable trading partners without the capacity to develop and export products and natural resources, pay for essential medicines and vaccines or pay debt, and require increased financial aid and humanitarian assistance. In short, a foreign policy that seeks to ameliorate health threats in poor countries can benefit public and private countries in developed as well as developing countries.

Extremely poor health in other parts of the world can also affect the security of the United States and its allies. Research shows a correlation between health and the effective functioning of government and civil society. The CIA for example finds that high infant mortality is a leading predictor of state failure. And the state department called AIDS a national security threat. States with exceptionally unhealthy populations are often in crisis, fragmented and poorly governed. In the most extreme form poor health can contribute to political instability, civil unrest, mass migrations and human rights abuses. In these states there is greater opportunity to harbor terrorists or recruit disinfected people to join in armed struggles. Politically unstable states require heightened diplomacy, create political entanglements and sometimes provoke military responses.

Diseases of poverty are overwhelmingly concentrated in sub-Saharan Africa so it's no surprise that many of these political and military entanglements occur in that region. But it's also true that Africa has weak political military and economic power so it can too easily be ignored. The same cannot be said about the burgeoning health crisis emerging in pivotal countries in Eurasia, such as China, India and Russia. These countries are in the midst of a second wave of AIDS with prevalence rates rising twentyfold in less than a decade. In the decades ahead the center of global AIDS is projected to shift from Africa to Eurasia. And recall that infant mortality is a prime predictor of state instability. Russia's official infant mortality rate which is thought to be vastly undercounted is three to four times higher than in North America and Western Europe. Nearly two-thirds of children born in Russia will be unhealthy, many suffering life-long illness and disability. Yet Eurasia has more than 60 percent of

Redressing the Unconscionable Health Gap:

the world's inhabitants, one of the highest combined GNPs and at least four massive armed forces with nuclear capabilities. But due to extreme health hazards Eurasia will suffer economic, political and military decline. Political instability in a region with such geostrategic importance will have major international ramifications.

Governments, therefore, have powerful reasons based upon narrow or enlightened self interest to ameliorate extreme health hazards beyond their borders. But do political leaders acknowledge and act on this evidence? The answer is that political engagement in global health is relatively limited. As UK now Prime Minister, then Chancellor of the Exchequer, Gordon Brown said when launching the International Finance Facility for Global Health, "Rich countries just don't care enough." Well, it's no surprise and we saw this with the Haiti telethon the other night that rich countries, philanthropists and even celebrities have announced with great fanfare breathtaking gifts to the poor, unprecedented. OECD countries increased global health assistance, rising from two billion in 1990 to twelve billion in 2005. The Gates Foundational Loan will donate up to three billion dollars per year. And this development assistance for health may appear substantial but it actually sits modestly beside the one trillion dollars spent on military expenditures annually and three hundred billion on agricultural subsidies. If you were to ask me, for example, what is the most destructive thing the United States does for international health my answer, and even here in the Midwest, it would still be my answer would be the Farm Bill.

The increase in development assistance, moreover, is largely attributable to extensive resources devoted to a few high profile problems: the AIDS pandemic certainly with the Global Fund and PEPFAR, pandemic influenza, the Asian tsunami, the Haitian earthquake. But even factoring in these new investments most OECD countries have not come close to fulfilling their pledges of giving 0.7 percent of GNI per annum. OECD countries would have to invest in an additional one billion dollars by 2015 to close the investment gap. And with these additional dollars WHO projects tens of millions of lives would be saved every year. And although I know we consider ourselves a very generous people in America and we are, nonetheless we do fall near the bottom even with PEPFAR in terms of our global health assistance as a percentage of GDP. Notably and thankfully I noticed that President Obama has announced that in the spending cuts for discretionary spending the global health initiatives are going to be exempt.

Well, perhaps it does not or should not matter if global health serves the interests of the richest countries. After all there are powerful humanitarian reasons to help the world's least healthy people. But even ethical arguments have failed to capture the full attention of political leaders and the public. The global burden of disease is not just shouldered by the poor but disproportionately so, such that health disparities across continents render a person's likelihood of survival drastically different depending upon where she is born. These inequalities have become so extreme and the resultant effects on the poor so dire that health disparities have become an issue no less important than global warming or the other defining issues of our time. The current global distribution of disease has led to radically different health outcomes. Disparities in life expectancy among the rich and poor are vast. Average life expectancy in Africa is 30 years less than the Americas or Europe. Life expectancy in Zimbabwe or Swaziland is less than half that of Japan. A child born in Angola is 73 times more likely to die in the first years of life than a child born in Norway. And a woman giving birth in Africa is a hundred times more likely to die in labor than a woman here in America. While life expectancy in the developed world has increased throughout the twentieth century it actually decreased in the least developed countries and in transitional states such as Russia. And as little as one concrete example offers a sense of proportion about the global health gap. In one year alone 14 million of the world's poorest people died while only 4 million would have died if this population had the same death rate as the global rich, ten million avoidable deaths a year.

Redressing the Unconscionable Health Gap:

The diseases of poverty are endemic but barely get noticed among the wealthy. Diseases such as elephantiasis, Guinea worm, Malaria, River blindness, schistosomiasis and trachoma are common in poor countries but many are virtually unheard of here. Beyond morbidity and premature mortality the diseases of poverty cause physical and mental suffering. For example, when a two-foot Guinea worm parasite emerges from the genitals, breasts, extremities and torso with excruciating pain. Alfilaria worms cause disfiguring enlargement of arms, legs, breasts and genitals. Or River blindness leads to unbearable itching and loss of eyesight, all preventable.

Well, human instinct tells us that it is unjust for large populations to have such poor prospects for good health and long life simply by happenstance of where they live. And although almost everyone believes that it is unfair that the poor live miserable and short lives, there's little consensus about whether there is an ethical let alone a legal obligation to help the downtrodden. What do wealthier societies owe as a matter of justice to the poor in other parts of the world? Well, perhaps the strongest claim that health disparities aren't equal is based upon what I call a theory of human functioning.

Health has special meaning and importance to individuals and communities as a whole. Health is necessary for much of the joy, creativity and productivity that a person derives from life. Individuals with physical and mental health recreate, socialize, work and engage in family and social activities that bring meaning and happiness to their lives. Perhaps not as obvious health also is essential for the functioning of populations. Without minimal levels of health people cannot fully engage in social interactions, participate in the political process, exercise rights of citizenship, generate wealth, create art and provide for the common security. Amartya Sen famously theorized that the capability to avoid starvation, preventable morbidity and early mortality is a substant to freedom that enriches human life. Depriving people of this capability strips them of the freedom to do what they want to do and to be who they want to be

A Proposal for a Global Plan of Justice, 2009

and have a reason to value. Under a theory of human functioning health deprivations are unethical because they unnecessarily reduce one's ability to function and their capacity for human agency. Health among all other forms of disadvantage is special and foundational and that its effects on human capabilities impact one's opportunities in the world. And I can think of no place other than the University of Michigan and its medical and public health research and dedicated people who live by that motto.

But unfortunately Amartya Sen's theory does not answer the harder question about who has the corresponding obligation to do something about global inequalities. Even the most liberal egalitarians that believe in just distribution such as Nagel, Rawls and Rotzler frame their claims narrowly and rarely extend them to international obligations of justice. Their theories of justice are relational and apply to fundamental social contracts. But positing such as relationship among different countries and regions is much more difficult.

Well, suppose that states were convinced of my arguments so far that amelioration of global health hazards was in their national interests or they otherwise accepted the claim that they have an ethical responsibility to act. Would the consequent funding and efforts make a genuine difference? Well, if past history is any guide the answer is no. Most development assistance is driven by high profile events that evoke public sympathy such as a natural disaster in the form of a hurricane, tsunami, drought, hurricane or famine or an enduring crisis such as AIDS. Or even worse yet, and America is really bad at this, we lurch from one frightening disease to the next irrespective of the level of risk ranging from anthrax to smallpox to SARS to influenza H5N1, to influenza H1N1, to bioterrorism.

What is truly needed, and this is what I believe most passionately, and what rich countries like America do instinctively, maybe not adequately as Peter Jacobsen and Harold Markel will know, they do for their own citizens what I call basic survival needs. By focusing on the major determinants of health the international community could dramatically improve prospects for good health. Basic survival needs include

Redressing the Unconscionable Health Gap:

sanitation and sewage, pest control, clean air and water, tobacco reduction, diet and nutrition, essential medicines and vaccines and well functioning health systems. Meeting every day survival needs may lack the glamour of high technology medicine or dramatic rescue. But what they lack in excitement they gain in their potential impact on health precisely because they deal with the major determinants of common disease and disabilities across the globe. Mobilizing the public and private sectors to meet basic survival needs comparable to a Marshall Plan could radically transform prospects for good health among the world's poorest people. And meeting basic survival needs can be disarmingly simple and inexpensive if only it could rise on the agenda of the world's most powerful countries. It does not take advanced biomedical research, huge financial investments or complex programs.

Consequently what poor countries need is not foreign aid workers power shooting in to rescue them. Nor do they need foreign run state of the art facilities. Rather what they need is to gain the capacity to provide basic health systems and services themselves. Well, if meeting basic survival needs can truly make a difference and if this solution is preferable to other paths then can international law structure legal obligations accordingly? The answer is that extant health governance has been lamentingly deficient. Everyone agrees with this. And a fresh approach is badly needed.

The WHO was founded in 1948 as an incredibly powerful normative institution. But its potential has never been realized. The WHO constitution empowers the agency to adopt conventions which unlike normal treaties affirmatively require states to take action. And despite WHO's impressive normative powers modern international health law is remarkably thin with only one significant regulation and one treaty in 60 years of existence. The international health regulations which were revised in 2005 in light of SARS originally applied only to cholera, plague and yellow fever. The same diseases originally discussed at the first International Sanitary Conference in Paris in 1851. The WHO did not create a treaty until it adopted the Framework Convention on

A Proposal for a Global Plan of Justice, 2009

Tobacco Control in 2003. And although a laudable achievement, the FCTC is almost generous because it regulates a vilified industry that had denied for years and decades scientific realities about health, engineered tobacco to create dependence and targeted youth women and minorities. And it still does in developing countries.

Although norms created by the WHO are sparse there is a much larger body of international law that affects global health ranging from food safety, arms control and the environment to trade in human rights. I'm currently finishing up a book on global health law for Harvard University Press so I've been really steeped in it. The WHO should be a leader in creating or at least influencing many of these norms, but that has not happened. The agency has shied away from the high politics of international law because it sees itself principally as a scientific technical agency. Thus WHO is comfortable developing technical standards for food safety but it has not ventured into the harder terrain of WTO rule making and dispute resolution. It ought to have a great deal to contribute and sway over the traded goods and services, sanitary and fidosanitary measures and intellectual property rights, all of which clearly affect global health. Yet its influence is nowhere to be found. As a result social activists have increasingly turned to the language of human rights to articulate their fondest hopes and dreams for global health.

But recasting the problem of extremely poor health as a human rights problem, which I actually heartily support, isn't good enough either for a number of reasons. First, the legal obligation for the right to health falls primarily on each state to protect its own population. Although the international covenant of economic, social and cultural rights, which by the way the United States hasn't ratified, posits that all states have duties to cooperate in achieving economic and social rights. The obligation to assist states cannot become primary. Secondly, the right to health itself is expressed as progressively realizable so there is little agreement as to when a state has reached an obligation to its people let alone reached an obligation to people in faraway places. And finally, even if some obligation to offer financial and technical assistance could be read in to human rights documents there's no systematic method of implementation and enforceability. In short, human rights don't do what we need which is to obtain scalability and sustainability of health systems.

This leaves us with the very problem that I have posited throughout this lecture. That the duty to improve the health of the world's most disadvantaged falls primarily on those who lack the means to do so. This is undoubtedly an untenable position if global health is to be taken as a solemn issue of international concern. If the law is to play a constructive role then innovative models are essential. And here I make the case for a framework convention on global health. I am proposing a global health governing system incorporating a bottom up strategy that strives to build health system capacity, set priorities, meet basic survival needs, engage stakeholders to bring to bear their resources and expertise, harmonize the activities among proliminating a proliferating number of actors operating around the world in a fragmented way and to evaluate and monitor progress so that goals are met and promises are kept. The framework convention approach is becoming an essential strategy of powerful transnational social movements to safeguard the environment and, of course, with tobacco control.

A framework convention on global health would represent an historical shift with a broadly imagined global governance regime. The initial framework would establish the key modalities with a strategy for subsequent protocols on the most important governance principles. This would include the framework's mission, objectives, its engagement and coordination, state parties and stakeholder's obligations, institutional structures, empirical monitoring, enforcement, ongoing scientific analysis and guidance for subsequent law making processes. I detail these in quite specific ways in an article in the *Georgetown Law Journal* and in a shorter way in a two-part series in *JAMA*.

The framework convention approach has a number of advantages based on its incremental nature and its ability to evolve over a long period of time and to engage stakeholders. The process of creating international

A Proposal for a Global Plan of Justice, 2009

norms and institutions also provides an ongoing and structured forum for states and stakeholders to develop a shared humanitarian instinct on global health. A high profile forum for normative discussion can help educate and persuade states and influence public opinion in favor of decisive action. A framework convention, however, will not be a panacea and it cannot easily circumvent many of the seemingly intractable problems of global health governance: the dominance of economically and politically powerful countries, the deep resistance to creating obligations to expend or transfer wealth, the lack of trust in international legal regimes like the UN, and the vocal concerns about the integrity and competency of countries and governance in the world's poorest regions.

But given the dismal nature of global health governance I believe that a framework convention on global health is a risk work taking. It will at a minimum identify the genuinely important problems in global health. It will target the major determinants of health. It will prioritize and coordinate currently fragmented activities. And it will engage a broad range of stakeholders from business, media, foundations and states. It will also provide a needed forum to raise visibly for one of the most pressing problems facing humankind.

So this evening what I have sought to demonstrate is why politically and economically powerful countries should care about the world's least healthy people. It may be a matter of national interest so that helping the poor makes everyone safer and more secure. Or global health assistance simply may be ethically the right thing to do to avert an unfolding humanitarian catastrophe. Or there may be a growing sense of legal obligation whether through WHO treaties and regulations or the international human right to health. Although no single argument may be definitive in itself the cumulative weight of evidence is now overwhelmingly persuasive.

Whatever the reasons perhaps we're coming to a tipping point when the status quo is no longer acceptable and it is time to take bold action. Global health like global climate change may soon become a matter so

Redressing the Unconscionable Health Gap:

important to the world's future that it demands international attention and no state can escape the responsibility to act. And if that were the case states and stakeholders would need an innovative international mechanism to bind themselves and others to take an effective course of action. Amelioration of the enduring and complex problems of global health is virtually impossible without a collective response. No state or stakeholder acting alone can avert the ubiquitous threats of pathogens as they rapidly spread and change forms. And if all states and stakeholders voluntarily accepted fair terms of cooperation through a framework convention or another mechanism then it could dramatically improve life's prospects for millions of people.

But it would do more than that. Cooperative action for global health like global warming benefits everyone by diminishing our collective vulnerabilities. And think about this, the alternative to fair terms of cooperation is that everyone would be worse off and particularly those who suffer from compounding disadvantages. Absent a binding commitment to help, rich states might find it politically or economically easier to withhold their fair share of global health assistance hoping that others will take up the slack. Major outbreaks of infectious disease including extensively drug resistant forms would become increasingly more likely. And even if the economically empowerful escaped major health hazards themselves as the rich often can do we would all still have to avert our eyes from the mounting suffering among the poor. And we will have to live with our consciences knowing that much of this physical and mental anguish is preventable. What is more important is that if the global community does not accept fair terms of cooperation on global health soon there's every reason to believe that affluent states, philanthropists and celebrities simply will move on to another cause. And when they do the vicious cycle of poverty and endemic disease among the world's least healthy people will continue unabated. And that is a consequence that none of should be willing to tolerate. Thank you very much for inviting me.

Old and New Ethical Problems in Innovative Stem Cell Research, 2010

Bernard Lo, M.D., Director in Medical Ethics, Professor of Medicine, University of California at San Francisco

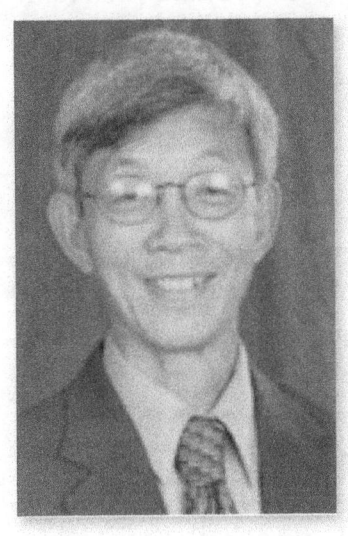

Thank you very much. That's a very gracious introduction. I'm delighted and honored to be here. I'm honored to give a talk in the memory of Dr. Waggoner who is really, I think, a leader in academic medicine. He chaired a department and really built it into a major department over a long period of time. I think that kind of commitment to academic excellence is something to really respect.

I'm going to talk today about stem cells. I'm going to keep my formal remarks relatively brief, about 40 minutes or so. I'd like to have a lot of time for questions and discussion at the end.

So as is customary I'm going to tell you about my conflicts. I don't have any financial conflicts. I have no relationships with companies. But I do have two sort of intellectual commitments you need to know about. First, in California I chair the standards working group of the California Institute for Regenerative Medicine. That's the group that allocates state funds. The tax payers voted three billion dollars in funding for stem cell research and our committee recommended the regulations under which those funds were given out to researchers and the restrictions on the kinds of research that could be done. I also serve on the NIH human embryo working group. That's the group that Dr. Collins and I each convene to go over stem cell lines that want to be qualified for NIH funding. And we determine on a case by case basis whether a line meets the standards that NIH has set up for its funding.

So what I'm going to do today is talk about a number of topics. First, I'm going to review with you the ethical concerns in public policy debates surrounding human embryonic stem cells. And as Dr. Margolis said this is highly controversial in the U.S. But it may be both less controversial and more controversial than we think. But moving beyond embryonic stem cells I want to talk about induced pluripotent stem cells, the stem cells that can be derived by reprogramming adult somatic cells as for example from a skin biopsy into pluripotent cells. And also talk about stem cell clinical trials which are now taking place in the U.S. and abroad.

So I'm going to start with just a quick review of some stem cell biology. So a pluripotent stem cell, doesn't have to be an embryonic cell; it can be an IPS cell, has two very important characteristics. First, it's self-renewing. It can create daughter cells that are also pluripotent and that stem cell line can remain in existence through many passages. But a stem cell line also has the potential to differentiate into all the lineages of the adult body and all the specific tissues. And one of the real goals of stem cell research is to try and figure out how to drive a pluripotent cell into end organ cells and to use these cell for replacement therapy.

So there's a lot of interest now in driving pluripotent cells into pancreatic beta islet cells, cells that produce insulin, for replacement therapy in people with type one diabetes. There's also a lot of interest in driving stem cells to neural stem cells and neural precursor cells. And there are three clinical trials now in the U.S. with neural stem cells derived from pluripotent cells including a new trial that's just started recently for patients with acute spinal cord injury. There's active research in my institution on using stem cell derived cellular therapies for adult respiratory distress syndrome, failure in adults. So the hope is that not only will we understand how to derive cells to a more committed state, but also to be able to use those cells for therapy.

This is an enlarged photo micrograph of a human embryo slightly beyond the stage which it ordinarily implants into a woman's uterus. And if it implants and develops normally it becomes a fetus and can become a live born child. This is a picture of a slightly earlier stage of embryonic development. And what we've done here is we've opened up the blastocyst. And in the inside of a blastocyst, or embryo, there are cells whose colors are reversed called the inner cell mass at one end of the embryo. And if you take those cells out and culture them in the lab under the right conditions those can become embryonic stem cells. And I think this image, which is courtesy of the Welcome Trust, shows that to derive an embryonic stem cell line you actually have to disrupt, destroy an embryo. And once these inner mass cells are taken out that embryo no longer can be used for reproduction. There's no way of putting it back together and using it for reproduction. And this sort of fundamental fact of stem cell biology is the scientific root of the moral controversy we have which is really quite prominent in this country.

So one question that is asked is what is the moral status of this embryo? I think we need to say that clearly it's a potential person, that if that embryo were implanted into a woman's uterus at the right stage in her cycle it could implant, develop and become a live born child. So it's certainly a potential person. And there are many people in this society who actually go many steps beyond. They say that's not a potential person that group of cells on the head of the pin I showed you is more than a potential person. It's a person just like you or me or a child that's delivered in the obstetrics suite. And so based on that belief people draw very strong conclusions about stem cell research. So if you ask is human embryonic stem cell research morally acceptable, if you believe that embryo is a person with all the rights that a person should have, the answer is clearly no. That to derive that stem cell, to take it apart, make it no longer usable for reproduction in the eyes of those people is tantamount to murdering a person. And so that sense of outrage at doing that, that drives the opposition to embryonic stem cell research.

So this is a *Newsweek* magazine cover from 2001 when President Bush at that time was considering whether to allow federal NIH funding for embryonic stem cell research. *Newsweek* summarized it as the stem cell wars. Here's a picture of a blastocyst. "Embryo research versus pro-life politics: There's hope for Alzheimer's, heart disease, Parkinson's, and diabetes but will Bush cut off the Money?" So this is how it's often posed, research versus pro-life politics. But actually I think that's really an oversimplification. There are a number of, quite a few, very prominent conservative, pro-life politicians who are stem cell research supporters: former First Lady Nancy Reagan, remember her husband President Reagan developed Alzheimer's and lived for many years as it declined, she supported stem cell research. This is Senator Orrin Hatch, republican from Utah, one of the most powerful, influential men in the Senate, staunch conservative who says on his website referring to embryonic stem cell research, "This research is consistent with bed life, bed rock, pro life, pro family values. Stem cell research facilitates life, abortion destroys life." He goes on to say, "I cannot equate abortion with the simple act of disposing of a frozen embryo," left over after a woman has completed her IVF treatment and decided she doesn't want to use it herself or give it to another woman or couple, "disposing a frozen embryo that will never complete the journey towards birth." And Senator Hatch actually started out as an opponent in the stem cell research. And over the years has changed his position, has co-sponsored bills in the Senate supporting federal funding for certain types of stem cell research. So I go into this to say that it's easy to sort of say there's a polarization and it's an irreconcilable conflict. In fact, people can change their minds and I think we should be open to trying to listen to people who disagree and to try and persuade them.

So President Bush in 2001 set federal policy for embryonic stem cell research funding. He said there'd be no federal funding for the derivation of new embryonic stem cell lines. So no U.S. dollars would be used to support

Old and New Ethical Problems in Innovative Stem Cell Research, 2010

research that takes embryos and renders them unusable for reproduction but derives stem cell lines from it. Now that derivation is permitted in almost all states under either private funding or in some states under state funding. But what President Bush did is he said he would allow federal NIH dollars for research using existing stem cell lines, lines that were in existence in August 2001 when he set this policy. He said we will allow federal funding for research using those lines. And the argument that he made was that those lines are already in existence. Nothing can go backwards in time and recreate the embryos from which those lines were derived. And his argument was since those embryos were irreparably destroyed for reproductive uses why not allow the stem cell lines to be used for research that might benefit future patients in this society. Now it's important to note that other types of research have always been permitted under federal funding. Adult stem cell research and cord blood stem cell research which do not involve embryos are eligible for funding and for derivation of new lines.

So a lot of things have happened. This is the election of 2004 where my state, California, passed a bond measure to set aside three billion dollars for state funded stem cell research including the derivation of new lines. Other states have followed. I think Michigan has a similar program. In Congress the Stem Cell Research Enhancement Act was introduced in 2005 and 2007. And that would allow by legislation federal funding for research on additional embryonic stem cell lines that were derived from embryos originally created in infertility treatment, IVF treatment, but not needed for that purpose and the women in treatment decided not to give them to another couple, not to destroy them, but to allow them to be used for research. That passed both houses of Congress in 2005 and 2007, but it was vetoed by President Bush and there were not enough votes in either the House or Senate to override that. So as you remember at those times they were a Republican controlled congress so despite a clear Republican majority in Congress and a lot of conservative members of Congress these bills were passed. So how this would shake out now after yesterday's election, I don't know.

Well, after the 2008 election interestingly both Senator Obama and Senator McCain were supporters of this increased federal funding for stem cell research. After the election in March 2009 President Obama issued an executive order allowing broader NIH funding for embryonic stem cell research. And these are the guidelines that are in place and are now under challenge. And under those guidelines NIH may fund research on a wider range of existing embryonic stem cell lines. These are lines that were derived after informed and voluntary consent from the IVF patient who donated an embryo to derive that line after being informed of all the options for the embryo that she no longer needed for her reproduction. And this committee that I sit on adjudicates whether these and other criteria are met.

Now in the news you'll hear a lot about the Dickey-Wicker Amendment which is a rider to the Appropriations Bill that's been passed every year by Congress since 1996. And what this amendment does is it bans federal funds for being used for the creation of human embryos for research and also it bans research in which a human embryo is destroyed or discarded. So that's the plain language of the act. And the current lawsuit, which I'll tell you about in a minute, rests upon an interpretation of this amendment.

Now under this amendment the Department of Health and Human Services, NIH, has allowed federal funds to be used for research on human embryonic stem cell lines that have been derived with non-federal funding. And this was allowed under both the Bush administration and the Obama administration. And what that rests on conceptually is distinction between the derivation of human embryonic stem cells, which the researcher that does that actually actively is involved in the destroying the embryo for reproductive purposes. But the thing HHS and congress has not objected has allowed that to be distinguished from research that uses the line that was created through that stem cell derivation but does not of itself destroy additional embryos.

A lawsuit brought by two researchers, one of whom is named Shirley, Sibelius is the nominal defendant as the secretary of the HHS, was brought and is not being litigated in the courts. And two adult stem cell researchers sued to overturn the Obama guidelines. And they made the argument that these new guidelines violated the Dickey-Wicker Act. They said that that act, properly interpreted, should ban not only the funding of the derivation but any downstream research that relies on embryos having been destroyed to create the stem cell line. So this now turns on legal issues of what is the meaning of the Dickey-Wicker Amendment. It is under review. There are going to be oral arguments made before the D.C. Court of Appeals in about a week or so.

Shirley and the other plaintiff advanced another interesting argument, which is that the NIH guidelines caused those two plaintiffs irrefutable harm because they said funding for human embryonic stem cell research harms them by taking funds away for scarce NIH dollars and making less money available for people doing the type of research they are doing. And they actually persuaded a trial judge to issue an injunction to stop the NIH to continue to fund stem cell research because they said they were suffering irreparable, serious harm. Now the Court of Appeals has rejected that injunction, but that's all part of a complex legal battle. So this will continue to be in the headlines pending the final results of this litigation.

So what can we expect? Certainly the case can be decided in the courts. There has been some talk, Dianne DeGette, a representative from Colorado, has talked about introducing a bill in both houses to clarify Dickey-Wicker to make it clear that Congress did not mean to cut off funding from stem cell lines derived without federal funding, whether that and the new Congress will be introduced, whether it will work its way through committee to the floor and be passed is, I think, anybody's guess. Obviously the elections yesterday caused a major realignment in Congress. So we'll just have to see.

But I want to turn away from embryonic stem cell research to talk about some work that is less controversial in many ways. But I also want to sort of suggest to you that it raises another totally different set of controversies that we need as scientists and policymakers to pay attention to and to try and fix. So let me step back to other kinds of stem cell research.

One of the goals of many stem cell researchers is to create a pluripotent stem cell line that's matched to a specific phenotype, clinical characteristic or patient or specific DNA. Now why might we want to do that? Two reasons, the first is what excites many scientists which is to create a stem cell line from a patient with a known disease to create a model for studying that disease in the lab. You'll hear the phrase disease in a dish model of illness. And the reason they want to do that is first to elucidate the mechanisms, the pathophysiology of the disease state. Secondly is to identify new targets for drug therapies, not stem cell therapies, but by understanding the mechanism of disease we can identify potential new targets for therapy and it also may be a way to evaluate potential new therapies. In a minute I'll show you a dramatic example of how that might work. In the popular mind there's a lot of talk about personalized medicine, personalized stem cell therapies. So if I can take one of my own cells and make it into a stem cell line and dry therapy from that I will be able to have individualized therapy and I won't reject those cells because they're genetically identical to my own.

So how might this work? So this is a scheme of induced pluripotent stem cells. You can take an adult stem cell, most of this work now is done with skin fibroblasts from just a skin biopsy of fibroblasts. And in the lab you reprogram it. You manipulate it in the lab to take it from a differentiated adult cell back in development to a pluripotent cell. And originally this was done by viruses introducing first it was six factors then four, but now stem cell scientists have gotten much more adept at this reprogramming back to a pluripotent state. There were a lot of problems with using viruses. You can use it with plasma, people have done it just with proteins and now with small molecules. So scientists are able to reprogram adult cells back into the pluripotent state. And if you think about how that might work once you have a pluripotent cell derived from a committed cell you can then go back and try and differentiate it into other cell types. And so the notion is you start with the skin cell, derive an IPS cell and then turn that into a pancreatic islet cell, a cardiomyocyte or whatever. In fact, there's now evidence that you can directly reprogram one adult committed cell to a different type of adult cell without going back through the IPS pluripotent stage. So this is all revolutionary. It certainly contradicts everything I learned as a medical student or I taught medical students, so dramatic advances. And my guess is that Shinya Yamanka who developed this IPS technique originally will someday almost certainly get a Nobel Prize for this.

This is a banner article in the *New England Journal* just this past summer. And it's a big group from Munich, "Patient specific induced pluripotent stem cell models for Long QT syndrome. So Long QT syndrome is a cardiac disorder, an arrhythmia that is a cause of sudden, unexpected death in athletes. So the Long QT interval in the EKG is prolonged and that predisposes these patients to arrhythmias, torsade de pointes, fatal ventricular arrhythmias. And they're particularly likely to happen with exercise because of catecholamine induced stress.

So what do these researches do, they took IPS cells from a family with Long QT syndrome and they derived IPS cells, induced pluripotent stem cells. They then drove those stem cells into cardiomyocytes. And they took individual cardiomyocyte cells and studied them in the lab and studied the action potentials of those single cardiac cells. So it's just amazing to think of measuring the action potentials in single cells. And what they showed was they compared to control lines from normal volunteers. These cardiomyocytes from this IPS family were susceptible to catecholamine induced tachyarrhythmias. So when they bathe them in a catecholamine solution they could worsen the abnormalities and the action potential. Then they went a step further. One of the treatments for this pathophysiology in Long QT syndrome is if it's catecholamine induced you give beta blockers to try and reduce the effect. And what they showed is that if you pretreated these individual cardiomyocytes with beta blockers you've blonded the abnormal response to catecholamines.

So they really did recapitulate in their very elegant laboratory model the path of physiology of this genetic variant of Long QT.

Now you can see one very interesting thing here. If you had another new candidate drug for treatment of this particular type of Long QT what you might do is see if pretreatment with that new candidate drug abolished the abnormal response to catecholamines. And if it didn't you might say what's the point of going further in drug development on this, why bother going through animals and preclinical testing. Let's move on to another candidate drug. So you might short circuit a lot of time and expense in sort of screening drugs for this condition. So I think this has a lot of promise. This is really a very, very intriguing proof of principle for how IPS cells might be used to help understand and to develop better treatments for a really awful condition causing unexpected sudden death in otherwise healthy, young people.

So I've said a lot about is this a new era in stem cell research. So the derivation of IPS cells avoid sidesteps, all the controversies with embryonic stem cell research. There's no embryo involved, none of this involves pluripotent cells. Moreover, there's actually very little difficulty in obtaining somatic cells to derive IPS cells from. To create embryos through IVF it's a very long process with hormonal retrieval. It's a lot for the woman undergoing IVF. In comparison a skin biopsy is a relatively minor procedure and most people are perfectly happy to undergo a skin biopsy for this kind of research. In addition, sitting in freezers all around the country, probably in the Michigan Cancer Center, there are well-characterized frozen specimens, well annotated, that could be used to derive additional stem cell lines. And under current federal regulations if there is existing human biological materials already out of someone's body, in the freezer, if those are de-identified or if they were given under a very blanket consent those can be used for any other type of downstream research without additional consent. So a lot of specimens available for derivation of IPS lines for a host of diseases. So this sounds great, but my colleagues and I at UCSF said yes, but. And the but is what I'm going to talk about in the next couple of minutes.

Old and New Ethical Problems in Innovative Stem Cell Research, 2010

So there's nothing problematic ethically provided you get informed consent. There's no coercion or undue influence, it's pretty straightforward. But there's some downstream research that you can do once you've got a pluripotent stem cell line, and it could be an IPS line, it could be an embryonic stem cell line, which I think can cause a lot of ethical controversy. And I think we need to look ahead to that downstream research. So first from a lab researcher's point of view, I was always a klutz in the lab even in organic chemistry. And so some stem cell lines are really easy to work with that even someone like me is not going to ruin them. They're very forgiving in terms of temperature, culture media. They don't die on you. And those are the lines that researchers like to work with. And when you're deriving a new IPS line you don't know if you're going to be lucky and get a line that's easy to work with or if yours is going to be very finicky and hard to work with. If you happen to have a line that's easy to work with and particularly if it's well-characterized a lot of other researchers are going to want to use that line and you as a scientist will want to share to the--remember these are pluripotent lines that can regenerate new pluripotent cells. And you're not going to know what those other researchers are going to want to do with those lines. You may have said to the people who donated those skin cells this is what we're going to do, but what those future researchers may want to do might be very different.

One thing that already we have seen protocols for at UCSF is to use IPSC lines to derive gametes and to use them for reproduction. Now why might people want to do that? Well, if you think about women who undergo cancer chemotherapy and are cured of cancer but the therapy has destroyed their ovaries and rendered them incapable after therapy of conceiving that's a really big issue. Now there are other approaches, oocyte freezing, ovarian tissue freezing. But this is something that is of interest to many cancer survivors and even if it's not something that's clinically useful we might learn a lot about how oocytes mature. So we've had protocols to do just in vitro derivation of pre-gamete cells from IPS cells. This has already been done in mice and other non-human models.

But you can see where this is going, right? That if you say to someone we think that we can take a skin biopsy, derive an IPS cell and now derive an oocyte. And we look at it in the lab and it has all the markers, it looks like an oocyte. The real question is does it function like an oocyte, will it work in reproduction. So that might be one option in addition to the frozen oocytes, the frozen ovarian tissue.

Now if you really start to think ahead so you might derive what look like mature gametes do you want to just put them into clinical use? Give them to the IVS clinicians? You're going to say wait a minute let's do a little more. Let's make sure that somehow in this reprogramming we haven't done something horribly awry and reprogrammed in a way that can have some very severe genetic problems. So one thing you would certainly do in an animal model is to fertilize those oocytes in the lab, see what the embryos look like and do the embryos develop normally. So now I'm starting to get right back into a lot of ethical controversy. So if you start to create an embryo in the lab not for reproduction yet, but to see if it's safe to proceed with the next step of reproduction, is that ethical? To create an embryo that won't be used for reproduction itself, even if the purpose of doing that is to move to the next set of experiments which are reproductive experiments. If this happens we are going to have to think about what our ethics are with regard to creating embryos for research purposes because if you don't do that in humans what you--then offer to patients is either we don't do this at all as an option. So if a woman didn't freeze oocytes or didn't freeze ovarian tissue before cancer or chemotherapy she may be cut off from this option. Do you then say to her we don't know if this would work, but we also don't know if it would go horribly awry if we use it for reproduction? Is it ethical to offer her that without some more preclinical evidence? These are tough decisions and they're going to be hard decisions.

Now I want to sort of take it another step back. Remember I talked about these IPS lines that are easy to work with, that are widely used. A lot is known about how to grow them, they are very forgiving. For proof

Old and New Ethical Problems in Innovative Stem Cell Research, 2010

of principle can you derive gametes from IPS cells? My sense is many scientists will want to use existing lines that they know are easy to work with and have been well characterized by other researchers. But if you think about the somatic cell donor whose fibroblasts were used to derive that line, if you went back if you could find that donor, it may be even impossible to do so because they are not de-identified, but if you said to them we originally talked to you about this cardiology syndrome and we said we might also use it for cancer, diabetes and you said fine. But you know, we had no idea that we might also want to derive not cardiac cells or pancreatic cells, but to derive gametes, oocytes from those cells my guess is there are going to be some donors who would say I have no problem with donating it for the cardiology research, diabetes research is fine, Alzheimer's is fine, but now you're talking about deriving gametes that's--you didn't tell me and had you told me I'm not sure I would have agreed to that. So we've been very, very concerned about this notion of getting blanket consent to do research in general. So I don't know what the situation is in the University of Michigan, but the standard consent form at UCSF, and I think this is true in many other major hospitals, is when I got in and have a biopsy done, in that consent form there's an option that leftover tissue no longer needed for my clinical care may be used by Doctor Loan and associates for teaching quality assurance and research. And that's all it says. Now a lot of institutions now put it in a separate box so it's not buried in the surgical consent. But when you just say it that way I'm just wondering what do people think you're talking about in terms of research. And if you said, oh, in that research is stuff like that what would they think. So these are some of the dilemmas that we're trying to grapple with now at UCSF. We are concerned about this broad or open-ended consent which is typical in many institutions. It's good to have broad consent because it facilitates the use of IPSC lines for lots of different types of research. But you can't specify what people are going to do in the future. So how do you get consent for something that you can't even explain? We've sort of tried to suggest a middle ground which is you have to be as informed as the circumstances permit. And one of the things we think that might be very relevant to the decision to donate cells for IPS research is that these cells if successful might be widely shared and used by researchers for all kinds of things that we might not be able to conceive of. And if some donors may find some of that downstream research objectionable. And we've actually tried to think about the kinds of research that if you told people about some people might say, I didn't realize that's what you're going to do. So sharing with other researchers what you don't know.

Injection into animals. We had a visiting professor from Finland a couple of years ago and she said I don't know what you're concerned about. In Finland and Europe people are concerned about their cells being injected into animals. And she actually studies cardiac arrhythmia and she says some families say you can manipulate these cells in a laboratory, but I don't want you injecting them into animals to show that they actually function, for example, like cardiomyocytes. Patenting commercialization with no plans to share royalties with the donors, whole genome sequencing will almost certainly be done if the one thousand dollar genome, where every single base pair could be identified, becomes reality. And we think that predictably some donors will object to some of this downstream research.

So we've said first you've got to explain before you ask for permission what this might involve and the fact that some of this may be objectionable to some people. After you do that disclosure we say then you may request broad permission for future research but not open-ended permission because we think that we should exclude from a broad authorization studies that we can foresee that a sizeable percentage of donors might object to. And we particularly thought about the kind of reproductive research I was talking to you about involving IVF fertilization and actually it's certainly possible using IPS cells in non-human animals, particularly mice, to use it for reproductive cloning through a sort of technical wizardry called tetroployed complementation. You can create a live-born mouse that's genetically identical to the donor of the somatic cell donor. Now whether you should even try that in humans at all is a huge question. My own personal view is no, we shouldn't do that. But if you just have broad, open-ended research to all research, that's not precluded. And we also thought, and this would be a change, that research with existing tissue for IPS, even these cells are anonymized has to have some sort of oversight to make sure that researchers aren't doing something that would be that controversial in the eyes of some donors or people like the donors.

So what we are proposing is to allow broad use of IPS cells for research under a broad consent, but not open-ended, to facilitate research into lots of diseases, not just a single disease that's of interest to the original scientist deriving IPS cell lines. But it's not open-ended. We want to put some boundaries around it so donors can say, okay, within all that that's fine. And the empirical evidence is that most donors if they're particularly interested in diabetes they don't care if you then use those cells for cancer research or Alzheimer's research as long as it's really focused on curing those horrible diseases.

So I'm going to sort of move on now and sort of talk for a minute about clinical trials. So this is a gentleman with a spinal cord injury. And these can be devastating even with rehabilitation. A lot of people have severe long-term permanent impairments. This man has a high injury and requires some ventilatory support. And as I said there's now a stem cell trial for acute spinal cord injury. And obviously this is an example of if a therapy really worked in resorting function the way it does in some of the mouse models it would be a real boon for people with this kind of devastating injury.

But there are some potential problems with using stem cells for therapy. Remember I said that a stem cell is pluripotent. It can get to all kinds of sort of end differentiated cells. When you're giving what you think is a neural precursor cell there's some potential problems. One is if there's any impurity and you've actually also included in that therapeutic transplantation some undifferentiated pluripotent cells, they might differentiate into another line that you didn't want. And, moreover, there's now increasing evidence that adult stem cells are more plastic then we thought. That you might be able to take a parasite and convert it into a blood for example or vice versa. Maybe what you think is a neural precursor cell might also differentiate into other cells.

There are some case reports that suggest this actually happens. So this is a case report, a very special case. It is a young child with Wiskott-Aldrich syndrome who had multiple stem cell transplants in Russia. It's not really clear what was injected where, what it was. But he went home to Israel and developed a lot of new neurological problems. And he was found to have multiple tumors all along his spinal cord which were shown to be of donor origin or at least not of his origin. So this is an example and you can say, well, this is totally different from what would happen in a clinical trial. But cells differentiating into the wrong kind of cells and integrating into tissues where you didn't want them to integrate. This is not just isolated.

Here's a report from Toronto where some researchers were studying injection of adult stem cells, autologous adult stem cells, cells derived from the donor's peripheral blood, re-injected into the kidneys of patients with renal disease. That patient developed multiple angioloma periphery of lesions in the kidney, again cells honing into locations where they weren't supposed to and differentiating into cells they weren't supposed to. So that's the flip side of plasticity. You can get things you didn't want. And the other thing just to say, unlike drug therapy if you have a side effect you can stop and hope the patient recovers, with a stem cell transplantation once you've injected it, once you've transplanted it it's going to be very hard to remove the cells to make them stop proliferating although there's some talk about how that might be done.

So if we're talking about diseases that are now long-term chronic diseases we have to be concerned about the long-term adverse effects. So, again, we've thought a lot at UCSF about ethical issues in clinical trials. This is an article I published with some colleagues. We think this is one example of clinical trials of really highly innovative new interventions where the animal models are just not very predictive of what might happen in humans. And we suggested some safe guards that might be put in place and particularly thinking of stem cell clinical trials of stem cells derived from pluripotent stem cells.

First, there should be combined scientific and ethical review simultaneously by the same group because certainly our experience with a couple of clinical trials we've reviewed is that combined review comes up with a lot of suggestions on how to reduce risks for the first recipients of these transplants. And that includes excluding people of inappropriately high risk and also thinking about better ways to detect adverse effects so you don't go on and keep injecting transplants when in fact you've already had some adverse effects in the first several patients.

We also suggested, and I don't know if this will take traction, that it would help and IRB reviewing a stem cell clinical trial to have access to reviews of other IRBs that have reviewed similar clinical trials. Because frankly none of us is as smart as we'd like to be and we may not think of things that another review body thought of but we wouldn't know unless we have confidential access to their reviews.

Second is we think that there needs to be real thought to detecting unintended differentiation and integration of cell therapies derived from pluripotent or actually even multi-potent stem cells. One thing we identified in one of the studies we reviewed is even though it was for a very serious lethal childhood neurological disease there were no plans for autopsy studies in humans who were almost certainly going to die within a year of transplantation. And that it struck us was foregoing an opportunity to see on a pathological postmortem exam whether there was unintended integration and differentiation. And given the nature of the special studies that need to be done we suggest that you need to think about that in the planning of the trial so you set up how the autopsies are going to be done. And we said you should talk to the parents of the children enrolling to see if they have objections to autopsy per se where they would never consent to a postmortem. And if so we said maybe you're not going to get the maximum scientific value if you forego the autopsy.

There's also a large problem with unrealistic patient hopes, a lot of hype and a lot of people are, I think, unrealistic about what might happen. Remember phase one studies are for safety. You're not going to be able to assess ethicacy in an uncontrolled phase one trial.

And finally, we were very concerned about failure to publish negative results. So unfortunately in innovative therapies negative results may not be published promptly even though that might have a lot of value to other scientists and to future participants in clinical trials. And you might say, well, wow, that doesn't happen anymore. That there's clinicaltrials.gov and you have to post both the protocol and the results on clinicaltrials.gov. Well, it turns out there's a loophole in clinicaltrials.gov. If you're studying an intervention that does not get FDA approval, for example, because the sponsor abandoned it because of adverse effects, they don't have to publish on clinicaltrials.gov. So other scientists might not know about that.

Now why might a company want to keep silent about negative results? Well, if you think about a biotech company who has one product and it turns out not to work they might want to have a little time to think about shifting gears, developing other products and to not tip off their competitors that they need to go in a different direction because a bigger company might say, we'll avoid all their mistakes we'll go a different direction. Now as an academic scientist if you're doing a clinical trial not to publish results that have a big impact in the field I think really goes against the grain of what we hope science is in terms of open transfer of information.

So we have insisted at UCSF that if these kinds of clinical studies are done the contract or grant include very strong language giving the scientist complete control over the data and the right to publish. Now there's a clause to sort of show the sponsor a draft of the manuscript and let them comment and stuff like that, but the decision to publish is with the academic scientist not with the sponsor.

So let me summarize and we'll leave some time for questions. Stem cell research is a field that is progressing rapidly. I think some of the discoveries are just, frankly, mind boggling and really sort of open the doors to lots of new things. Ethics and public policy not only need to keep pace with science, I've tried to argue the ethics and public policy need to be a step ahead or two of the science and that's what we're trying to do now with consent for biopsies to derive stem cells.

Physicians and researchers need to be involved in this policy process. Stem cell research is highly politicized, I think, scientists and physicians need to be involved in helping explain to the public what this science will do, what realistically it's going to do and the time frame in which it's going to take place. So I leave with you the hope that, I know Michigan has a lot of great stem cell research, a lot of public interest trying to develop spinoff companies and the like, that not only does the research continue but we create a policy environment where the public has trust that the research is being done with high ethical standards and it is acceptable today.

On Becoming A Physician: Stresses and Strengths of Physicians-in-Training, 2011

Laura Roberts, MD, Professor and Chair, Department of Psychiatry and Behavioral Sciences, Stanford University School of Medicine

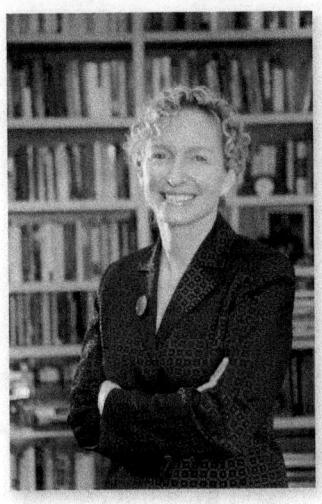

Thank you. Thank you for being here late in the day. And who are you? Do I have medical students? Thank you for entering the profession, working so hard, taking on debt, doing all that you're doing. Who are my residents? I have some residents? Thank you for coming. And who are my faculty? Thank you for dedicating your life to academic medicine because you had other choices and yet here we are. And thank you to all of the rest of you who are friends of this institution, of Dr. Waggoner and all that we will talk about today.

So the first thing I'd like to ask is for people to remember. For medical students it just means remembering like yesterday, maybe earlier today but physicians who have been in practice for awhile and faculty, please think back to what it was like when you were a resident and when you were a medical student. And I'll just give you an illustration. I sat down last night and I thought about what it was like for me. By age 24 when I was a second year medical student, third year medical student I had watched one of my classmates sneak alcohol in the anatomy lab. I had taken care of about a dozen patients who were on clinical trials, many of whom did beautifully

On Becoming A Physician:

and went home and had extended life and an extended quality of life. But a couple of whom died, one of whom died on a Texas trial, an African American patient with cell carcinoma. Terrible prognosis who was in a trial who believed that he was in a study to extend his life but actually it was just to determine how big of a toxic burden his body could carry.

I held the hand of one of my patients who was 15 years old in a life threatening asthma attack all through the night, completely exhausted because I hadn't slept the night before. I went up scouring the wards for patients so I could interview them. It was part of what we had to do when I was in medical school. Got up very early in the morning, went up to the coronary care unit and encountered one of my classmates who had taken a tricyclic overdose the night before. I quickly went off hoping that he didn't see me.

I saw a classmate who kept on going to the student health center because he had terrible, terrible GI symptoms before exams and the attending physician there said, "You know, I had that too. Isn't it terrible? It's really awful." Well when he had ravaging Crohn's Disease that had gone without being diagnosed that led to him nearly bleeding out he then dropped out of medical school. I occasionally see him modeling in catalogs from time to time which is like, I think it was a good ending.

I had my first child. I had my first child in medical school. I gave birth in front of the resident who later graded me on my OB/GYN rotation, oh my God. My classmates read my chart and I was mortified because they knew my weight but they also learned kind of my family history, all kinds of stuff because that was back in the day. I put patients on involuntary holds. I took care of two patients who were concentration camp survivors. I performed urologic procedures with my, you know, obviously attending physicians on children and elders who then had devastating cancer. We snuck homeless patients in and had them stay overnight in the hospital and give them a little bit of medicine just to kind of keep them in from the cold Chicago cold in the middle of the winter.

Stresses and Strengths of Physicians-in-Training, 2011

So this is all by the time I'm 24 and this is after just sitting down for just a couple of minutes last night and thinking about these incredibly powerful interactions. But you saw in the midst of those were the issues that my classmates had, not just my patients, really significant health issues. And that inspired a whole line of work which I'm going to share with you today.

So first let's think about medical students. There are many thousands and I think I will use this pointer. Right here, about--more than 40,000 students who apply to enter medical school. If you look at the pattern over time it's growing to be more equal proportions of men and women but not everybody gets in. Those are the applicants. There are roughly 16,000 or greater applicants or graduates every year and again, a little bit greater proportion of men but really a closer disparity now. And if you then look at the total number of applicants in the match, in the overall pattern, you see that there are many, many applicants but really the number of positions is only growing just a little bit. And part of the big reason for this as you'll see and I think is evident is that these are all of the applications in the residency match, right? So you've got seniors of U.S. medical schools as the majority. U.S. citizens who went to international medical schools is another large group and then that second is non-U.S. citizen student graduates of international medical schools. So you see over time there's a much greater proportion of internationally trained or international origin individuals. And you can see there are many different areas and our interests and the different areas of medicine are populated by people with different strengths and performance records.

So this past year there were 23,000 PGY1 positions offered and 15--more than 15,000 were filled with U.S. seniors. The 96 percent fill rate was one of the most successful on record and of the U.S. seniors who matched 81 percent went to one of their top three choices. So right now our medical students are really driving the decisions. And there were more overall residency slots. Internal medicine had more than 100 new positions. Family medicine had 100 more positions, pediatrics, a handful and emergency medicine. So you can see that there is an increment in these primary interfaced areas.

So I don't know if you really remember but this is a really great summary of what it's like to be in medical school. You've got to start sometime. Why don't you operate on this one? I know, I'm going to let that one sink in a little bit. It's hard. It's like way hard. It's unbelievably anxiety producing. I'll never forget the first day I went on my third year rotation and my resident said, "Pick up a patient." And I was like, "Pick up a patient?" "Pick up a patient. Pick up a patient. What does pick up a patient mean?" I was terrified. So this idea of really starting and assuming the identity as a physician, you are the one. You are the one who becomes so profoundly responsible for the well being of another person is a very intense, very, very challenging thing. And what we've learned over the last few years is that there is a cost. There's a cost in the psychological well being of our trainees.

We know from studies that have been done over a number of years that psychiatric symptoms are emerging in both medical students and residents, that they're linked with particular training stresses and milestones and they're much higher at certain periods of training. But the proportions are very great. About a quarter of medical students have anxiety symptoms and about 40 percent, nearly half will have significant depressive symptoms. So the point is these are measurable, clinically meaningful findings. And we know that there's suicidal ideation that is being experienced by our medical students. I mean it's unbelievable. The most unbelievably talented, important individuals and as a resource in our country and the world really and to have our young people be so distressed that contemplating suicide is something that is becoming almost ordinary. And it is greater than in the general population and it is greater than age matched, gender matched comparison professional students. And it's greater among under represented minority physicians in training.

It appears to heighten, the suicidal ideation in particular, this pattern appears to be greater during high stakes kind of transitions and high stakes evaluations. And it's greater among students with preexisting illness and it's very prominent, in fact your own senior associate dean has done some of this very beautiful work looking at how dropping--students who are contemplating dropping out or do leave medical school are a particularly important at risk population.

So let me walk you through a few of these studies. This was a six school study of depression and suicidal ideation, large number 2,193 physicians in training. By that I mean both medical students and residents just for simplicity of presentation. Twelve percent overall met criteria for probably major depression, nine percent overall met criteria for probable minor or moderate depression at that time. So it's a cross section. Greater among medical students than residents which is interesting. Greater among medical students than residents, I have a hypothesis about that, and greater among women than among men. In this study six percent overall have reported recent suicidal ideation and suicidal ideation as I mentioned in this particular study was greater among underrepresented minority students than majority of physicians in training. So Alaska native, Native American, Pacific Islander, and African American physicians in training, this is a very huge burden of suicidal ideation that people are living out. And Hispanic and Asian physicians in training, these percentages are not as overwhelming, given other demographic and other comparisons, these are very high numbers.

There was a study in the United Kingdom of more than 2,000 medical students and a vast majority of the doctors, meaning the residents and 54 percent, a little bit over than half of the medical students reported their own personal illness experiences. They felt less prepared for their work. They felt more anxious and performed less well on examinations.

There's also been this talk about burnout and I have to say this was not a concept that I embraced readily. It seemed a bit vague but what they--the model is a combination of what's referred to as emotional exhaustion I think has intuitive meaning, depersonalization which has in this context the meaning of distancing, kind of objectifying and distancing. And then a low sense of personal accomplishment, so how effective we feel. And it was not meant to be just a simple marker of depression. And of these more than 2,000 students 50 percent met criteria for burnout, 46 percent for depression, and 11 percent astonishingly had contemplated suicide in the prior year. And when you looked at quality of life scores they were lower than comparison populations.

So I like this slide too. This is Calvin and Hobbs and he says, "Want to see something weird? Watch. You put bread in this slot, push down the lever and in a few minutes toast pops up. Wow. Where does the bread go? Beats me. Isn't that weird?" So I like to do this as the sense of wonder bread and at the end we become toast, okay? It's really--it's been--it can be hard. And when I think as a psychiatrist though if we are defended, we are exhausted, we are shut down, we are toast, it's hard to be flexible and responsive and resilient and problem solving and to meet the next person with a sense of joy and kind of the sense of the privilege we should feel when we take care of patients.

So this study was very interesting and it kind of looked at this issue. If you had a great deal of burnout, emotional exhaustion, depersonalization, and low sense of self efficacy and then you look at what are referred to as unprofessional clinical behaviors and I'm going to go through them in just a minute, is there a connection? And these are the examples of "unprofessional" clinical behaviors: signing an attendance sheet for a student who wasn't present say at a lecture like this, copied from a crib sheet of another student during an exam, permitted another student to copy from you during an exam, taking credit for another person's work, reporting a laboratory test or x-ray is pending when you really weren't sure if it was ordered if you knew it hadn't been, ever reporting a result as normal when you knew that really it had been omitted from an exam, ever saying you ordered a test when you actually have not, and endorsing one or more of these--more than one of these.

So the idea is these are kind of softer signs of unprofessional behavior and is there a connection? And those researchers, one of whom is in this room, did find a connection. There was an association between a number of cheating or dishonest clinical behaviors and the scores on these measures related to depersonalization and emotional exhaustion. So the idea here is that when we become kind of defended, distanced, we're interacting with patients as if they're objects, we're kind of detached from the humanity, the humanness of the experience, it's a little easier to take shortcuts. It's just a little bit easier.

This study though had some good news which is that there were higher physical quality of life scores in similar aged individuals in the general population and actually with time burnout seems to ease up. So there's something about the entry, the entry into certain kinds of duties that really creates a vulnerability. It's a vulnerability developmentally in the training process. So situational stressors rather than fundamental attributes of the individual may be at play and there may be really ripe intervention points that we can work with. And I'm going to tell you about my work which was really inspired by my early experiences. And I also want to use it as an illustration of how you can do shoestring research. We did this study, literally I told earlier of the story about how we gave M&M's as reimbursement to people who took the survey. I went to a bunch of my buddies and said, "I'm really concerned about this. There's almost nothing in the literature. Let's do a study together." So I got colleagues at multiple places to do this totally cheap. We literally had 1500 dollars to pay a statistician to help us with this. So you really can do these important labors of love and pursue ideas, even if it isn't on somebody else's funding agenda if you see the importance of it.

Anyway in this study we had over 1,000 medical students who participated from nine different schools. Ninety percent expressed need for healthcare. Fifty-four percent identified a need for physical healthcare and 46 identified a need for mental healthcare. However the majority of students didn't seek necessary care. They encountered difficulties in obtaining care about half of the time. They felt that it was too difficult to take time off and they were very worried about the cost of care. And a majority of the students in this study kind of crab walked up to a resident they knew and asked them for a prescription or crab walked up to an attending who they knew was a softie and asked for some medical help rather than going and seeking care from a doctor, having a traditional doctor/patient relationship and all that that involved. It was convenience and cost.

The other thing that we looked at is what kinds of concerns do people have that stop them from seeking care that aren't related to convenience and cost? And really academic jeopardy emerges a huge issue. There was significant concern expressed by the students in our study that academic status might be jeopardized if the dean of students learned that they had different health issues. They also thought that on individual rotations if their supervisors learned that they had health issues they would get worse grades, even if their performance was the same, that they wouldn't be seen as the tough, fierce physicians that they needed to be. There was obviously greatest concern expressed for stigmatizing health issues, drug and alcohol issues, HIV, serious infection, the mental health issues, and also interestingly cancer, relationship issues. And there was a very strong preference for off site care, so care not received at your training institution for a stigmatizing health issue. And 90 percent of respondents wanted insurance permitting off site care which I don't know what the standard is but I don't think that that is typical across the United States.

We asked a subset to almost 1,000 to respond to a series of vignettes depicting severely ill student peers. So in the context of a suicidal classmate and I've got to tell you, these vignettes were really vivid. I mean, these were bold probes. It wasn't an ambiguous suicidal classmate. In this, 45 percent said that they would tell no one or take no action. And the range across schools was 19 percent to 70 percent. What I would say is at the school where it was 19 percent they were doing some things right. And the school where it was 70 percent, boy, there must have been some harsh issues in that culture. Thirty-seven percent, about a third would seek advice and really a small proportion would tell the dean's office or intervene actively.

Stresses and Strengths of Physicians-in-Training, 2011

With a student with known alcohol, amphetamine use, and erratic behavior endangering patient care on a clinical rotation 53 percent would tell no one. Thirty five percent would seek advice and only 12 percent would tell the dean's office. So very significant issues and wait, let me just finish up. I mean remember that the essence of professionalism is that we belong to a profession that have two components to it. We have the privilege of serving this role, acquiring expertise, serving patients and serving society but there are obligations to it which is like we've got to be really good at what we do and we've got to assure that our profession, our colleagues within the profession fulfill these responsibilities well too. And if we have potential for impairment or compromise in our colleagues that is as much of an ethical obligation that we have in the profession as making sure that we take very good care of patients. So it's two pieces to it. So this, I thought, was very concerning data.

We then did a smaller study. It was funded by the Arnold Gold Foundation, again, shoestring research but we wanted to look at these same questions in residents. And we found a smaller percent reported frequent health problems but it was definitely worse among the women. Sixty-five percent of residents in this particular study reported a health decline over the course of residency and again, worse among women. Residents identified healthcare needs but again, avoided or delayed care. Time constraints, privacy concerns, expense, discomfort with the dual role interestingly were offered as reasons. And there was also concern about quality of care and how to access care. Our trainees who are in our midst have difficulty accessing care sometimes. Resident also endorsed informal consultation or curb siding is a common practice due to schedule, cost, and confidentiality.

We then talked--asked people how much--basically how much trash talking is going on in your culture? How much of a problem is it if a person is sick? And we asked about private health issues of residents and were they perceived as being discussed a lot? Kind of is there a lot of gossip or isn't there not? And really the residents responded by saying it was only sometimes brought up. But interestingly after being absent from work residents were perceived as being treated a little bit more negatively and some empathy among--from some colleagues and some ostracism from some colleagues after they've had to miss work. The residents felt that their fellow residents fell into two categories, either more empathetic or more inclined to ostracize than attendings. There was kind of a bi-modal response. And it was a more pronounced pattern among women respondents and among women--or residents in specialty training really conveying a greater sense of stigma and negative impact and the importance of special care pathways for these areas.

And I'm sorry, I was noticing it didn't come across quite as well but on the top what this graph shows is whether people would have concern if anybody learned about them having different illnesses. And what you see is basically a perfect stacking of more stigmatizing illnesses to less stigmatizing illnesses. Again, would you like to have your care inside or outside of the institution? Again, it isn't as easy to see but again we have kind of a perfect stacking that people would prefer to have outside care for stigmatizing illnesses and they're comfortable receiving care inside for things like pain or allergies.

And cost, time, and quality are the kinds of things that lead people to want to stay at their training institution but embarrassment and confidentiality drives people out. This was what we found with both residents and medical students.

So these are some of the major issues that we're facing right now. What are some of the causes? Well there was an important study about medical student abuse done and I would say that this is good news and bad news. This landmark study that was published in 1990 was at University of Colorado and there was an 83 percent response rate for this large study of 400 students. And the medical students there reported abuse as nearly universal. Seventeen percent of students had been abused by supervisors and residents, most commonly by residents interestingly by the end of first year, 33 percent by the end of second year, 68 percent by the end

Stresses and Strengths of Physicians-in-Training, 2011

of the third year and 81 percent by the end of fourth year. The highest incidence was in third year with 20 percent of the students experiencing at least five episodes of abusive treatment that was of major importance and very upsetting. And these were not soft, pastel descriptions of abuse.

In more recent times the AMC graduate questionnaire has really been asking very deeply about mistreatment and abuse. And I'm sure that we've made a great deal of progress. And yet 12 to 17 percent of graduating students reported mistreatment in the context of medical school and 18 percent of graduating students had witnessed mistreatment of a peer from the most recent data. And as I say the things that we're talking about are being publicly belittled or humiliated, being required to perform personal services. I don't know about you but I was asked to babysit and do--pick up dry cleaning. Receiving unwanted sexual advances, not as common but it should be zero, being subjected to personally offensive remarks, should be zero, being denied opportunities for training due to gender, should be zero, receiving lower grades due to gender, still unbelievable. So what you see is this kind of dynamic tension of the preexisting strengths, incredible resilience, incredibly positive motivation, the intelligence and tenacity of a remarkable group of people who have joined us in our profession, positive experiences of being inspired by role models, feelings of being effective and doing something of importance, trying to adapt in the context of the stresses of medical school and really the potential positive environment. These are all things that could really strengthen and enrich the experience of medical students. But we also know that students come with some preexisting vulnerabilities. There's a reason why we're here, many of us. They may have negative experiences and stressful experiences in the course of their training. There may be the emergence of more maladaptive behaviors than we would like to see as a profession. Really disproportionate and inappropriate stresses and can be kind of a negative professional environment that can hold people down.

So we've come to kind of a crisis. It says either cheer up or take off the hat. I didn't mean that about you guys. Cheer up, we're getting there.

On Becoming A Physician:

It's okay. But it is--I think either cheer up or take off the hat was kind of the mindset when I was in medical school. I think it's a little bit more sophisticated, a little bit more nuanced thankfully in this time. And I guess I want to say that we cannot make the experience of human suffering easier. We can't make holding a child's hand as they try to struggle through the night and not die from their life threatening asthma any easier. This is the reality of life and death and illness and disease and unfairness that we work with and work with every day. That's why we joined our profession was to try and do good for these very, very people. And I love this poem. It's by Emily Dickinson. It says, "On the bleakness of my lot, bloom I strove to raise. Late my acre of rock has yielded grapes and maize." So in other words some of our patients are going to have a very hard path and that's the nature of it and there's nothing I can do to make medical school make that go away. I don't want it to. That is the nature of the profession. However what we can do is we can recognize the issues for their reality, what the stresses and the impact on our young colleagues and we can support them. We can help them through this. There are ways that we can take this very difficult set of issues and transform them, I think, into a source of compassion and a sense of motivation and a reason for being in our profession.

So let me tell you about what I think are the really positives in all of this. If--I'm going to have you look at me. If any of you have ever been ill and have also been a caregiver you know that you can never treat a patient like an object. If you yourself have ever lived through an illness or someone you deeply love has lived through an illness you know what it means to suffer, to feel kind of scared and helpless. And so the power of that as a compassion inspiring experience is one that I think that we need to recognize. And actually in our study residents do recognize this. Personal illness experiences have been seen overall as giving rise to greater feelings of empathy and more compassionate clinical practices, enjoying talking with patients, feeling compassion for patients, valuing a thorough understanding of your patients, sitting with them, helping them bear what they're going through, providing more effective pain management. And this was seen as more relevant, more critical for people with personal illness experience. Women and men saw this a little bit differently. It was a very strong result for women who have had personal illness experiences as seeing the power of the compassionate lesson in that.

And that isn't just our work. This study that was done in the United Kingdom where they found that people who were physicians in training who were stressed and felt ill and felt like they weren't performing as well still felt that they were better prepared overall for their medical training. They understood the realities of illness. They conveyed more empathic attitudes, deeper sense of motivation, patient centeredness, and attentiveness to the personal implications of clinical practice for their patients. And in our study I had these beautiful, beautiful gifts of stories that I'm going to read a few of them to you. These were the comments of medical students to open into questions about family experiences with illness and empathy and their intentions about being physicians.

So one student wrote, "I would hope to be like the physician who cared for my father when he was passing away." Another student wrote, "My mother had stage four ovarian cancer. I had many opportunities to interact with her oncologist, respect them for their knowledge but determined that my own bedside manner would be markedly warmer than the vast majority of house staff and attendings." Another student said, "My brother underwent ten neurosurgeries. Mistakes made by physicians and the lack of technology convinced me to enter and advance the field." Another student wrote, "Seeing many family members die from cancer has had a profound effect on my becoming a physician. I would not allow anyone to die in a hospital surrounded by overworked, impersonal staff."

I think every patient who dies in a hospital is surrounded by overworked, I hope not impersonal but I think overworked staff. This is another student. He wrote, "I had a skin graft for a lesion on my head and the day of the surgery at 6:30 am I was consented for a possible skin graft. I was alone and nervous so I signed this consent. Now I have a five centimeter by six centimeter bald spot on my head. I didn't think clearly. I was without support. It was not an appropriate time to obtain consent. The experience made me very cynical and skeptical towards physicians. I think that very often doctors do what's easiest and efficient with little concern for their patients' well being." Another student wrote, "I have osteoarthritis in my right hip which was removed from me many joys and stress relief activities in the past year. I am learning how far reaching a disease can be into someone's life and the need for good communication from healthcare workers to alleviate fear and anxiety."

I think these are going to be amazing doctors. I think these individuals who have lived through this who understand. I had another example where a wonderful medical student wrote, "I had to take antibiotics four times a day. Do you know how hard that is!!" I just thought it was a wonderful insight. So I think there's power and something very positive that we can capture with some of these concerns but we have to be smart enough to see it. And we have to be prepared and we have to help our early career professionals be prepared to see this.

So let me just offer some solutions and a few other comments. I think we do really need to express our concern palpably. We need to elevate the topics of self care and wellness within our curriculum and within our culture. We have to recognize the stresses, the predictable stresses that occur that are completely kind of embedded in the architecture of our individual curricula at different medical schools. We have to recognize illness, educate people about symptoms, not normalize some of these things when they actually have reached a clinically concerning level. We also have to think about life cycle and stress issues, role and significant issues that our medical students are experiencing in residents. We have to have really realistic policies and routines, procedures. It shouldn't be invented every time a student or a resident has a concern. And we have to make consistent efforts in support of a positive training environment that affirms people's overall well being. In our curricula we need to develop opportunities for self reflection, motivation, the importance of

Stresses and Strengths of Physicians-in-Training, 2011

self care, kind of deconstruct the hidden curriculum of the superhuman, super macho physician to one where it's okay to be human and here we are together. But it's very important that you take care of yourself so that you can be here in our profession to help serve our patients.

There appear to be setting specific and specialty specific--I hesitate to say gender specific but perhaps some very particular targets that we might want to think about with our teaching. I think small group, case based discussions so that it becomes very real for people will be valuable. Targeted content related to recognition of symptoms of illness. Addiction appears to be a significant concern, different treatment modalities and the optimism that we have when we give people accurate information about mental health and physical health treatments, self care skills training and coaching and mentoring initiatives for the faculty because they're the ones who are going to need to implement this. We also need safeguard pathways to care, policies and procedures to protect confidentiality, accurate information to students and residents about what happens when they seek care. Who is going to see the record? Who is going to know? They're terrified that it's going to damage their ability to get into a residency or to get a good job. They're afraid that it's going to influence the grades that they receive. Protected access points and role separations, you don't have the wrong pairing of clinicians who provide care for medical students and the people who actually grade them. Values informed approaches to insurance and services, not just cost driven. This is a battle I've had at every institution I've been at. We have to be smart enough to offer insurance options to students and to residents so that they are able to seek the care that they need. And it shouldn't just be driven by cost. We may need resources to help subsidize care and non-punitive approaches to early recognition and self referral.

Now I'll tell you a story. These are Roma, Roma people in Europe, perhaps the most marginalized community in all of Europe. And there was a beautiful study done by some of my colleagues at Medical College of Wisconsin who recognized the huge issue of sexually transmitted diseases in the Roma population. So what they did was they went and instead of scolding people to engage in different sexual behaviors or to behave badly--not so badly, instead they went and gently talked with people and tried to find out who were the opinion leaders? Who were the people who set the social norms? Who were the people who were like the emotional metronome, the drivers of the culture within the Roma population? And they identified, say, a dozen people and they went and sat with this dozen people. And they talked with these natural leaders in the community about the importance of HIV recognition, sexually transmitted disease recognition, working with these opinion leaders on safe sex practices, all of the things that would decrease transmission of disease. And then they turned them loose. They let them go and do the heavy lifting in the community. They just inspired them and informed them and they had these opinion leaders go and deal with what was probably the most radical and serious public health issue that this community was living with. Okay? And then they looked at zero prevalence of HIV, incident of new infectious diseases and not only did the problem go down with these diseases, over time the protective effect of these conversations improved the community's health with the longer--the longer you looked at it the more the improvement occurred. Okay? So I'm trying to explain to you the importance of us. If we are the ones who influence our community whether we have the proper title for it or we're just the go to people, the people who live out and are role models and are important in influencing the social norms and behaviors within the culture here at the University of Michigan and my places that I've worked at, we can transform this problem, serious problem that it is now and have it improve not with like a lot of interventions. You do something today and it decays over the next several months. Instead, if we can put this in the hands of the opinion leaders in our culture then we can inspire and really bring about significant culture change that will grow and the social norms themselves will change. And I'm telling you, if you can do it with the most impoverished, marginalized, and severely

Stresses and Strengths of Physicians-in-Training, 2011

ill subpopulation, vulnerable subpopulation in Europe I'm pretty sure we could do it here. I'm pretty sure that we could accomplish the kind of cultural change that is absolutely necessary.

But I will tell you that it's going to be serious and hard. This was a study that was just published in the archives of *Surgery* and it had to do with suicidal ideation among surgeons, American surgeons. And what they found in this study of more than almost 8,000 surgeons is that 15 percent had had thoughts about taking their own life. Seven percent had had thoughts about taking their own life in the prior year and 39 percent were reluctant to get help because they were afraid they were going to lose their license.

So I tell you about--I tell you about the Roma and I hope to inspire you that we can change things through this very on the ground, very deep opinion leader kind of approach where you, each and every one of you take responsibility to talk with others about the importance of these issues and the ways of seeking care, the importance of recognizing these problems in our culture. But I will tell you, we have to start with ourselves first. We will have to look at our own issues with great courage. So this is the kind of issue. We have to create a culture of courage, compassion, and belonging. It accepts the harder aspects of medical training while also creating a culture in which people are valued. They have a sense that they deeply belong and are engaged in meaningful work that will never be easy. Being a doctor will never be easy but it should be meaningful and you should have a sense of purpose and a sense that you belong. And these are very strong protective factors in people's lives. We have to get clarity about our professionalism responsibilities which is first around serving patients, building expertise, building new knowledge, assuring that the future is better for the people that we serve, but also, making sure that our colleagues are doing okay. We need to engage in professional development for faculty and staff, really do honest inquiry scholarship and the sharing of best practices across the country and leadership and role modeling on every single level. And those of you

On Becoming A Physician:

who are students who feel very relatively disempowered, you're students, you are important influence leaders, those of you who are residents who are really critical to this and those of you who are faculty, we are in this together and need to help support all of our colleagues.

So with that, I'll say that professionalism is this social contract. And as Bob Dylan, the great moral philosopher said, "A hero is someone who understands the responsibility that comes with his freedom." We have the most immense privilege by serving our patients and working on science and engaging in education, working in communities, being leaders in this profession that serves others and helps others bear their suffering. Sometimes we get a cure or remission but mostly we should be here to help people bear their suffering. But it comes with a little bit of a price and I thank you for your listening tonight.

Fixing Health Care the Ethical Way, 2012
Jeremy Lazarus, M.D. President, American Medical Association

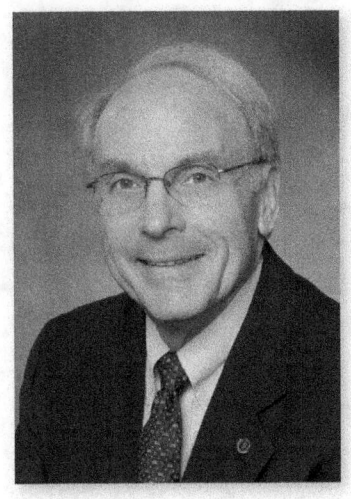

Well thank you so much to both of the introductions It is a real pleasure, an honor, and a privilege to be here at the University of Michigan. I actually haven't been up here since I was in college down in Northwestern and came up here to play the Wolverines.

I am both humbled and honored to speak to you on this wonderful Waggoner lectureship. And as you've already heard Dr. Waggoner was a great teacher, a great psychiatrist, and a great man, and whether as an administrator or as president of the APA he was a true visionary. He was also the consummate optimist and a strong believer that with the right ethics and values physicians could accomplish great things.

Today I want to talk about ethics in the context of our evolving healthcare system. With so many challenges and so many changes taking place how can physicians ensure that our core obligations are upheld? And how can we, like Dr. Waggoner before us, bring both the human and the humane to our healthcare system? How can we fix healthcare the ethical way?

Now let me start by taking a step back and looking at the big pictures. Scholars have weighed in on the topic of ethics for centuries. "We do not act rightly because we have virtue or excellence but we rather have those because we have acted rightly," Aristotle. "Man without ethics is a wild beast loosed upon this world," Albert Camus. "Relativity applies to physics, not ethics," Einstein. Now all three of these quotes testify to the need for an agreed upon set of principles governing behavior, a code that separates man from beast. And this code serves for all of us as a moral compass when we make decisions. And we are relying on it not only in our personal lives but certainly in our professional lives as well.

Of course in certain professions, especially in medicine where life and death are at stake and perhaps that's why we at the AMA have such a rich legacy in ethics dating back originally to Hippocratic Oath. And then in 1847 the AMA built on that foundation by publishing the first code of medical ethics in the country. We detailed the obligations of physicians to their patients, to their colleagues, and society and we've been updating that code ever since. And for those of you psychiatrists in the room you may remember that the APA's code was first published around 1972. It had annotations, especially applicable to psychiatry.

If we were to summarize that code as it stands today we could use the words of Georgetown University professor, physician Edmond Telegrino. He says, "Our charge as physicians is to work with patients to arrive at a right and good healing decision." And in order to do that we have to keep six core commitments in mind. First to put patients' interests above our own, to be compassionate and candid, to help patients understand their medical situation and treatment option so they can make informed decisions, to seek to understand each patient's values and goals for healthcare, to work with patients to develop treatment plans that align with those goals and values, and respect the autonomy of patients to make decisions.

Now in the past the majority of ethical questions in medicine have revolved around the bedside, whether it's physician assisted suicide or palliative sedation. And while many of these challenges still persist today we're also faced with a new set of ethical challenges, challenges that involve not just our relationship to the individual patient but to the larger healthcare system as a whole.

Fixing Health Care the Ethical Way, 2012

Now we've got lots of difficulties in this country. One is we've got soaring healthcare costs. As this chart shows our healthcare costs are generally at least double and in some cases even triple those of our first world counterparts. We spend more than two trillion each year on healthcare. And that comes to almost 18 percent of our GDP or 7,681 dollars for every single man, woman, and child in this country.

So where's all the money going? Well 448 billion dollars is going to treat patients with heart disease and stroke. One hundred seventy four billion to treat patients with diabetes and the list goes on as you can see up there on the slide. And today a full 75 percent of healthcare spending can be attributed to a second major challenge for our healthcare system, the epidemic of chronic conditions.

So more than two thirds of adults and almost one third of children are either overweight or obese. The number of Americans with diabetes has tripled since 1980 with 18 million diagnosed cases and another seven million undiagnosed cases. Every 40 seconds someone in the United States has a stroke which is the leading cause of long term disability. And the American Cancer Society estimates that 1.6 million new cancer cases will happen in 2012 alone. So the fact is that there's an epidemic of chronic conditions sweeping this country and caring for patients with complex, long term illnesses is costing us more than a trillion dollars every year.

Now on top of these problems there are of course numerous other challenges that we all face. The lack of access to insurance which forces millions to neglect their health until a worst case scenario and sends millions more to the emergency room for services that could have better been provided at a doctor's office. We have a fragmented and disjointed delivery system where physicians, nurses, hospitals, and nursing homes basically operate independently rather than in some coordinated effort.

Our healthcare outcomes often lag behind those of many of our first world counterparts as I mentioned and hundreds of billions of dollars is lost in administrative waste. And to add on to this are certainly the social determinants of health which I will not talk about in great detail, things like poverty, unemployment, access to healthy food, access to transportation to get to see the doctor and education. These all add to the complexity of what causes the healthcare situation we're in right now.

Now as you know the Affordable Care Act seeks to address many of those problems and while it isn't perfect it is a historic first step in reforming our healthcare system. And since I was told by Mrs. Margolis that she didn't realize that the AMA supported the healthcare act, the Affordable Care Act, if you don't know that, the AMA supports the Affordable Care Act. So if this is news to you I hope that's good news. It might not be good news to some of you but it was good news to a lot of patients.

So what are the key provisions in the law? Well it expands coverage to 30 million Americans, about half in Medicaid, about half in private insurance. It reforms an array of insurance practices from lifetime coverage limits to pre-existing condition denials. It invests in new delivery models such as accountable care organizations, medical homes, bundled payments, other forms of payment delivery. It supports prevention and wellness efforts. It promotes quality and the use of comparative effectiveness research. It streamlines administrative processes and it invests heavily in health IT.

Now today during the third year after the ACA was passed many of these provisions are already underway and the quest to engineer a better healthcare system has begun. But how can we be sure that it's going to be an ethical system? What commitments need to be made at the system level and what commitments need to be made at the personal level? And what is the AMA doing to help create an ethical healthcare system?

So let me begin with the system level. As physician practices, hospitals, insurance companies and other stakeholders across the country begin transitioning towards large integrated systems such as you have here at the University of Michigan there are five core ethical elements and commitments that have to guide our way. Now first we have to have open communication between physicians and patients. If managed care taught us one thing it's that physicians should never be incentivized to withhold information from patients. And as physicians we always have to feel free to treat patients with a particular drug even if it isn't on a health formulary or a specialist--refer to a specialist who isn't in the plan network. But given the current pressure to reduce spending we certainly should keep costs in mind when we compare different treatment alternatives. And I'll talk more about that in a few minutes. But ultimately all the options, not just the cheapest ones, must be communicated to patients. And for some of you who have been following the news down in Florida and the issue down there where the Florida legislature passed a law that pediatricians and family physicians could not ask parents of kids whether they had gun, gun safety in their homes, the AMA appealed that ruling and that's now on hold. So that was a gag clause that was initiated by unfortunately the state government.

Going on with commitments at the system level we have to make sure that an ethical system must base its guidelines for resource use on real, hard data about the practices involved. We have, for example, a family practice has a different kind of patient population than myself as a psychiatrist. And just as academic medical centers tend to see patients with more complicated conditions than the average community physician, so resource expectations have to be set accordingly. They must focus on the specific demographics and needs of the patients that they serve.

Number three, an ethical healthcare system must employ well designed incentives. It has to promote efficiency but never at the expense of patient needs. Just as physicians should not be incentivized to withhold information from patients, we shouldn't discourage the ordering of a clinically useful diagnostic test solely because it's expensive. And by the same token we shouldn't be encouraged to order extra diagnostic tests just because we'll be reimbursed for them.

In addition incentives need to be based on sound data about care and costs. They should be collected from large populations of patients and multiple physician practices. They should be over long periods of time, at least a year instead of six months so that periods of high utilization of services are more likely to be balanced with periods of low utilization and give a more accurate picture of what the actual costs are. And they should provide ways to compensate physicians when they treat patients with unusually complex or extensive needs.

Now well designed incentives should also limit the magnitude of financial risk faced by any individual physician. The more timely an incentive ties a financial outcome to a specific treatment decision the more problematic the incentive is. And they should be implemented even handedly across all physicians participating in the organization. So for example they shouldn't be deployed in a way that favors specialists over primary care physicians. It's also important that incentives don't encourage cherry picking, that they don't disproportionately affect patients with chronic illness, complex healthcare needs or other special populations and that they don't disadvantage physicians who care for these patients. And of course it's crucial that incentives are developed with physician input through a mechanism analogous to a hospital medical staff or health plan pharmacy and therapeutics committee on which physicians are representative--represented.

Finally, an ethical healthcare system must allow physicians to be advocates for patients. It must build exceptions into resource utilization guidelines. It has to make it easy for physicians or their staff to appeal a denial of coverage on a patient's behalf and it has to be transparent, fair, and consistent in reviewing these appeals.

Now to summarize an ethically strong healthcare system or organization takes a physician's core commitments into account and promotes their integrity as professionals. And it achieves this by supporting a physician's focus on their patients' welfare, their fundamental commitment as healers, by respecting the patient/physician relationship and the process of developing treatment plans that compared with the patient's values and goals, that promote treatment recommendations that are both patient centered but also cost conscious and minimizing conflicts of interest.

Now this last point about conflicts of interest, that warrants some further examination because the fact is all models of payment and care delivery including those that we're looking at now and experimenting with raise some conflicts of interest for physicians and systems be they financial or otherwise. For example under a fee for service system there's a built in incentive for physicians to over-utilize healthcare resources whereas under capitation system there's a built in incentive to under utilize resources in order to stay within a fixed rate of per member per month that's paid for capitation.

Now that brings me back to the individual physician and what we can do to help create an ethical healthcare system. One thing we can do is to think of ourselves as responsible and prudent stewards. That is, we can balance our commitment, our commitment to care for each individual patient with our responsibility to use common healthcare resources in a wise and prudent way. Someone once quipped and I'm sure you've heard it that the most expensive technology in healthcare is a doctor's pen. And there's certainly some wisdom in that. And for example, in 2010 Consumer Report surveyed nearly 1200 healthy 40 to 60 year old men and women with no known heart disease, risk factors, or symptoms and found that 44 percent had received screening tests for heart disease. Now obviously physician treatment recommendations aren't the only drivers of healthcare costs as I mentioned before. But our decisions do play a significant role in healthcare costs and how we utilize the resources we have. So that's why this past June the AMA, our house of delegates, passed ethics policy advising physicians to be prudent stewards of the resources that society entrusts to us as healers.

Clearly there is no magic bullet here when it comes to being responsible stewards. Like all ethical issues it's complicated. And as one of my former mentors in ethics told me when asked about an ethical situation he said, "It depends." So it is complicated. But the AMA has laid out some basic guidelines that we can keep in mind.

First we always have to ensure that treatment recommendations are based on medical need. That is, we should not order, recommend, or participate in care that does not offer reasonable likelihood of medical benefit. We need to listen closely to what our patients and family members tell us and to understand their goals for their healthcare. We need to make sure that our treatment recommendations should always be scientifically grounded. Existing data and research should help us to assess the potential benefit of a proposed intervention. And fourth, when alternative causes of action offer similar likelihood or degree of benefit we should recommend the lower cost option. So for example, not ordering a serum pregnancy test when a less costly urine test would be just as appropriate clinically in the patient's circumstances or using a generic SSRI instead of a name brand SSRI if we think they are equivalent. And fifth, we have to clearly explain our thinking to patients, the differences between alternatives including costs, and why we think a less costly alternative will meet their healthcare goals.

Now as you probably know the AMA is not alone in advocating this kind of cost conscious decision making. In January the American College of Physicians published an updated version of its ethics manual that advises doctors to deliver parsimonious care that utilizes the most efficient means to effectively diagnose a condition and treat a patient. And in April the American Board of Internal Medicine Foundation unveiled a list of 45 overused tests and procedures that nine specialty societies say doctors and patients should think twice about before they order them and perform them.

So now these organizations are responding to the reality that a large percentage of healthcare being delivered today and some experts say it's as much as 30 percent is either duplicative or unnecessary. Now as the nation strives to reign in healthcare costs physicians can actively contribute to the solution. Another thing we need to do to support a more ethical healthcare system is to embrace a new set of values, four core values. One's better suited to integrated and coordinated care and let me explain that a little bit more.

For years one of the values that we as physicians have cherished most is autonomy and there's good reason for it. As Atolga Wondey put it, "The core structure of medicine, how healthcare is organized and practiced emerge in an era when doctors could hold all the key information patients needed in their heads and manage everything required themselves." And those who trained at about the time I went through know that that's exactly the case. We had to have all the information in our heads. We had those little black books but everything was in our heads when we needed to take care of our patients. But those were the days before insurance company hassles, medical malpractice and multiple government regulations. It was also before physician shortages, aging populations and the kind of complicated chronic conditions we have and before we had more than 6,000 drugs and 4,000 clinical procedures at our disposal. In those days it really did make sense for physicians to value things like autonomy, independence, and self sufficiency. But today those values really don't suffice.

We have come a long, long way since the days of a doctor with a black bag holding the tools of his trade. I still got my old bag that I got from Lilly and here's a doctor looking at an iPad viewing their medical history, coordinating the care with a team of physicians and other professionals. So whether it's in medical homes, accountable care organizations or a system like you have here at the University of Michigan collaborative care models are the wave of the future. That is the way things are going. It doesn't mean everything is going to go in that direction but likely going to head in that way in a more accelerated way.

Now in order for team based models to work there needs to be a shift in some of the fundamental values we have. So for example instead of autonomy we need to value teamwork to recognize that no one person can provide all the answers or all the care that a patient needs. We need to cultivate mutual trust, recognizing that each medical team member has unique skills and knowledge to help the patients that we take care of, that the general practitioner has a different set of skills to offer the Alzheimer's patient than the neurologist or the psychiatrist who's treating that patient's depression or the caregiver who delivers the daily regime of medications to that patient. We have to support this trust with open and timely communication among all healthcare providers so that all members of the care team are on the same page.

We also need to admit that on rare occasions admittedly we do make mistakes. And discipline at times is necessary but a willingness to use guidelines, checklists, standard procedures can help us to avoid those problems so that hopefully we don't end up in medical boards. And finally we have to fully commit to improving the quality of healthcare for our patients in this country. That means keeping an eye on the larger healthcare delivery system and it means collecting, sharing, and analyzing data so that we can leverage that for the care of all the patients in this country.

Now here at the University of Michigan I know that you're already functioning in a large, integrated system. But as I travel across the country and I've traveled across east and west, north and south, on behalf of the AMA you would be amazed how many physicians vehemently resist this notion of collaborative care. And it's not just that they want to maintain a private practice but the idea that I am autonomous, I still have all that information and I'm doing the best I can resonates with some physicians in this country. They think that being part of a team and following guidelines and best practices somehow robs them of their ability to think or create or to do good by their patients. And I think that in general they are wrong and a great example of the kind of creativity and impact of integrated healthcare teams can have and I talked about it a bit this morning at Grand Rounds is the South Central Foundation which is based in Anchorage. It's run by and for Alaskan natives up there. And they have garnered national attention for their success at reducing health disparities through a coordinated approach that they call the NUKA, N-U-K-A, system of care. And here's how the system works.

Patients are assigned to a healthcare team. It might be, for instance, a physician, a nurse, two medical assistants, a behavioral health therapist and an administrative assistant. They're connected to a nutritionist, pharmacist, and various specialists, sometimes even including traditional healers in their facility. And then through emails and texts physicians can keep tabs on their patients, reduce unnecessary visits to both the office and the emergency room. So today South Center serves 60,000 Native Americans with just 1400 professionals. It offers 65 programs to tackle domestic violence, suicide, obesity, substance abuse, diabetes, heart disease and a host of other issues and all delivered in the context of cultural sensitivity and understanding. Basically they built from the ground up and as a matter of fact they call their patients consumer owners. They don't call them patients. They call them consumer owners.

But the proof really is in the numbers. So in the last decade South Central has achieved a decrease of 40 percent in ER visits, 75 percent in hospitalizations, and 30 percent in routine doctor visits. Moreover they have successfully accommodated an annual increase in the number of patients of seven percent while receiving only a two percent annual increase from the Indian Health Service. And they've made significant inroads in addressing major health disparities among their population. So today up in Alaska binge drinking, strokes, heart disease, and cancer rates for Anchorage area natives are now about the same as the national average which is a major victory for this particularly demographic area of our country.

Another example of this and I spoke a bit about this this morning is the Diamond Initiative up in Minnesota. This is in an integrated care setting where it's a Minnesota based program that helps primary care clinics more effectively care for patients with depression. And they used six key components. They used a screening tool, the PHQ9 for the diagnosis and ongoing management of depression. They do systematic tracking of their patients using that PHQ9 and they use a registry to track any changes in those PHQ scores. They use evidence based guidelines and a stepped care approach for treatment modification. They have relapse prevention planning for patients. They have a care manager who educates, coordinates care, troubleshoots for the patients and they have psychiatric consultation and case load review.

Again, the proof is in the numbers. By the beginning of 2012 more than 8,000 adult patients with major depression or dysthymia had participated in the Diamond program. The clinics reported that 30 percent of their patients with depression were in remission within six months of their initial assessment. That's a rate that six times higher than the results reported for primary clinics statewide. The 12 month remission and response rates for Diamond patients were at 53 percent and 70 percent respectively which shows that over the course of time they have been successful in terms of relapse prevention also. And due to the success they've had with depression they're looking at expanding that to other mental illnesses as well and really to provide a foundation for the design of a very good healthcare home for the patients that those clinics take care of.

So I hope you see that from our point of view that integrated care models provide lots of room for innovation. They can achieve dramatic results in a relatively short period of time. And by incentivizing different members of the healthcare team to work together they can improve patient outcomes. They can lower healthcare costs and they can increase patient safety and satisfaction. So from an ethical point of view they make it easier for physicians to actually fulfill not only our obligation to our individual patients but also to society or the community of patients that we're taking care of. So we can say that they create a win/win situation for everyone involved.

Now of course I'm a psychiatrist and I realize the last statement about win/win sounds a little bit optimistic but even, maybe, a little Pollyannaish. So lest you think that I've started playing the glad game here or self medicating, let me temper that statement with the following observation that the transition that I am talking about is very big. It is very big. It's very complicated and it is not going to be easy. As a matter of fact it's going to be very difficult. No matter what's happening with the Affordable Care Act my presumption is that it's going to be implemented, our hope is that it's going to implemented. We have a very long and difficult hill to climb to make that integrated notion of care actually take place across the country for those who want to do it. And that takes me to the last topic that I want to talk with you briefly about and that is the work the AMA is doing to try to tackle a number of these big, big problems. And as our new CEO Jim Adari says--calls this, these are moon shots. These are extraordinarily difficult things that have been difficult for systems, for our country to actually undertake in the past. But we think we're going to work at trying to create an efficient, more-efficient and effective and a more equitable healthcare system.

So we recently developed a five year plan to help America's patients and physicians actually thrive and do well in the 21st century. So our goals are threefold. First, to improve health outcomes, second to improve payment and delivery models and third to improve medical education. First let me tell you a little bit more about the health outcomes.

As I mentioned before at the beginning of this presentation today the United States spends twice and in some cases almost three times as much per capita on healthcare compared to other similar counties, Australia, Canada, Germany, and the UK. Yet when we compare the care that we deliver at--and what we have available to members of our population we're the last or next to last. If you can take a quick look at that slide you'll see we're at the bottom there on most of these measures that we have dealt, obesity, heart disease, mortality, AIDS incidents and so on. You can--if you want a slide we can get it for you. But it's pretty clear that we are down low in all of those measures.

Now it's not that we don't have the capability. I mean you have the capability right here at the University of Michigan to do many of these things and I'm sure on many of these measures you do quite well. We have the foremost training and great physicians and great training but there are a number of variables, as I mentioned before, that contribute to those poor outcomes including the social and environmental determinants and accessibility to healthcare that I talked about. In addition to that medicine is becoming more and more complex, as you know. Today there are more than 13,600 diagnoses. There are 6,000 drugs and 4,000 medical procedures to keep track of. So ensuring that all the patients in this country get all the care they need at the right time and at an appropriate cost is a big and Herculean task to undertake. So as physicians we have to work to deliver the best care to our patients on an individual basis each and every day. And now at the AMA we are harnessing our resources to help our medical profession do the same collectively across the nation.

So we have already begun analyzing outcomes data and speaking to leaders in the field to identify clinical conditions that impact a large segment of the U.S. population. Next we will develop a national dashboard on specific health topics. We'll work with partner organizations to reduce both the disease and the cost burdens associated with them. We'll establish national goals for improvement and facilitate the adoption of strategies that achieve the triple aim of better care, better health, and lower costs. And we'll track our progress and tweak our strategies as necessary to ensure we're having the biggest impact.

Now in a couple weeks I think we'll know a couple of disease entities we'll be taking a look at, maybe diabetes and maybe depression and maybe congestive heart failure. But I can tell you that they're going to be the big disease entities that will have a dramatic impact hopefully on the population at large.

Next, improving payment and delivery systems and I talked about a little bit about that before. For decades both health plans and the government have attempted to reign in excessive costs, reduce fragmentation, and improve quality but to date it really hasn't worked except in pockets around the country. So in both the public and the private sectors there is a consensus that the current system no longer meets the needs of physicians and patients in this country. Of course as physicians we know that identifying what's broken is generally far easier than fixing it. So for example this morning I talked about the broken Medicare payment physician--payment formula, the SGR which I'm sure some of you are familiar with. We're trying to get it repealed but we're also trying to find a way to replace it with something that will work better because no one has presented a formula that's going to work better than it yet. So when it comes to fixing something as complex as healthcare delivery one size definitely doesn't fit all because what works for organizations and physicians in Detroit is probably not going to work for physicians and organizations here in Ann Arbor.

So over the coming years at the AMA we will analyze current and emerging payment and delivery models from the physician perspective. We've already been partnering with a variety of physician organizations across this country. We have 25 physician organizations from small practices to middle size practices to large integrated systems like you have here at the University of Michigan. We will work with them to identify which models best provide both high quality patient care and physician satisfaction because what we hear from a lot of physicians and I talked about this a little this morning is physicians in a lot of areas of this country feel burned out. They don't like what they're doing. They get depressed. They're suicidal. There's a lot of stress in the system based on what's going on now.

So what we want to do is present models to physicians that--so that they can pick the kind of practices that will be best for them. And for example what's the best way for a small practice to incorporate health IT? How can a large hospital based practice use nurses effectively? Which models offer the most autonomy if that's what a physician wants to have and what about the relationships with payers? How can we deal with payers in a different way? So these are just some of the questions we're going to ask. I'm not going to get into the weeds on this because we've just started this process but -what we hope to do is leverage the findings that we have. We already have a physician innovator group. We have groups that are already working in new models of delivery and then we'll get tools and resources out to physicians across the country so that physicians can choose the kind of system or practice that they want to be in likewise can be better educated about what kind of physicians can work best in their particular setting.

And finally our third strategic goal is to improve medical education. I think as many of you know it was the work of the AMA's Council on Medical education in the early 1900's that led to the Flexner report and the implementation of standards for physician training in the U.S. But it's been over a century since medical training was evaluated and updated in any comprehensive way. In 2005 the AMA launched the initiative to transform medical education to examine the gap in current physician training and the future needs of our healthcare system. And what we found was a clear need for reform in medical education, more flexibility and individualized learning, training and teamwork and professionalism. So medical students and residents were already trained to go into those systems that I talked about and to have measures to promote continuous improvement and increase patient safety.

Over the next five years the AMA will convene a national team of healthcare leaders to help us develop innovative models and new education models. We are going to work with selected medical schools across the country to begin implementing these ideas and an RFB's going to be going on--out shortly if it hasn't gone out already.

Now while we are just beginning this process, again this is a very early stage of this, let me just tell you about some of the goals of this process. We are hoping to help students better understand how healthcare is financed and delivered. We want to promote flexible and competence driven medical education rather than calendar driven training. We want to promote skill development that emphasizes performance improvement, patient safety, and team based care. We want to enhance the development of professionalism throughout our medical environment. And in short we're going to be doing everything within our capabilities to make sure the 21st century medical education meets 21st century healthcare system needs. So if we can actually do these things and again, these are big, audacious goals, we think that we can influence healthcare--the healthcare in this country in very significant ways. We think it can actually shape a brighter future, both for physicians and for the country as a whole. So just imagine the possibilities if all of this works out wonderfully.

We're going to have improved health outcomes and have those achieved at a lower cost. We're going to have healthier patients who are more engaged in their own well being. We're going to have physicians working in a more coordinated, efficient environment that they themselves have helped create. We call the leader of this strategic team our physician satisfaction doctor and we're going to have a new generation of doctors trained to transition seamlessly into this world of 21st century medicine. So again, big, big goals. You're going to be hearing more about these as the strategic plan gets implemented. I hope we can reach maybe 80 percent, 90 percent. If we can reach 100 percent, that's good. But it took us a long time to get to the moon and it's going to take us awhile to get to these big goals also.

So given everything I have described it's clear that we do have significant ethical challenges facing us as physicians. These are perhaps greater than we ever had before when we focused mainly on the individual patient that was in our exam room when we're looking at the needs of our whole society. And so every time a patient walks into a room there are a number of obligations that we have to be thinking about now. We have to have an obligation to that individual patient that's in front of us. We have an obligation to the collective patient, to the larger healthcare system and we have an obligation to do as much as we can to fight the challenges of the day from cost to chronic conditions to sub-optimal health outcomes. And none of us need to face these obligations alone and when there's a troubling issue that comes up we can consult our colleagues and refer to ethical guidelines.

I'm sure you have an ethical committee and group here but I do want to refer you to three AMA resources if you're not familiar with them. Certainly the AMA medical code of medical ethics which comprises our principles in medical ethics and the opinions of our counsel on ethical and judicial affairs, our virtual mentor which is a monthly online ethics journal with articles, case studies, analysis of relevant health law. It focuses on a single theme like confidentiality or shared decision making. The virtual mentor is especially good for medical students and residents. It really provides a case vignette, a real time case which has ethical experts talk about it. And then we have the ethical force program which explores ethics for healthcare organizations rather than for individual physicians.

Fixing Health Care the Ethical Way, 2012

So finally in the midst of the details of the last 45 minutes or so I hope I've gotten a few core messages across. One, this is a time of really historic change. And it's been, for me as AMA president, it's really been a privilege to be riding this crest. It's a difficult time in many ways. We'll have a better idea, again, about what's going to happen next week after the election but clearly whatever happens in the election, things are changing very dramatically and how healthcare is delivered in this country.

Second, while there are significant challenges that I talked about, significant challenges on the ethics side, on the resource side and how we think about how we're going to treat patients and work in the healthcare system there also are terrific opportunities available to us that we didn't have before. I just touched the surface about accountable care organizations. The fact that CMS has put up 170 million dollars to get these accountable care organizations going or the fact that we have the Center for Medicare and Medicaid Innovation which has ten billion dollars available in grants for pilot programs across the country. Three thousand programs have already applied for those. We've never had that kind of funding for innovation in healthcare before. Maybe some on the private side but have never gotten that kind of financing. We've got the comparative research effectiveness arm of the Affordable Care Act which actually will help us to compare the kind of treatments that we render and make sure that we render the kind of treatments that are cost effective. And three, right now today we really do have an unprecedented opportunity to shape healthcare in this country as physicians.

So right now we are at a crossroads. I think we are defining who's getting healthcare, how they get it and how we pay for it. So if you haven't done so already I hope you'll consider to--if you're not a member of the AMA that you will join us. We need your help. We need your voice. We need your input because I think together we can create that ethical healthcare system that I talked about, a system that's effective, a system that's efficient, and a system that is ethical. So thank you and I look forward to your questions.

Myths and Misconceptions in Biomedical Ethics, 2013
Robert M. Sade, M. D., Professor of Surgery, University of South Carolina

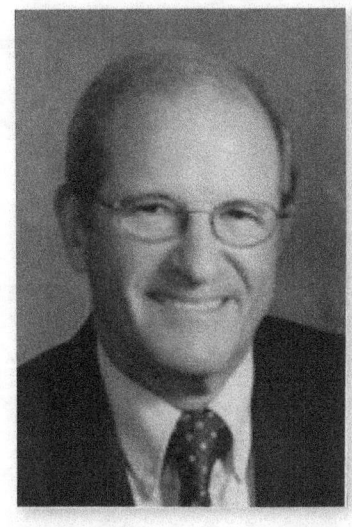

Thank you very much for the kind introduction, Dr. Margolis. I'm truly honored and grateful for having been invited to be the Waggoner Lecturer for 2013.

Previous speakers in this series are an illustrious group, and I hope to live up to the high standards they've set.

Some of you know that I'm a native of Boston, which I called home for 37 years. Although I've been living in Charleston for 38 years, I've remained a loyal fan of Boston sports. The last decade has been incredible for Boston. The Celtics won their 17th NBA Championship, in 2006, their first in 22 years, thanks to the "Big Three." The Red Sox finally broke the "Curse of the Bambino" by winning their first World Series in 86 years in 2004, and have added two more since. And the Patriots won the Super Bowl for the first time ever in February, 2002, with a thanks to the University of Michigan for sending to us their quarterback, who led the Wolverines to victory in the Orange Bowl, over always tough Alabama, in 1999. We got him at the end of the 6th round, the 199th pick in the NFL draft and he became the fourth string quarterback with the Patriots. In his second season, Tom Brady replaced the injured Drew Bledsoe and led the Patriots to the championship in Super Bowl 36, and two more NFL championships after that. So, from this Bostonian, a great big Thank You to the University of Michigan.

So, to get to the topic at hand: The history of medicine is filled with misconceptions and myths that in retrospect have been surprisingly persistent both in science and in ethics. The history of medicine has been described as a "grand narrative of progress,"[1] but that may be the biggest myth of all. There was virtually no progress in our understanding of human physiology from the time of Galen in the second century AD for nearly 1500 years, when modern medical science began with the experimental investigations of William Harvey on the circulation of blood, published in 1628.

Scientific progress after that point was nearly continuous, as depicted in this partial list of scientific achievements in the 18th and 19th centuries, but that wasn't true of clinical medicine. The practice of medicine continued to be mired in the ancient myths and misconceptions of Hippocrates and Galen for more than 200 years after Harvey's seminal work. Textbooks of medicine were essentially restatements of Hippocratic and Galenic therapies until the late 19th century. For example, the Hippocratic therapies of bloodletting and cauterization persisted for 2,000 years. Bloodletting was still in common use well into the 19th century.

Although modern scientific investigational methods were introduced in the 17th century and still flourish, modern clinical practice arguably didn't begin until after Louis Pasteur's publication of his studies of germs in 1861 and Joseph Lister's incorporation of these ideas into the clinical practice of antisepsis in 1865.

Lister documented decreased infection rates when carbolic acid antisepsis was used during surgery, shown here as carbolic acid (what we now call phenol) is being sprayed on the surgical field. The persistence of misconceptions in medical practice is illustrated by the fact that Lister's antisepsis was not generally accepted and his methods were not widely adopted for decades, because the idea of bacteria and antisepsis was

Myths and Misconceptions in Biomedical Ethics...

mistakenly believed to be wrong-headed in the medical and surgical communities. Lister's experiences were well known in the United States because his ideas were refined and popularized by William Halsted of Johns Hopkins, shown here with another giant of 20th century surgery, Harvey Cushing. Nevertheless, it took over 40 years for antisepsis in surgery and the consequent reductions in infection rates to become widespread in this country. I'm sure you can think of other examples of slow adoption of successful new medications, technologies, andmethods in your own field.

Myths and misconceptions have been as widespread in bioethics as they've been in science. Maybe the most persistent misconception originated with Hippocrates, who said this some 2500 years ago: "Perform these duties calmly and adroitly, concealing most things from the patient while you are attending to him… revealing nothing of the patient's future or present condition." Underlying this instruction was the mistaken belief that patients are harmed by knowing the truth about a bad prognosis, that is, by hearing bad news. It wasn't until the late 20th century that this paternalistic culture changed.

For example, a survey of physicians that was done in 1961 asked this: "The following questions apply to your policy about telling patients they have cancer. For the purpose of this questionnaire, assume that the diagnosis is certain and that though treatment may be possible the eventual prognosis is grave." "What is your usual policy about telling patients?" 88% of the responses were not to tell the patient. The same question was asked in a survey of physicians in 1979. This time the answer was to tell the patient in 98% of the responses. Clearly a major cultural shift had happened. It was based on the realization that most patients actually benefit and prefer to know the truth about their condition and their prognosis.

Lots of other myths and misconceptions are common in medical ethics. Although we're doing a lot better about being honest with patients, many physicians still have trouble dealing with the emotional stress of delivering bad news, so we tend to avoid doing it, on the pretext of protecting our patients.

A large majority of physicians believe, "Gifts from industry influence the prescribing practices of many of my colleagues, but they don't influence mine."

"Industry controlled continuing medical education biases the practice of many of my colleagues, but I personally am untouched."

"I deceive insurance companies only to benefit my patients — I don't do it to serve my own interests."

There's a widespread belief that informed consent exists on a form signed by a patient, that this form is ethically necessary. Many residents believe this, especially surgical residents who get patients to sign operative permits every day. As clinicians, we believe that the informed consent form is ethically necessary and often don't realize that it's only a piece of evidence to be used in a courtroom if it becomes necessary; informed consent is a process, not a form.

When we declare a potential organ donor dead by either brain criteria or circulatory criteria, we believe that the patient is actually dead, and legally, they are. But the death of these patients is arguably a legal fiction that's designed to allow donation of viable vital organs by satisfying the Dead Donor Rule. The debate over abandoning the Dead Donor Rule has heated up in recent years; the most recent salvos were fired in the New England Journal of Medicine just a month ago, in the October 3 issue.

In a move that demonstrably decreases the availability of organs for transplantation, we accept the misconception that altruism is and should be the only acceptable motivation for organ donation. This misconception has cost the lives of thousands of patients with end organ failure: over 10,000 patients in 2012 alone.

Finally, there's a misconception that health professionals are guided by a single set of ethical principles that apply throughout the field. This mistake can have serious consequences for both the care of patients and the operation of hospitals.

I have only a limited time to talk about myths and misconceptions in biomedical ethics, and we could go on all day with this list. But I'll spend the rest of the hour talking about only two of them: the myth that altruism is the sole acceptable motivation for organ donation and the misconception that certain ethical principles are of equal importance for all health professionals.

I'll start with the myth that altruism is the sole acceptable motivation for organ donation. I'm going to argue that this policy was built on soft ground from the beginning and that prohibiting the use of economic incentives for organ donation is an incoherent, unjust, and lethal policy.

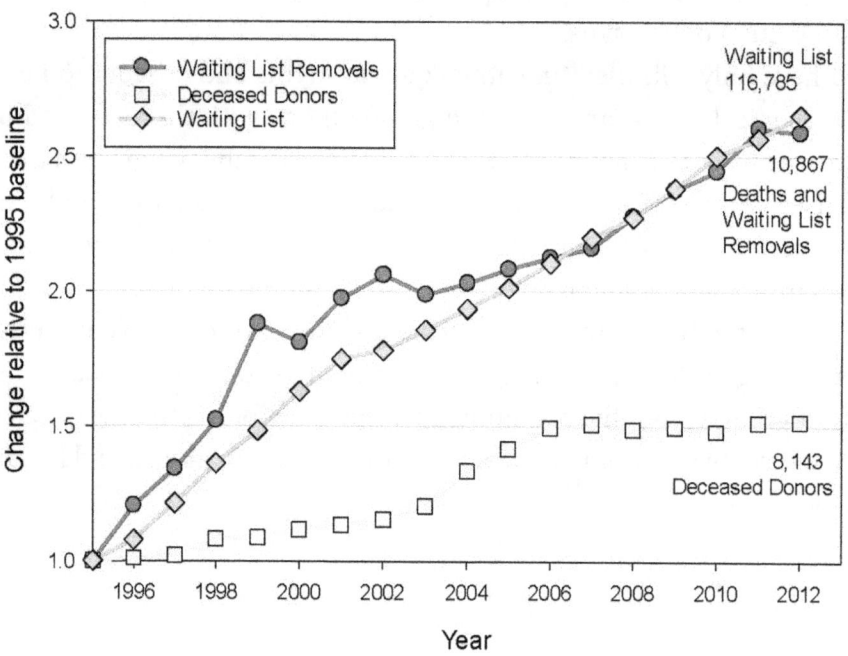

Relative change in transplant data

This graph depicts the fundamental problem with organ donation and transplantation. Taking 1995 as the base, the rate of growth of the waiting list for organs has grown at a linear rate that's 3--1/2 times faster than the rate of increase of deceased donors. While the waiting list and deaths continue to grow, the number of donors has essentially stabilized over the last seven years. This accounts for what's come to be known as the organ gap. Economists from the University of Florida and Auburn University have calculated that it would take on the order of $1000 of financial incentive per donor to reduce the waiting list to essentially zero over a period of a few years.

Why don't we simply do that? There are reasons, and, in my view, they're not good ones. In fact, I believe the origin and continuing existence of our dysfunctional organ procurement system is founded in both myth and misconception, as I'll explain now.

Motivation is important in determining what people do. The National Organ Transplantation Act of 1984 made it a federal felony to provide or accept any "valuable consideration" for an organ. Thus, over the last 30 years, the only motivation that's legally acceptable is altruism, that is, providing organs for no reward other than the satisfaction of doing something good. But is the reasoning underlying this view justified? In my view, this position is based on misconceptions, namely, that payment is intrinsically wrong because it violates justice, and that payment for donated organs would exploit the poor.

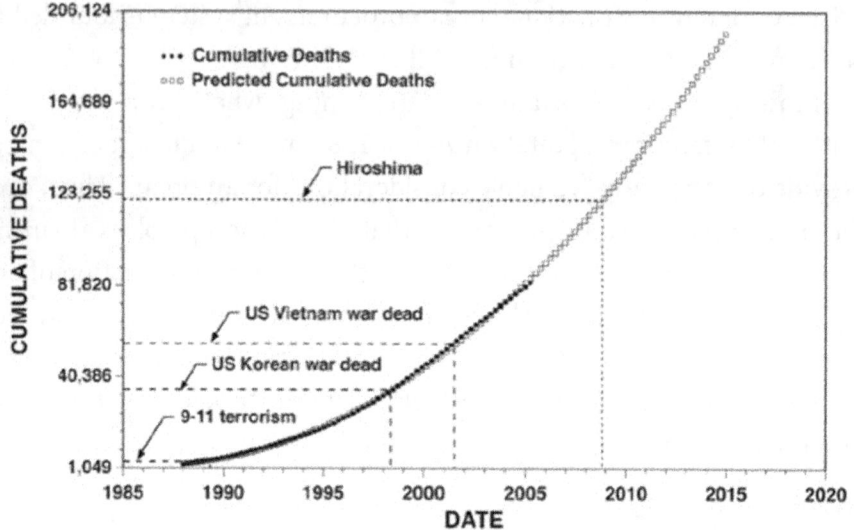

FIGURE 5

Cumulative Deaths
1988 to 2015

Beard TR, Jackson JD, Kaserman DL. Gathering Storm: The Failure of US Organ Procurement Policy. Auburn University. 2007.

These misconceptions have led to what amounts to a massive loss of life over the last few decades. The number of deaths on organ transplant waiting lists exceeds the number of Americans killed in action in the Korean War and the Vietnam War. We passed the 123,000 dead from the Hiroshima atomic bomb in 2009. The death rate has shown no signs of slowing down over the last few decades, as you've already seen.

When people are restricted to only one acceptable motivation to donate organs, they find many reasons not to donate.

- Many think that bodies should be buried intact, based on their religion or personal beliefs.

- We all avoid thinking about or confronting the loss of loved ones and certainly our own mortality.
- In some communities there's a distrust of the medical community that seems entirely justified on historical grounds, such as the horrific 40--year Tuskegee study, which understandably still influences the attitudes of many in the African--American community.
- Some believe that allocation is inequitable and some mistakenly believe that transplantation is ineffective.
- There's widespread misunderstanding of what brain death means — "The doctors say Uncle John is dead, but he looks exactly the same as he did yesterday when he was still alive; is he really dead?"
- And there are serious stresses at the time of the sudden unexpected death that's always true in the case of organ donors whose brains were severely damaged by a catastrophic medical event such as stroke or a ruptured aneurysm, or severe head trauma.

What about reasons to motivate donation? When there's only one acceptable motivation to donate —service to others — We're not all angels, so it's not surprising that half of the potentially available organs are buried or cremated.

By way of history, the first successful human transplant took place at the Peter Bent Brigham Hospital in Boston in December 1954, when a kidney was transplanted from an identical twin into his brother. Joe Murray, the surgeon and researcher, won the Nobel Prize for Physiology or Medicine in 1990.

Because of problems with immune rejection, the field of transplantation developed slowly after that. In 1968, the first version of the Uniform Anatomical Gift Act, which intended to help increase organ donation, had no ban on selling or buying organs, although the matter was discussed and no consensus was reached. Cyclosporine was tested in 1979, and came into clinical use in 1982. It was the first truly successful immunosuppressive agent.

Transplant developed rapidly after that and became a growth industry. A Virginia physician, Dr. Barry Jacobs, proposed that financial incentives be provided to deceased donors, and saw the need for someone to serve as an intermediary between people who wanted to donate and those who needed an organ, so he set up a brokerage firm for organs. At the same time, a committee of the US House of Representatives was drawing up a bill that came to be known as the National Organ Transplantation Act. The committee members were so outraged at the idea of buying and selling organs that they added a draconian clause to the bill that forbade any "valuable consideration" for donating an organ. This clause disallows all incentives for donation other than a good--hearted public spirit, excluding such incentives as paying for funeral expenses, tax credits to the estates of donors, and other potential incentives, in the belief that the harms of incentives substantially outweighed the benefits.

Let me illustrate how counterproductive the prohibition is, with a story about a problem we had when I was Medical Director of LifePoint, our state's Organ Procurement Organization. We had a potential organ donor who was brain dead after a fall from a ladder, and was an undocumented alien from Mexico. When we were finally able to reach his family in Mexico City, they were willing to consent to organ donation, but only on the condition that we pay for transporting his body back to Mexico — his body minus a heart, 2 lungs, 2 kidneys, and a liver — at a cost of about $3000. We couldn't do it, because paying for repatriating a body is a "valuable consideration" and would therefore be a federal felony. Six people died on waiting lists because the man's organs were buried rather than transplanted. When the same thing happened a year later with a potential donor (from Michigan, as it happens), I was able to persuade the OPO administrators that we ought to just do it. This, of course, was a clear violation of NOTA, but neither I nor the OPO was worried about prosecution. No prosecutor was likely to pursue the case, and for sure, no jury would convict on the basis of paying $3,000 to save multiple lives. I haven't counted how many patients we ultimately saved while committing federal felonies.

The balance of harms and benefits of organ donation have changed a lot in the last 30 years. For example, in a well--known and often cited book in 1972, The Gift Relationship, Richard Titmuss argued that paying for blood donation was not a good idea because it provided an incentive to lie about infection with hepatitis B virus, which would lead to an increased infection rate in the blood pool. He also said that payment was going to lead to a decrease in donation. There was only anecdotal support for these assertions, but Titmuss's work has been repeatedly cited as an important reason not to allow payment for organ donation.

A review of the recent literature from 2001 through 2012 was published in Science this past May, and provided strong evidence from several controlled studies that economic motivation increases blood donation, with no increase or change of any kind in the infection rate. There was zero evidence of a decrease in motivation to voluntarily donate blood. Because of NOTA, it's not possible to do any direct studies of financial incentives for organ donation without a waiver by an act of Congress, but these recent studies suggest that some of the most frequently cited arguments against allowing financial incentives have been purely mythological.

A case can easily be made that tax credits or paying for funeral expenses should be allowed as incentives for deceased donors. But I'm going to make the much tougher case: paying cash to motivate living donors to provide kidneys, by regulating the price of the incentive at some nonzero level that's sufficient to meet the need for organs. I hasten to point out that when financial incentives are available to donors, it's still perfectly possible to have altruistic donation, for example, to family and friends, and also to strangers. Designated donation, that is, naming a person to whom your kidney should be given, would also not change.

Since I'll be talking about living donors, I'm going to focus on kidney donation.

I'll make the case for paying people to donate a kidney starting with a few claims. First, is the Donation Is Good claim, which I'll designate as DG — meaning that donating a kidney is both legal and is praiseworthy. The second claim is that Payment for Tissue is OK, which I designate as PT--OK, since we don't have a problem with payment for sperm, eggs, or hair. We also don't have much of a problem with paying for blood donations, which isn't particularly praised, but also isn't awful. While there's a huge difference in pain and recovery time, there appears to be no morally relevant difference between donating blood and donating a kidney.

So, my prima facie case is this: if my two claims —Donation Is Good and Payment for Tissue

Is OK — are true, then paying people to donate a kidney is not problematic.

I want to explain why the ban on financial incentives for kidneys, which I'll call kidney sales, is inconsistent. If we oppose selling kidneys because it's too dangerous, then we ought to oppose kidney donation as well.

But we don't oppose kidney donation because we know that the risk of donating a kidney is very low. So it's inconsistent to oppose paying for a kidney because it's dangerous and at the same time support the idea that donation is a good thing.

If we oppose paying for kidneys because we shouldn't sell body parts, then we ought to oppose commercial blood banks. But we don't oppose commercial blood banks because by producing blood components, they save lives. Therefore, it's inconsistent to both oppose kidney sales and support paying for tissue donation. To be consistent, we have to support paying for kidneys.

There are two main objections to this prima facie case. They are that paying for kidneys is intrinsically wrong because it's unjust, and that paying for kidneys would exploit the poor. Let's consider first the assertion that paying for kidneys is unjust.

Respect for autonomy is a principle that's highly regarded in both law and in ethics. There are two ways of thinking about autonomy — the first is that autonomy consists in making decisions rationally, what we might call the "thick" version. Here, autonomous acts are those in which the choices that are made are consistent with self--respect and one's own humanity. The thin version of autonomy holds that autonomous acts are those in which choices are made without interference by others, no matter the rationale underlying the choice.

Now, the law protects autonomy in the thin sense because law is not used to enforce self-- respect or humanity. For example, in the process of informed consent, the goal is to prevent imposition of a thick morality — patients can make any choice they want. So protection of autonomy that comes from the thin version supports the selling of kidneys.

Also, even if the law were to protect autonomy in the thick sense, that is, respect for one's dignity and humanity, our humanity is not vested in every one of our essential body parts. Rather, our humanity comes from our mind, located in our brain, not from our kidneys. Removing a kidney doesn't affect our overall well--being, and it doesn't affect our essential humanity.

To many people, the prohibition on paying for kidneys is justified because motivation by money indicates greed, and our emotional response to greed is revulsion. But observe that the seller's motivation could be noble, because she could be motivated both by saving a life and paying,, for example, for her child's education. Also, the unpaid donor's motivation could be anything but noble; for example he could be motivated by an irrationally low self-- worth or by a desire to generate indebtedness in order to manipulate someone else. The impulse to do good is not binary — it's not either there or not there. Motivation is highly variable. And law, such as NOTA, is too blunt an instrument to separate noble from base motivation.

The arguments that intend to show that paying for kidneys exploits the poor often use the fact that there's an international black market in kidneys, in which wealthy people from industrialized countries pay for organs that are of uncertain quality, and the donors from the Third World are poor people who desperately need the money — but after they donate a kidney, they go back to a miserable life in which there's little or no follow-up care. These practices are and should be condemned.

But where do black markets come from? They appear when free markets are suppressed, and a regulated market for organs would do precisely the opposite — it would prevent a black market. In this country, transplantation is safe and medical care is sophisticated. There's careful screening and selection of donors and follow-up care is standard for all donors regardless of economic status. What I'm suggesting is a regulated market: the amount of the payment for a kidney is predetermined. There's no bazaar with people standing on street corners selling kidneys to the highest bidder. Rather, allocation of organs remains as it is today, through the United Network for Organ Sharing. Only the donation side would be affected.

The exploitation argument also suggests that although the financial benefits would be equal for the well-off and the poor, the burdens are unequal, because the poor are desperate, which makes paying for kidneys unreasonable and irrational. The seller is coerced into selling a kidney, so the argument goes, and the market exploits that vulnerability. But if it's true that donation is a good thing, then paying for kidneys may be reasonable and rational because the poor seller may gain exactly the same satisfactions as the unpaid volunteer donor, but in addition get a financial reward for doing so.

It's also argued that financial incentives for kidney donation is a slippery slope because commodification of body parts will lead to degeneration of the social fabric. It's been argued that paying for a kidney will lead to the breakdown of generosity and friendship and love, but consider that most donations are between family members, while most sales are likely to go to strangers. Furthermore, people who receive money for a kidney are unlikely to love their family or friends less or to be loved less because of accepting money.

If the arguments for prohibiting the sale of kidneys are so weak, why is there such widespread support for them? I believe it's because selling a body part produces an emotional response — repugnance — which generally resists rational argument. Yet if we consider repulsive ideas and technologies of former times, we see that they often have led to valuable outcomes, such as transplantation itself and in vitro fertilization that were vilified at one time, as was the threat of recombinant DNA research to human health, which led to the formation of the Recombinant DNA Advisory Committee, the RAC, of the 1970s, charged with reviewing and approving all recombinant DNA experiments. Yet the revulsion that was felt toward recombinant DNA research resulted in therapies of major importance, such as the creation in the laboratory of human insulin, streptokinase, human growth hormone, erythropoietin, hepatitis B vaccine, human interleukin, alpha and gamma interferon, Factor VIII, and 500 other therapies that are used widely in treating serious diseases.

In considering the issue of prohibition of any valuable consideration for organs for transplantation, we shouldn't ignore the whole story. The donor is only half of it. The other half is the 10,000 people on the waiting list who died last year because not enough organs were available to replace their failing vital organs. In my view, those who support the ban on payment for organs have to bear some degree of moral responsibility for those thousands of deaths that could be prevented by motivating millions of people who have two kidneys but need only one, to give up one of them in exchange for around $1000 to $5000.

I've already talked about some issues of justice. There are lots of different views of what justice is, but one widely held view, certainly in this country, is that justice means equal treatment under the law. With regard to organ transplantation, it's interesting to note that everyone in the system, from beginning to end, is paid for what they do, including organ procurement organizations, surgeons, hospital employees, and drug and device companies. With one exception. The one participant who's critical to the transplant process is the source of the organ, the organ donor, and it just doesn't make sense that everyone in the system is paid except for this key participant. Justice demands that organ donors should be paid for their critical contributions.

All efforts to increase organ availability in our purely altruistic system have failed. The current system is based on myths and misconceptions — the 40-year-old myth that paying for blood donation decreases voluntary donations and contaminates the blood supply. It's based on the misconceptions that payment for organs is intrinsically wrong because it's unjust and it exploits the poor, none of which holds water. A system that provides financial incentives would not only substantially increase the supply of organs, saving thousands of lives every year, but it's ethically preferable to the donation system we currently have and, even more importantly, it would eradicate all of the rationing problems that comprise 90% of the ethical dilemmas of transplantation by wiping out the waiting list, which now stands at 120,000 patients at risk of early death.

Both law and bioethics in this country place a high priority on human well-being and autonomy. If we intend to be truly serious about these values, then a regulated market for organs is not just acceptable, it's a moral imperative.

The following words were written over two decades ago and are stunningly prophetic about the outcomes in our current system: "We have never encountered a single policy more at odds with public welfare than the current altruism only organ procurement policy in the United States… If the current policy is maintained the shortage will continue to grow worse as will the needless suffering." This is from the Yale Journal of regulation 1991. As long as we continue the current policies, the slope of these lines won't change, the death rate will grow.

Ethics for the Emerging Health Care System

I'm going to change gears now and talk about something a little more abstract. A few months ago, I was asked to address my medical school's faculty on the topic, "Ethics for the Emerging Health Care System." In that talk, I identified two misconceptions: that all health professionals are guided by a single set of ethical principles, and that the shape of the health care system will be determined by the Affordable Care Act. I'll place the ethics of health care in the context of the huge changes that the ACA has brought about and is going to continue to bring about in the next few months and years. We don't know what the emerging health care system is going to look like down the road because of the current political climate and because, like Yogi Berra, I think, "It's difficult to make predictions, especially about the future." Anyone who predicts the form of the emerging health care system is likely to follow in the footsteps of Charles Duell, US Commissioner of Patents, who said, in 1899, "Everything that can be invented has been invented."

And don't forget Harry Warner, one of the Warner Brothers, who famously said, in 1927, the era of silent movies, "Who the hell wants to hear actors talk?" Or, Dr. Stephen Paget who wrote about my own field, in his book, The Surgery of the Chest, in 1896, in the opening sentences of Chapter 10, Wounds of the Heart: "Surgery of the heart has probably reached the limits set by Nature to all surgery. No method, no new discovery, can overcome the natural difficulties that attend a wound of the heart." ... So much for open heart surgery.

Or, Dr. Lee DeForest, the electronics pioneer, so--called "Father of Radio," who said, in 1967, "Man will never reach the moon — regardless of all future scientific advances." Two years later, Neil Armstrong was walking on the moon. So ... no predictions from me about the future form of our health care system.

Now, I said that it's wrong to think that there's a single ethic for all who work in the health care field and that the shape of the health care system will be determined by the Affordable Care Act. Here's what I meant by that.

It's not news that the health care enterprise is very complex and has a lot of different players, including clinical professionals, teachers, scientists, and administrators. Each of those groups has different purposes and goals, and each works toward achieving those goals guided by ethical principles. Of course, in pursuing our goals, we have to stay within the law, and, in health care, federal law is going to determine the health care system's broad outlines.

But it's important to realize that the law isn't the only determinant of the shape of the emerging health care system. Regardless of the successes and failures, of the ACA, we workers in the trenches of health care will still be responsible for caring for patients, maintaining facilities that we use to provide that care, teaching and training future generations of health professionals, and innovating and discovering toward enhancing our ability to prevent and cure disease. Each of us will also help to shape the coming health care system, guided not only by the law, but even more by our respective ethics.

I say "respective ethics" because I believe that there's not a single health care ethics to guide decision making. Rather, I believe that there're different ethical guides for at least four distinct groups — clinical professionals, teachers, research scientists, and hospital administrators. It's not unusual for one person to serve in more than one of those roles, or even all four, all at the same time. Back in my callow youth 25 years ago, I was at the same time a practicing pediatric cardiac surgeon, a teacher of medical students and surgical residents, a research scientist, and Medical Director of the University Hospital. According to the AMA's Code of Medical Ethics, I had the same ethical obligations in all those positions. Here's what it says:

"Assuming a title or position the removes the physician from direct patient--physician relationships does not override professional ethical obligations... Adherence to professional medical standards includes ...

Myths and Misconceptions in Biomedical Ethics...

placing the interests of patients above other considerations, such as ... employer business interests." I think this is a misconception. I'll explain why.

But first, I want to be very clear. The ethical principles for clinicians, teachers, researchers, and administrators are the same —we're all human beings, and each of has a human nature that requires certain kinds of responses to daily challenges. But, although the principles are the same, their order of importance is critically different, because the problems that each group faces are different. Let me back up and explain.

Every day, each of us has to make thousands of choices, from deciding whether it's healthier to use butter versus margarine on our toast for breakfast to whether to recommend medical treatment versus open heart surgery to a patient with coronary artery disease, or whether life support has become futile and it's time to discontinue the ventilator. To navigate those choices successfully, we need certain principles as guides. A partial list of the principles that're important for all of us includes respect for the right of every patient to decide what happens to their own bodies, honesty in all professional interactions, integrity, that is, consistency between what we believe and what we do, work-- related competence, compassion for suffering patients, and an attitude of benevolence toward others. But, the precise order of importance for the various principles, and these are only a few of them, is different for the different groups. That's because their goals and the problems they face are different. I'll describe what I mean for each of the four groups.

Hospital administrators are basically business people, so their ethical principles are essentially business ethics. To understand the relative importance of principles for administrators, we have to know, what's the goal of the business of maintaining hospitals. The central goal of hospital administrators is to preserve the hospital's long--term existence and flourishing. Given that, what does it take to preserve long--term existence? Well, for patients to be willing to come for treatment to my hospital or to yours, they have to trust that the hospital will treat them honestly, fairly, and respectfully, exhibiting what some have called "common decency". Administrators have the responsibility to make sure that their staff relates to patients in those ways.

Hospital administrators have to deal with problems related to the financial balance sheet. They have to keep revenues and expenses in relative balance in order to ensure long--term survival of the institution. Also, they have to create and enforce policies so that the hospital can accomplish its mission.

These administrative responsibilities aren't easy. For example, Emory University and its hospitals lost a huge amount of trust when a scandal erupted 4 years ago. Dr. Charles Nemeroff, chair of the Department of Psychiatry, was revealed to have accepted over $2½ million from drug companies ... while publishing papers and speaking on behalf of the companies' products. Clearly, Nemeroff handled his conflict of interest poorly. But, the university administration made it much worse by stonewalling the investigation. Administrators had an unambiguous responsibility to oversee conflicts of interest like this, they knew about Nemeroff's conflicts of interest for several years, yet they abdicated that responsibility. A number of similar scandals at the university level have taken place in recent years, for example, at Harvard, the University of Pennsylvania, the University of Wisconsin, and UAB.

The hospital's primary goal is its continuing existence and flourishing in the long term, so the administrator's role requires that their foremost ethical principles have to be to ensure honesty, fairness, and common decency.

The activities of science have an entirely different goal: the discovery or creation of new knowledge. Like all human beings, scientists should be benevolent toward others and have compassion for the human condition. But the ethical principles that're most important for successful achievement of the goals of science are not beneficence and compassion — they are integrity and honesty. Without absolute honesty and integrity in designing, conducting, and reporting results of their studies, the foundations of science can be undermined and even destroyed.

Right now, those foundations are at risk because of pockets of ethical wrongdoing in the biomedical sciences. A recent study of several thousand early-- and mid--career scientists asked whether they personally had engaged in any of 10 seriously unethical practices, including, for example, falsifying or fabricating research data. Fully 33% of the respondents admitted they had engaged in at least one of those 10 egregious behaviors in the previous three years.

Research misconduct of this magnitude seriously endangers the foundations of science, and, worse than that, they pose risks to patients whose doctors and other clinicians will be making patient care decisions that are based on false information.

These disturbing studies clearly show the critical importance for scientists to base their day--to--day behavior on the ethical principles of integrity and honesty, regardless of external pressures.

Teachers and trainers of future physicians, nurses, technicians, and other health professionals have their own special goal: to transmit to their students and trainees the knowledge and skills needed for successful professional practice — fully, accurately, and without bias. To do that, two ethical principles rise to the top: to accomplish their primary goal, teachers need to have competence in the knowledge and skills being transmitted to students and integrity in dealing with the asymmetry of power that exists in every teacher-- student relationship.

Imbalance of power is responsible for the occasional abuses of research trainees that I've seen in my role of ethics consultant, like when investigators take credit for the work of their graduate students and postdocs. Worse still are the scandalous results of sexual harassment that this year destroyed the career of Professor Colin McGinn at the University of Miami and last year resulted in a long prison term for Jerry Sandusky and catastrophic damage to Penn State University. But worse than both of those is a widespread stain on the culture of medical education.

In medical schools, professorial competence isn't usually a problem, but abuse of power is. My field of surgery probably has a reputation for more mistreatment of students and residents than other fields — I'm not sure that's true. A medical school dean of education put it this way: "It is with difficulty that I articulate the often dominant teaching culture of our profession, which is adversarial and based on intimidation, public humiliation, harassment, belittlement, and fear, especially in the clinical years. This is an international phenomenon, and one that includes not only physicians, but other professions in medicine as well."

Data supports this bleak view. The Medical School Graduation Questionnaire, administered to all students graduating from AAMC accredited medical schools, was answered by over 12,000 graduates in 2012. The questionnaire has a section devoted to medical student mistreatment, which lists abuses ranging from serious, such as public humiliation, to very serious, such as requests for exchange of sexual favors for grades. The percent of students who said they personally experienced at least one of those 15 abuses was 47.1% — nearly 6,000 of the more than 12,000 respondents. Maybe the descriptors of our teaching culture, "adversarial and based on intimidation, public humiliation, harassment, belittlement, and fear" aren't very far off--base.

To do our job as teachers well, we have to be aware of our primary goal: transmitting our knowledge and skills. To reach that goal, our most important ethical principles are competence and integrity. It should be obvious that we have to be not only competent in our disciplines, but also have to have integrity in the way we manage the special power we hold over our students and residents, as well as other trainees.

Now I'm going to talk about ethics for the clinical professions, taking medicine as representative of all of them, while recognizing that the ethical principles that guide the professional activities of physicians are in some ways different, but in many more ways, very similar to those of other clinicians.

The foremost professional goal of physicians is to work for the good of the patient. For the healing relationship to succeed, the first requirement is that patients trust that their physicians are acting in their best interest. There's good reason for this: successful medical care requires that physicians have access to intimate details of the patient's personal history, as well as intimate access to the body itself ways that are allowed to no one else, including the patient's minister, lawyer, and even the patient's husband or wife. Think here of physical exams of private body parts and surgical opening of body cavities in patients who're anesthetized and completely vulnerable. The fundamental need for those extraordinary intimacies means that patients have to trust that their doctors are acting in the patient's interest rather than the doctor's.

So for those reasons, the virtues required for physicians to serve the good of the patient come in two packages: what's good for the patient from the biological perspective and what's good for the patient in terms of their own value systems. First, to serve the patient's biological good, the physician has to have scientific objectivity and has to be competent in both medical knowledge and technical skill. Then, to serve the good of the patient from the patient's point of view — the physician has to respect the patient's personal values, has to be honest in disclosing the information patients need to make decisions that're consistent with their own values, and has to have compassion for the patient's humanity and suffering. To sum it up in a single word, the physician has to be trust--worthy — that is, has to have all of the other qualities I just mentioned to be truly worthy of the patient's trust.

But, there're problems in the house of medicine. When a medical error occurs and a patient is harmed, the doctor's first responsibility is to the patient and the patient's right to know what happened. Yet a survey of 1300 physicians found that only half of them, 50%, believed that a serious error should be disclosed to the patient. As a matter of honesty and personal character, physicians should not withhold information from patients.

To point to another problem, honesty requires that physicians shouldn't lie to insurance companies. Yet misrepresentation of diagnoses and procedures is commonly supported by physicians. Asked if they would approve of deceiving an insurance company to get coverage of an uncovered service, such deception was supported by 58% of physicians for a coronary bypass operation, and 56% for arterial revascularization. They do this ostensibly to help patients, but these deceptions may be self--serving, since the physician and the hospital often benefit by being paid for their otherwise unpaid services.

There are no doubt practical reasons for withholding from patients information about medical errors and for lying to insurance companies. But, it can be argued, as I do, that these acts are simply wrong, they're wrong because dishonesty diminishes personal character, and most importantly — it undermines trust--worthiness.

The ACA contains lots of penalties for violating the law. But, laws and threats of punishment are blunt instruments. They are far from the best way to address ethical misconduct. Doing the right thing depends on developing habits of doing the right actions in the given circumstances, and these habits have to be internalized for right action to be reliable in the long run. We internalize ethical behavior by doing what we know to be right deliberately every time we make a choice. These habits of chosen actions are what some have called virtues.

Albert Einstein said, in 1930, "I never think of the future. It comes soon enough." The emerging health care system is coming soon enough, but its form is hardly predictable. We need to be prepared for whatever emerges, and fortunately, as human beings with a human nature that's been stable for thousands of years, our responses to the coming challenges can rely on our internalized ethics — if you will, our virtues — to meet the upcoming challenges successfully.

For administrators, this requires consistently acting with fairness and common decency in the service of the institution's flourishing. For biomedical investigators, it requires exercising impeccable honesty and integrity in the responsible conduct of research in the service of science. For teachers, it requires competence and integrity in conveying knowledge and using power. And for clinicians, it requires being trustworthy in every way, in the service of unswerving, even ferocious dedication to the welfare of our patients. We owe them nothing less.

Thank you.

www.ingramcontent.com/pod-product-compliance
Lightning Source LLC
Chambersburg PA
CBHW051624170526
45167CB00001B/46